THE LEUKEMIA CELL

Editors

Arnold D. Rubin, M.D.

Director
Division of Medical Oncology
College of Medicine and Dentistry of New Jersey
Newark, New Jersey
Director, Division of Oncology
St. Joseph's Hospital
Paterson, New Jersey

Samuel Waxman, M.D.

Head
Cancer Chemotherapy Foundation Laboratory
Mount Sinai School of Medicine
New York, New York
Attending Physician in Hematology
Veterans Hospital
Bronx, New York

Editor-in-Chief
CRC Immunology and Lymphoid Cell
Biology Uniscience Series

A. Arthur Gottlieb, M.D.

Professor and Chairman
Department of Microbiology and Immunology
School of Medicine Tulane University

CRC Press, Inc.
2255 Palm Beach Lakes Blvd. · West Palm Beach, Florida
33409

Library of Congress Cataloging in Publication Data

Main entry under title:

The Leukemia cell.

Bibliography: p.
Includes index.
1. Leukemia. 2. Cancer cells. I. Rubin, Arnold D. II. Waxman, Samuel, 1936- [DNLM: 1. Leukemia, Experimental. 2. Oncogenic viruses. 3. Cell transformation, Neoplastic. 4. Cytogenetics. 5. Histocytochemistry. WH250 L655]
RC643.L39   616.1'55   77-16656
ISBN 0-8493-5009-3

© 1979 by CRC Press, Inc.

International Standard Book Number 0-8493-5009-3

Library of Congress Card Number 77-16656
Printed in the United States

PREFACE

The Uniscience Series in Immunology and Lymphoid Cell Biology was initiated in order to present selected monographs of timely importance in this broad area of biomedical science. Where appropriate, the series seeks to emphasize subjects from other than conventional viewpoints in the hope that this may stimulate new studies of controversial or poorly understood problems. Within the scope of each monograph and chapter, each subject is treated with sufficient depth to be of interest to those with detailed knowledge of the area, while serving the needs of biomedical investigators outside of the specialized area for an appreciation of the complexities of the issues involved.

In *The Leukemia Cell,* Drs. Rubin and Waxman have brought together a number of topics in this field which are of special interest and concern to lymphoid cell biologists, immunologists, and clinical oncologists alike. In addition to a detailed consideration of the questions concerning viruses and cancer, particularly leukemias, there are also to be found chapters on cytochemistry, cytogenetics, and cellular kinetics of leukemic cells, as well as considerations of some current hypotheses of the molecular pathogenesis of the leukemic state. Other chapters deal with characteristics of cell surface-associated antigens present on leukemic cells and the production of coagulation factors by leukemic cells. In the individual chapters, the authors have highlighted specific examples of active research in leukemia and related diseases, which are in turn based on important technological advances of recent years. The emphasis in writing the book has been on providing a basis for the interested investigator who is not expert in these subdisciplines to become familiar with current viewpoints and unsolved problems in these important areas of leukemia research.

A. Arthur Gottlieb
Editor-in-Chief
Immunology and
Lymphoid Cell Biology Series
November, 1978

THE EDITORS

Arnold D. Rubin, M.D. is the Director, Division of Medical Oncology, College of Medicine and Dentistry of New Jersey — The New Jersey Medical School, Newark, New Jersey, and Director of the Division of Oncology, St. Joseph's Hospital, Paterson, New Jersey.

Dr. Rubin received his B.A. (cum laude) in 1956 from Harvard University, Cambridge, Massachusetts and obtained his M.D. degree with honors in pathology from the New York University School of Medicine, New York, New York in 1961. While at New York University, he received the American Society of Clinical Pathologists Award for Meritorious Student Research, among other honors.

Dr. Rubin is a member of Alpha Omega Alpha, the American Society for Clinical Investigation, American Society of Hematology, American Academy for the Advancement of Science, Sigma Xi, American Association for Cancer Research, New York Society for the Study of Blood, and the Bergen County Medical Society. He is a Fellow of the American College of Physicians and the New Jersey Academy of Medicine.

He has served as a Surgeon in the U.S. Public Health Service, as Head of the Lymphocyte Research Laboratory of the Mount Sinai School of Medicine, and as Vice-President, New York and New Jersey chapter, of the Leukemia Society of America Medical Advisory Board, as well as in other distinguished positions.

Dr. Rubin has published numerous works in the areas of Immunology, Hematology, and Leukemia research.

Samuel Waxman, M.D., is Associate Clinical Professor of Medicine and Head, Cancer Chemotherapy Foundation Laboratory, Mount Sinai School of Medicine, New York, New York and an attending physician in Hematology, Veterans Hospital, Bronx, New York.

Dr. Waxman received his B.S. degree from Cornell University, Ithaca, New York in 1957 and was awarded his M.D. degree (summa cum laude) from the State University of New York, Downstate Medical Center, Brooklyn in 1963.

Dr. Waxman is a member of Alpha Omega Alpha, the Harvey Society, the American Society of Hematology, American Federation for Clinical Research, American Society for Clinical Nutrition, American Association for Cancer Research, and American Society for Clinical Investigation. He is a Fellow of the American College of Physicians and has served on the Board of Internal Medicine and the Subspecialty Boards in Hematology.

Dr. Waxman has been active as a professor, physician, and researcher in his career at Mount Sinai and was Mead Johnson Scholar in Medicine there from 1965 to 1968.

CONTRIBUTORS

Shyam S. Agarwal, M.D.
Department of Medicine
K. G. Medical College
Lucknow, India

William G. Baxt, M.D.
Assistant Clinical Professor of
  Medicine
Assistant Research Biologist
University of California, San Diego
La Jolla, California

John M. Bennett, M.D.
Head
Medical Oncology Unit
Associate Director of Clinical
  Oncology
University of Rochester Cancer Center
Professor of Oncology in Medicine
University of Rochester School of
Medicine and Dentistry
Rochester, New York

Joel Buxbaum, M.D.
Chief
Rheumatology Service
Manhattan Veterans Administration
  Hospital
Associate Professor of Medicine
New York University School of
  Medicine
New York, New York

Stephen Davis, M.D.
Chief
Oncology Section
Veterans Administration Hospital
East Orange, New Jersey
Assistant Professor of Medicine and
  Pathology
College of Medicine and Dentistry of
  New Jersey — The New Jersey
  Medical School
Newark, New Jersey

Norman Gabelman, Ph.D
Albert Einstein College of Medicine
  and Yeshiva College of Yeshiva
  University
New York, New York

Michael L. Greenberg, M.D.
Associate Professor of Medicine
Division of Hematology
Mount Sinai School of Medicine
New York, New York

Lillian Y. F. Hsu, M.D.
Director
Prenatal Diagnosis Laboratory of
  New York City
Professor of Pediatrics
New York University School of
  Medicine
New York, New York

Ernest Lieber, M.D.
Chief
Division of Human Genetics
Long Island Jewish Hospital —
  Hillside Medical Center
New Hyde Park, New York
Associate Professor of Pediatrics
State University of New York at Stony
  Brook
Stony Brook, New York

Lawrence A. Loeb, M.D., Ph.D.
Director
Joseph Gottstein Memorial Cancer
  Research Institute
Department of Pathology
School of Medicine
University of Washington
Seattle, Washington

Murray Nussbaum, M.D.
Professor of Medicine and Director,
Hematology Division
College of Medicine and Dentistry of
  New Jersey — The New Jersey
  Medical School
Newark, New Jersey

Harvey Preisler, M.D.
Associate Chief
Department of Medicine A
Roswell Park Memorial Hospital
Buffalo, New York

Carolyn E. Reed, M.D.
Assistant Surgeon (2)
The New York Hospital
New York, New York

Marc. E. Weksler, M.D.
Wright Professor of Medicine
Director, Division of Geriatrics and
  Gerontology
Cornell University Medical College
New York, New York

TABLE OF CONTENTS

Chapter 1

A BRIEF HISTORY OF LEUKEMIA CELL RESEARCH

Arnold D. Rubin

TABLE OF CONTENTS

I. INTRODUCTION

Significant additions to scientific knowledge depend, to a large extent, on the design of new research techniques. The history of understanding of the leukemia cell has followed some of the more important technological advances in biological research. This concept is brought into focus by considering the evolution of thinking concerning etiology and pathogenesis. As scientists have been able to analyze or measure various phenomena relating to cell growth and function, a trend toward building the results of these studies into a comprehensive theory to explain the mechanisms of disordered cell growth has developed. Table 1 outlines the evolution of concepts regarding the nature and pathologic defect characterizing the leukemia cell.

II. EARLY RESEARCH

In the 19th century, research was entirely dependent on descriptive analyses.[1] Meticulous descriptions of the clinical and gross pathological changes observed in leukemia patients typified research at this time. The application of light microscopy to pathologic analysis led to detailed descriptions of histologic and cytologic anatomy. Conclusions drawn from these data were organized into a scheme, tracing the blood cell morphologically from birth to full maturation. The concept of the hemocytoblast as a stem cell evolved from the assumption that a completely undifferentiated cell must give rise through maturation to the functional entities known as granulocytes, monocytes, lymphocytes, and erythrocytes. Furthermore, it was assumed that the degree of maturity could be gleaned from the appearance of the cell under the light microscope. Thus, a pattern of fine, lacy chromatin containing a prominent nucleolus and surrounded by a rim of deeply basophilic cytoplasm correlated well with immaturity and ability to multiply. In a series of steps, the cell would mature and be characterized by increasing pyknosis of nuclear chromatin, disappearance of a visible nucleolus, decreasing basophilia of the cytoplasm, and inability to di-

TABLE I

History of Leukemia Research

Era	Technicological Advance	Ramifications in Leukemia Research
Mid 19th century	Light microscopy	Detailed descriptions, clinical and morphological
Late 19th century	Improved staining techniques	Controversies regarding relationship between leukemia and lymphoma
Early 20th century	Methods for studying radiation biology	Discussions regarding environment and heredity; somatic mutation theory, cell autonomy theory
	Enzymology and intermediary metabolism	Aerobic glycolysis theory
1920—1940	Animal virology and viral manipulation	Viral etiology
1940s—1950s	Tissue culture	Viral transformation and chromosomal alterations
	Immunochemistry	Antigenic markers
1950s—1960s	Molecular biology	Gene regulation, viral messengers
	Immunobiology	Immune surveillance; autoimmunity and cancer
1960s—1970s	Nucleic acid annealing	Reverse transcriptase and the oncogenic virus; oncogene-virogene theory; protovirus theory
1970s	Primate virology	Viral genetics and complexities of viral role in leukemogenesis; viral infection vs. transformation
	Cell biology of the surface membrane	Differentiation and cell origin in lymphatic leukemia

vide. Since leukemia cells manifested varying degrees of maturity, the forms of the disease were categorized with respect to their place in normal differentiation. In addition, the greater the morphological immaturity observed, the more acute was the disease from a clinical standpoint. Thus, discrete entities could be defined: acute granulocytic and acute lymphocytic leukemia where the cells resembled immature granulocytes and lymphocytes, respectively, and chronic lymphocytic and chronic granulocytic leukemia for those diseases exhibiting mature forms of these cells. With the development of stain technology, further categorization into morphologic subgroups resulted in raging controversies regarding clinical significance. For instance, the variegated appearance of the lymphocytes in the lymphoid malignancies stimulated speculation regarding origins of the cells and the interrelationships between leukemia and lymphoma.

Considering the lack of therapeutic methods at that time, most of the morphologic categorizations carried little practical significance and offered little insight into the nature of these diseases. Since the late 19th century, an intense curiosity has existed about the pathogenesis of leukemia. During the first half of the 20th century, research into enzymology and intermediary metabolism elucidated many of the key steps in biological chemistry. It seemed logical to assume that aberrations in these metabolic processes could result in disordered growth and maturation patterns. Perhaps this could explain the morphologic observations in the various forms of leukemia. Aided, to a large extent, by the measuring capacity of the Warburg apparatus, numerous types of cancer cells were analyzed for their capacity to consume oxygen. It seemed that cancer cells were selective in their tendency to undergo aerobic glycolysis. However, the lack of a strict comparison between a leukemia blast and its normal counterpart precluded any descriptive characterizations. Still, for many years it was assumed that neoplastic cells primarily depended upon aerobic glycolysis for their energy rather than oxygen consumption.

At the same time, investigators looking to the physical sciences explored the effects of high-energy radiation on biological systems. Since high-energy radiation could affect the growth pattern of living organisms from bacterial to mammalian, considerable speculation arose regarding environmental alterations causing somatic mutations in the genetic makeup of cells. This fit in well with existing knowledge of genetics whereby genes could be altered by chance or by certain mutagenic manipulations in bacteria. Perhaps the ordered maturation of blood cells could be altered in a similar fashion. There developed a concept of "dedifferentiation" characterized by reversion to immaturity and increased mitotic activity, phenomena reflected metabolically by the retention of aerobic glycolysis (Warburg phenomenon). By the middle of the 20th century, radiation became inexorably linked to the pathogenesis of leukemia when the Atomic Bomb Casualty Commission reported the markedly increased incidence of the disease in survivors of the atomic blasts of 1945.[2]

With newer techniques for laboratory manipulation of animal viruses becoming possible, forward thinking scientists such as Rous and Gross applied these to tumor systems. Gross, and later Friend, were able to transmit mouse leukemia by cell-free filtrates.[3] This phase of the research was greatly aided by two important technical advances — tissue culture and the electron microscope. With cell cultivation, it was possible to pass tumor cells infected with virus through many generations and to isolate large numbers of chemically analyzable viral particles. With the electron microscope, it was possible to observe the morphology of the particles in and out of the infected cells.

Meanwhile, the allied field of immunology was gaining sophistication, once free of the practical exigencies extant in the past antibiotic era. Through immunologic techniques, viral antigens could be identified independent of host cell antigens, thereby proving that an oncogenic virus may capture the cell's genetic machinery and be passed on from one generation to another — a true somatic mutation. The connection was thereby drawn between the various agents — physical (radiation), biological (viruses), and chemical (radiomimetic drugs) — as pathogenic in transforming the normal blood cell to a leukemic cell. All of these modalities seemed to interact with the genetic makeup of

the cell and might, in this interaction, alter patterns of growth and maturation.

III. INTENSIFIED ACTIVITY RESULTING FROM TECHNOLOGICAL ADVANCES

The 1950s marked a great turning point in biological research. The application of certain physical techniques such as X-ray diffraction by Watson and Crick led to the final proof and construction of a functional model of DNA as the hereditary structural entity. This model provided an easily validated explanation for replication, storage, and readout of genetic information. From this point, nucleic acid chemists and cell biologists began to devise a multitude of new techniques for analyzing native DNA and RNA molecules isolated from living organisms. In rapid order, descriptions of messenger RNA and the transcription of genetic information from the DNA template, of ribosomes, and of the protein-synthesizing systems in the cytoplasm were developed. Finally, the genetic code was broken by Nirenberg and colleagues. All of this had great impact on leukemia cell research. It was then possible to isolate nucleic acid from leukemia cells and analyze for evidence of abnormal information storage and possible transfer.

Following rather informative descriptions of how nucleic acids from virulent viruses such as the polio agent enter the mammalian cell and eventually replicate, the techniques of molecular biology were applied to oncogenic viruses by the mid-1960s. To account for the obvious fact that informational material (RNA) from oncogenic viruses establishes a permanent alteration in growth potential of the host cell, the information in the RNA must be integrated into a replicating structure. Temin and Baltimore predicted the existence of an enzyme and then identified it. This enzyme, reverse transcriptase, provided a mechanism for synthesis of a DNA strand complimentary to the infecting viral RNA. The DNA copy could then be operated on by a ligase and inserted into a stable replicating form in the host cell DNA through the agency of another enzyme, DNA ligase. True to the prediction, all oncogenic viruses contained reverse transcriptase. Nononcogenic viruses lacked it.[4]

Upon isolation of the reverse transcriptase enzyme it was possible to obtain DNA copies of oncogenic viral RNA for direct analysis. The technique of nucleic acid annealing involves comparison of base sequences by the degree of base pairing complimentarity between a nucleic acid of known origin and an unknown specimen, as from an oncogenic virus. Employing this technique, a DNA copy of viral RNA is synthesized in the presence of an isolated reverse transcriptase. This probe is then tested by annealing to calculate the degree of complimentarity with an unknown DNA. Thus, base sequences in the DNA of acute leukemia cells have been identified as similar to probes taken from viral RNAs known to be oncogenic in animals. This direction of investigation culminated in the isolation and characterization from oncogenic viruses of a 70S RNA which was bound to a reverse transcriptase. Furthermore, evidence of incorporation of complimentary DNA into the genome of leukemia cells, including some human leukemic cells, established a strong case for the viral etiology and provided models for understanding the infection of normal cells and their transformation into leukemic cells. The basis for the protovirus theory of Temin followed from these experiments.

The early 1970s saw intensified enthusiasm for isolating the human leukemia virus since molecular biologic techniques were suddenly available for verification that the virus met newly established oncologic criteria, e.g., they contained 70S RNA with a reverse transcriptase. However, investigators in this field continue to be frustrated by the inability to identify the virus as human in origin. Difficulties arose when it became obvious that some viruses which could be isolated from human tumor cells could transform cells from nonhuman species, but could not transform human cells. For instance, the ESP-1 virus isolated from cultured human lymphoma cells[7] probably reflected a contaminating mouse tumor virus. The RD 114 virus isolated from human sarcoma cells[8] seemed more likely to be an endogenous, non-oncogenic feline virus. A more promising prospect isolated from the bone marrow of a child with acute leukemia could actually grow in mouse and human cells in culture.[9] However, two viruses isolated from human acute leukemia cells[10,11] have stimulated most enthusiasm.

Both closely resemble known Simian Sarcoma Viruses biochemically, while the former will reproduce in continuously cultured cells from human as well as nonhuman species. Still, none of these viral isolates can be regarded with certainty as etiologic agents in human disease until Koch's postulates have been fulfilled. These require the agent isolated from diseased human tissue to produce similar changes by infecting normal cells from that same species. Presently the relationships between tumor virus and host cell have proven so complex as to preclude any simple statement of cause and effect. All this occurred at a time when the solution to the whole problem seemed imminent. Currently, attention has been focused on primate leukemia viruses as being similar or even identical to the putative human agent.

IV. CURRENT STATE OF LEUKEMIA RESEARCH

From the preceding discussion it is difficult to form a picture of leukemia research as a coherent effort. Clearly, this reflects the relatively primitive state of our approach to the problem. The discovery that leukemia could be passed by a virus should have established the etiology of the disease. However, there is no uniformity of opinion regarding this basic issue. As more sophisticated techniques were developed, the role of the virus as an etiologic agent appeared more elusive. A picture now emerges in which the virus blends into a complex relationship with the cell — a relationship which carries far beyond neoplastic transformation. If, in the larger scheme, the oncogenic virus may perform a beneficial service to the cell, then neoplastic transformation must represent an aberration of this relationship, to the detriment of the whole organism. It is even possible that the available animal models for studying the oncogenic virus are laboratory contrivances where infectivity and virility of transmissible agents are artificially high.

Thus, technological advancements have enabled investigators to identify phenomena, the significance of which cannot, as yet, be interpreted. Presently, techniques for settling the urgent question regarding the isolation of the agent which can both infect and transform the human blood cell are lacking. Attention must then focus back on the white blood cell in order to understand the basic nature of the neoplastic process. With this knowledge, the role of the virus would be clarified. On purely morphologic grounds, the various leukemias appeared to reflect faulty development from the precursor cell to the corresponding mature functional element. This is clear in the acute leukemias where the predominating form is a blast. It can also be appreciated in the chronic leukemias where the predominating cell may appear mature. As will be seen in the chapter by Davis and Rubin, chronic lymphocytic leukemia seems to represent a monoclonal proliferation of functionally inadequate immunocytes. Thus, understanding the mechanism of faulty maturation or differentiation of the leukemia cell may unlock the secret to the neoplastic process. Such an understanding has been the focus of much investigation.

The pioneering work of Till and McCollough[5] provided a system for analyzing the growth and differentiation of stem cells from the marrow. By lethally irradiating a mouse and then injecting cells from a known source, the progeny of these infected cells could be found growing in colonies in the organs, e.g., liver, of the immunologically unresponsive host. Analysis of the progeny from a known source reflected differentiation. The subsequent development of a semisolid suspension medium to grow individual marrow cells greatly enhanced the sensitivity of the stem cell studies. Differentiation could be analyzed directly through morphologic or cytochemical techniques. Applying these methods to marrow from granulocytic leukemia patients, it appeared that these cells had less capacity for differentiation into mature elements than corresponding normal marrow. Such findings might have been anticipated from the early works of Cronkite and others who, having developed methods for analyzing cell growth cycle kinetics in vivo, found that human leukemia marrow cells did not replicate faster then normal. In fact, many blast cells lay dormant, neither dividing nor differentiating.[6]

Additional information regarding differentiation came from an entirely separate area of endeavor. During the 1940s and 1950s, numerous investigators tried to understand the surface membrane of the cell. These investigators calculated the size of pores required to transport sodium and potassium and built models for the structure of the membrane — postulating a bimolecular leaflet of lipid interspersed with polar areas representing the pores. Much of their hypothesis was confirmed by the electron microscope, which enabled a more detailed picture to emerge. It appeared that the cell contained an elaborate structure of membranes which not only border the surface but are contiguous with subcellular organelles such as the Golgi apparatus and lysosomes. More recently, the technique of freeze-fracture of the cell membrane is enabling a much clearer understanding of these structures.

Simultaneous attention was focused on the polar areas of the membranes as the loci for enzymes, surface antigens, and other structures which clearly represented the vehicles for communication between extracellular stimuli and the cell interior in which execution of differentiated functions must be initiated. The techniques which made these studies possible in blood cells grew out of the fields of immunobiology and immunochemistry which were expanding at an exponential rate during the late 1950s and into the early 1970s. Progressing well beyond the limits of morphological analysis, these techniques employing immunofluorescence and radioimmune assay demonstrated that differentiated blood cells maintained certain surface markers which correlated precisely with their function. Such a phenomenon was significant in lymphocyte subpopulations where the cells appeared identical under the microscope, yet unique surface markers indicated that they had separate functions. As bearers of the gene products for both histocompatibility and the immune response genes, the surface of lymphocytes took on wider significance as markers for differentiation. Therefore, these studies were carried over to lymphocytic leukemia where specific markers were identified in both acute and chronic forms. Most interestingly, lymphocytes from chronic lymphocytic leukemia patients bore immunoglobulin markers of only one type, inferring a monoclonal origin. Here, the marker techniques were coupled with the methodology of immunochemistry which provided facilities for immunoglobulin characterization.

V. CONCLUSION

From this brief historical survey, there emerges a pattern illustrating how widely diverse disciplines have been brought to bear on the analysis of the leukemia cell. Technical advances in physics and chemistry, having brought forth the new discipline of molecular biology, have been applied to the biological phenomena involving the oncogenic virus. The descriptive phenomena relating to oncogenic viruses had been made possible by previously described methods for cultivating animal cells and for analyzing the chromosomes. Morphologic refinements took advantage of metabolic and enzymatic advances of previous years. Finally, modern immunology, one of the most eclectic of disciplines, opened up new possibilities for a better understanding of differentiation as reflected in surface markers and antigenic differences between normal neoplastic cells.

This book contains a series of chapters that will deal with specific examples of leukemia cell research, each based upon a technological advance of recent years. Since we have yet to form a clear picture of the nature of the leukemia cell, we must continue to watch developments from various approaches to the problem. The authors have been selected from a group of younger people actively contributing to their respective fields. I believe there can be gleaned a feeling for the leukemia cell as a pathologic entity. The cell appears to be arrested or attenuated in its differentiation. Genetic markers show signs of structural aberrations and may contain information derived from an etiologic virus.

We presently lack sufficient knowledge and understanding to concentrate investigations in this area to any one of the approaches exemplified in these chapters. We await the design of newer techniques for isolation of the leukemia virus and for a clearer picture of how it alters functional activity.

REFERENCES

1. **Dameshek, W. and Gunz, F.,** *Leukemia,* 2nd ed., Grune & Stratton, New York, 1964. 1.
2. **Bizzozero, O. J., Jr., Johnson, K. G., and Cicocco, A.,** Radiation-related leukemia in Hiroshima and Nagasaki, 1946—1964, *N. Engl. J. Med.,* 274, 1095, 1966.
3. **Gross, L.,** *Oncogenic Viruses,* 2nd ed., Pergamon Press, New York, 1970, Chap. 1.
4. **Temin, H. M.,** Malignant transformation of cells by viruses, *Perspect. Biol. Med.,* 14 (1), 11, 1970.
5. **Till, J. E., McCullogh, E. A., and Siminovitch, L.,** A statistical model of stem cell proliferation based on the growth of spleen colony forming cells, *Proc. Nat. Acad. Sci. U.S.A.,* 51, 29, 1964.
6. **Cronkite, E.,** The kinetics of leukemic cell proliferation, in *Perspectives in Leukemia,,* Dameshek, W. and Dutcher, R. M., Eds., Grune & Stratton, New York, 1968, 158.
7. **Priori, E. S., Dmochowski, L., Meyers, B., and Wilber, J. R.,** Constant production of type C virus particles in a continuous tissue culture derived from plerual effusion cells of a lymphoma patient, *Nature (London) New Biol.,* 232, 61, 1971.
8. **McAllister, R. M., Nicholson, M., Gardner, M. B., Rongey, R. W., Rasheed, S., Sarma, P.S., Huebner, R. J., Hatanaka, M., Crozlan, S., Gilden, R. V., Kabigting, A., and Vernon, L.,** Type C virus released from cultured human rhabdomyosarcoma cells, *Nature (London) New Biol.,* 235, 3, 1972.
9. **Nooter, J., Aarsen, A. M., Bentvelzen, P., Degroot, F. G., and Van Pelt, F. G.,** Isolation of infection C-type oncornavirus from human leukemic bone marrow cells, *Nature (London),* 256, 595, 1975.
10. **Gallagher, R. E. and Gallo, R. C.,** Type C RNA tumor viruses isolated from cultured human acute myelogenous leukemia cells, *Science,* 187, 350, 1975.
11. **Mak, T. W., Kurtz, S., Mamaster, J., and Housman, D.,** Viral related information and oncornavirus like particles isolated from cultures of human cells from leukemic patients in relapse and remission, *Proc. Natl. Acad. Sci. U.S.A.,* 72, 623, 1975.

Chapter 2
CYTOCHEMISTRY OF THE LEUKEMIC CELL

John M. Bennett and Carolyn E. Reed

TABLE OF CONTENTS

I. INTRODUCTION

Cytochemistry may be defined as the application of special histochemical stains to individual cells in order to determine the biochemical composition of the cell and, by doing so, to help in its identification. The justification for this discipline lies in two general areas. The first is to establish as exact and specific a diagnosis as possible within a given malignant hematopoietic category. The second is to aid in predicting the clinical course within this category and, if possible, to help in selecting discriminative chemotherapy. The employment of these techniques is designed to supplement the established methods of histologic and of morphologic diagnosis and in no way is meant to compete with or replace this approach.

We will begin by describing the various cytochemical stains, including their reaction in normal cells. The stains have been grouped into three categories: (1) cytochemical stains of diagnostic significance, (2) specialized cytochemical stains,

TABLE 1

Peroxidase Reaction in Normal Hematopoietic Cells with Light Microscopy

Myeloblast	0/+	Monocyte	0/+
Promyelocyte	++, +++	Lymphoblast	0
Myelocyte	++, +++	Lymphocyte	0
Segmented neutrophil	+, ++	Plasma cell	0
Eosinophil	++, +++	Megakaryocyte	0
Basophil	0	Mast cell	0
Monoblast	0/+		

Note: 0 = no activity, + = weak, ++ = moderate, +++ = strong.

and (3) cytochemical stains of limited value. Following these sections, we will examine the cytochemical characteristics of different types of leukemic cells. Methods of staining are detailed in the Appendix.

II. CYTOCHEMICAL STAINS OF DIAGNOSTIC SIGNIFICANCE

A. Peroxidase

Peroxidases are hemoprotein enzymes that catalyze the oxidation of a variety of substances by hydrogen peroxide (H_2O_2). The enzyme consists of a protein attached to a complex iron-porphyrin prosthetic group. There are many peroxidases that occur in animal tissues, but only myeloperoxidase is cytochemically significant. Granulocytes are rich in this enzyme, which imparts a green color to myeloblastic tumors. Myeloperoxidase and halide (chloride or iodide) enhance the antibacterial, antifungal, and antiviral activity of hydrogen peroxide produced in the phagocytic vacuole of polymorphonuclear leukocytes and monocytes following ingestion and degranulation. In the presence of myeloperoxidase and halide ion, hydrogen peroxide may generate bactericidal aldehydes by oxidizing bacterial constituents crucial for microbial multiplication.[1]

The principle of the peroxidase reaction is that of oxidation (i.e., loss of electrons and hydrogen ions) of a substrate that yields a highly colored and stable compound. The most commonly used substrate is benzidine, which yields a blue or brown compound upon oxidation at the site of peroxidase activity. In the normal granulocyte series, activity is seen first in the progranulocyte and persists through and includes the polymorphonuclear leukocyte. Eosinophils demonstrate a particularly strong reaction which is distinguish-

able from that of neutrophils by its greater activity at a lower pH and its cyanide resistance.[2] Basophils and mast cells are peroxidase negative. Lymphocytes and other cells of the lymphoid series (lymphoblasts and prolymphocytes) are nonreactive, as are platelets. Monocytes have a variable reaction from negative to weakly or moderately positive. The results are summarized in Table 1.

In granulocytes peroxidase activity corresponds with the primary or azurophil granules, which are formed only in the promyelocyte and myelocyte stage and bled off from the concave surface of the Golgi membranes. Specific or secondary granules, which are pinched off the convex surface of the Golgi complex beginning in the myelocyte stage, are peroxidase negative.[3] Monocytes contain two different kinds of primary lysosomes, and it is probable that peroxidase is found in the first storage or azurophil granule made during their developmental period in the bone marrow and continued cellular maturation in the blood. These azurophil granules are used in the initial stages of phagocytosis, and no additional formation occurs. In contrast, the second type of lysosome, the Golgi vesicles, contain and produce digestive enzymes.[4]

B. Naphthol AS-D Acetate Esterase Without and With Sodium Fluoride

Esterases catalyze the following reversible reaction: $R\text{-}COOR' + HOH \rightleftharpoons R\text{-}COOH + R'OH$. Studies using polyacrylamide gel electrophoresis and subsequent staining of esterase activity on the gel have shown that there are at least three groups of esterases that can be demonstrated cytochemically in human blood cells.[5] This esterase activity corresponds to nine distinct bands (isoenzymes) when mixed leukocyte extracts are

TABLE 2

Esterase Isoenzymal Pattern of Normal Hematopoietic Cells[a]

Cell	Band number
Mature neutrophils	2, 7, 9
Young granulocytes	2, 7
Monocytes	4, 5
Megakaryocytes and platelets	5 (3, 4)
Plasma cells	6

[a]Using polyacrylamide gel electrophoresis.

Adapted from Li, C. Y., Lam, K. W., and Yam, L. T., *J. Histochem. Cytochem.*, 21, 1, 1973.

electrophoresed. The chloroacetate esterases correspond to three major bands, 2, 7, and 9 in the system used. They are resistant to sodium fluoride inhibition but sensitive to a chymotrypsin inhibitor. The nonspecific esterases are sodium fluoride sensitive and consist of four major bands, 3, 4, 5, and 6. The third group of esterases, the aminocaproate esterase, is best revealed in human mast cells but has not been well studied in the gel system. The isoenzymal pattern of certain normal cells is summarized in Table 2.

Using naphthol AS-D acetate (NASDA) as the substrate and the diazonium salt Fast Blue BB as the coupler to produce a blue insoluble product, neutrophils exhibit a wide range of activity, from 1+ to 2+ to 3+, where 0 to 1+ = 0 to 5 granules, 1 to 2+ = 5 to 10 granules, 2+ = 10 to 20 granules, and 3+ = >20 granules. It is unusual to identify more than 30 grains per cell, with the average reaction being 2+. There is usually no (0) or, rarely, minimal (0 to 1+) reactivity in lymphocytes. With monocytes, a consistent 2 to 3+ reaction is observed. Utilizing sodium fluoride as an esterase inhibitor (NASDA-F), the only inhibition seen is in monocytes with essentially complete inhibition occurring, i.e., 3+ to 0. Occasionally a strongly positive monocyte (>30 grains) will be reduced to 0 to 5 grains (0 to 1+).[6] Plasma cells show strong activity, 2 to 3+, with partial inhibition.

In view of the zymogram study discussed above, it is apparent that the demonstration of activity in a wide variety of hematopoietic cells[7] is due to hydrolysis by isoenzymes from at least two esterase groups (including 4 and/or 5; 6; and 2, 7, and/or 9). The identification of a monocytic

component by using sodium fluoride[8] is responsible for the specificity, and, consequently, the value of this cytochemical reaction.

C. Leukocyte Alkaline Phosphatase

Polymorphonuclear leukocytes (neutrophils) contain an alkaline phosphomonoesterase. This enzyme was demonstrated first by Roche in 1931.[9] Subsequently, it was assayed quantitatively using biochemical techniques[10,11] and semi-quantitatively by a variety of cytochemical methods,[12,13] the majority of which employ azo dyes.

Clinical interest in leukocyte alkaline phosphatase (LAP) was stimulated initially because of the observation of low to absent activity in the mature granulocytes (stab and segmented forms) of patients with chronic granulocytic leukemia.[10,11] However, it must be emphasized that the identification of the level of LAP activity is also important in other clinical disorders.

In the method described in the Appendix, naphthol AS phosphate is used as a substrate because of the rapid rate of hydrolysis of the phosphate ester, high color density of the azo dye, substantivity, and low solubility in water and lipids.[14] The naphthol AS liberated by the enzymatic cleavage of the ester linkage is insoluble at the alkaline pH and couples promptly with the capture agent, in this case Fast Blue BBN, to yield an intense blue precipitate at the site of enzymatic activity. The brilliant granules can be easily counted and a scoring system devised.

No granulocytes earlier than "stab" forms are scored. Eosinophils are LAP negative and can be recognized by their large pale granules and should not be included in the count. One hundred consecutive neutrophils are graded from 0 to 4+ by the following criteria: 0 = no granules; 1+ = extremely few blue granules; 2+ = few to moderate number of granules; 3+ = moderate to numerous granules; 4+ = cytoplasm saturated by closely approximate granules. Each score is then multiplied by the corresponding number, i.e., 1+'s by 1, 2+'s by 2, etc. The normal range is 40 to 100 (includes two standard deviations). Three-plus reactions are seen in less than 10% of normals, and a 4+ reaction is most unusual.

Leukocyte alkaline phosphatase develops in the myelocyte stage and is associated with the formation of specific granules. The function of LAP in cell economy is not precisely known at the present time. Neutrophils from a boy with an abnormality of specific granule formation and absent LAP showed defective chemotaxis, abnormal formation of phagolysosomes, and defective staphylococcal killing.[15]

Unlike other cytochemical tests that help to identify certain cell lines, the major purpose of demonstrating leukocyte alkaline phosphatase is to help the clinician to identify a disease state. This will be discussed in greater detail in the section describing the cytochemical characteristics of the CML cell.

III. SPECIALIZED CYTOCHEMICAL STAINS

A. Leukocyte Acid Phosphatase

Acid phosphatases are a group of enzymes which hydrolyze phosphate esters in an acid environment. Almost all types of blood cells have acid phosphatase activity. Polyacrylamide gel electrophoresis studies reveal that the acid phosphatase in human leukocytes is heterogeneous.[16,17] The isoenzymes have been designated arbitrarily as 0, 1, 2, 3, 3b, 4, and 5 according to their electromobility, with isoenzyme 5 moving the fastest toward the cathode. Some of these isoenzymes are cell specific, i.e., isoenzyme 0 in Gaucher cells, 3 in lymphocytes and platelets, 3b in blast cells, 2 and 4 in neutrophils and monocytes. Leukocytes of normal blood contain isoenzymes 1, 2, 3, and 4. Fluoride, molybdate, and L(+) tartaric acid completely inhibit the activity of these four isoenzymes. Isoenzyme 5, which is very prominent in the "hairy" cell of leukemic reticuloendotheliosis (see discussion of hairy cell), is also inhibited by fluoride and molybdate but is not inhibited by L(+) tartaric acid. Thus, the resistance to tartrate is a specific marker for isoenzyme 5.

Many histochemical methods for the determination of acid phosphatase activity have been examined. The method described in the Appendix employs naphthol AS-BI phosphoric acid as substrate. The reaction product is seen as bright red granules. In peripheral blood smears, neutrophils and eosinophils are nonreactive with this substrate (n.b. positive with naphthol AS phosphate as substrate); platelets show occasional activity, particularly giant forms; reticulocytes are variable;

lymphocytes are strongly reactive ("T lymphocytes"), with 40 to 70% of cells reacting. The staining pattern is similar in bone marrow smears. Immature granulocytes and immature erythroids stain weakly. Megakaryocytes and plasma cells are intensely reactive.

B. Naphthol AS-D Chloroacetate Esterase

As was previously discussed, zymogram studies have shown that chloroacetate esterases correspond to three major bands (isoenzymes 2, 7, and 9) in the system used. They are resistant to sodium fluoride inhibition but sensitive to a chymotrypsin inhibitor.

The granulocytes, including promyelocytes and many myeloblasts, and mast cells show very strong activity for chloroacetate esterase. Monocytes and basophils show little or no staining. Eosinophils, lymphocytes, erythroblasts, plasma cells, and megakaryocytes contain no chloroacetate esterase activity. In the granulocyte series, the reaction parallels the peroxidase reaction except that the enzyme activity is detected at a somewhat later stage of the azurophil granule formation than with peroxidase. The special use of the chloroacetate esterase stain is its adaptation to paraffin sections. Using a modification[18] of Leder's method,[19] neutrophilic myeloid cells can be demonstrated in any tissue section.

C. Toluidine Blue

Toluidine blue is one of the most commonly employed metachromatic stains, staining mast cell granules and the specific granules of basophils purple to red (Figure G).* Stored and dilute solutions should be used to demonstrate the granules optimally. Stored toluidine blue undergoes isomerization, forming Azure A, which is responsible for the metachromatic staining.

The intense metachromatic stain is the result of binding of the Toluidine blue to the sulfate radicals of the heparin located in the mast cell (and basophil) granules.

IV. CYTOCHEMICAL STAINS OF LIMITED VALUE

A. Beta-Glucuronidase

Beta-glucuronidase is a lysosomal enzyme, the activity of which can be demonstrated bio-

---

*All figures in this chapter appear after page 23.

chemically in various tissues and cells. It has been shown to exist in blood with most of the activity in leukocytes. As with other acid hydrolases, β-glucuronidase activity has been demonstrated[20] in regions rich in T lymphocytes: the diffuse lymphatic tissue of the lymph node paracortical areas and around the central arterioles of the splenic pulp, whereas most of the lymphocytes in the lymph node germinal centers and in the lymphatic nodules of the splenic white pulp were negative.

Using Naphthol-AS-BI-β-D-glucoronide as the substrate and hexazonium pararosanilin as the coupler,[21,22] β-glucuronidase activity can be localized in various blood cells. Granulocytes may show a diffuse reddish tinge, with maximal activity in the intermediate stages of maturation. Erythroblasts and monocytes also may show a diffuse reaction. Plasma cells are strikingly reactive. In blood, β-glucuronidase activity is particularly evident in lymphocytes as discrete reddish granules in the cytoplasm.

Scoring systems have been set up by various investigators. In one such system,[23] one hundred lymphocytes are examined and graded on a 0 to 4 scale. Zero indicates no activity; 1+ indicates a single large granule or less than 5 small granules; 2+ indicates 5 to 10 small granules or one large granule and 2 to 5 small granules; 3+ indicates 10 to 15 granules; 4+ indicates more than 15 granules. With this method, a population of normal subjects had an average score of 197 ± 14 (range 140 to 230).

B. N-Acetyl-β-Glucosaminidase

N-acetyl-β-glucosaminidase is a lysosomal enzyme that hydrolyses β-glucosidic bonds formed by N-acetyl-β-glucosamine.

Using naphthol AS-BI-N-acetyl-β-glucosaminide as a substrate and fast garnet GBC as a coupler,[24] N-acetyl-β-glucosaminidase activity appears as discrete bluish-purple granules, enabling an actual count of the granules per cell.

In normal peripheral blood, monocytes consistently show activity throughout the cytoplasm and over the nucleus, while lymphocytes and neutrophils show only minimal reactivity. Occasionally, increased activity is observed in polymorphonuclear leukocytes, but the average number of granules per cell is still clearly higher in monocytes. Basophils and eosinophils are negative. Red blood cells and platelets show no enzyme activity.

In bone marrow smears, minimal reactivity is recognized in granulocyte precursors from promyelocyte through band forms. Enzyme activity is very strong in megakaryocytes, and variable activity is detected in plasma cells.

C. Periodic Acid Schiff

The periodic Acid Schiff (PAS) reaction has been employed widely for the identification of carbohydrates, together with glycol groups in the carbon chain, such as glycogens, mucopolysaccharides, mucoproteins, glycoproteins, and glycolipids. Periodic acid oxidizes glycols to aldehydes that then react with the Schiff reagent. The "fuchsin," so released, stains the cellular components containing the oxidizable material.

Glycogen is present in the cytoplasm of all granulocytes, most monocytes, and a few lymphocytes. In the neutrophilic myeloid series, the glycogen content increases with increasing maturity, a strongly positive reaction being seen in a segmented neutrophil. The erythroblasts of normal individuals are negative. Megakaryocytes and platelets are positive. A scoring system for the PAS positivity of 100 lymphocytes has been described.[25] The scoring technique is 0 for no cytoplasmic positivity, 1 for up to 10 red granules, 2 for 10 or more red granules, and 3 for large blocks of red material. Approximately two thirds of the positive reactions for PAS correspond to Type 1. Type 3 is not encountered in normal adults. The scoring of an individual cell becomes somewhat arbitrary, and the system is only useful if the score is definitely increased. A summary of PAS reactivity in normal hematopoietic cells is found in Table 3.

D. Oil Red O and Sudan Black B

Lipids are present in cells either as droplets, globules, or granules and have the common feature of being soluble in organic solvents. In leukocytes, one must distinguish between two classes of fats. Neutral or simple fats consist of mixtures of triglycerides that contain several fatty acids (i.e., oleic, palmitic, etc.). These acids are very susceptible to oxidation. The second class is that of phospholipids, one such example being lecithin (phosphatidylcholine). These latter lipids are much less prone to oxidation.

One can take advantage of some selective staining of neutral fats and phospholipids by Oil Red O for the former and Sudan Black B for the latter. The total lipid content of mammalian

TABLE 3

PAS Reaction in Normal Hematopoietic Cells

Myeloblast	0	Lymphoblast	0, +, ++, +++
Promyelocyte	0, 0/+	Lymphocyte	0, +
Myelocyte	0, +	Nucleated RBC	0
Segmented neutrophil	++, +++	Platelet	+, ++
Monoblast	0, +	Megakaryocyte	+, ++
Monocyte	0, +		

Note: 0 = no activity, + = weak, ++ = moderate, +++ = strong.

leukocytes accounts for approximately 2% of the total mass of the cells. Neutral fat accounts for 30% of this total, cholesterol for 20%, and phospholipid for 45%. Studies by Gottfried[26] suggest that granulocytes have considerably more phospholipid (highly concentrated in the membrane of lysosomes) than do lymphoid cells.

Oil Red O, a diazo dye of the sudan type, produces a positive reaction due to the presence of the dye within the lipid substance. This depends on the lipid solubility, which is determined by the partition of the dye between the solvent employed and the lipid substance. Positivity is judged by the presence of round orange-pink areas that do not display refractility as the microscope is focused up and down. In areas of the smear that are well stained, positive orange flecks on and between red cells are usually seen. In normal smears, Oil Red O positivity is restricted almost entirely to lymphoid precursors and to histiocytes.

In leukocytes, the degree of sudanophilia parallels the peroxidase reaction when Sudan Black B is used. Lymphocytes and lymphoid precursors are negative, as are plasma cells and erythroid precursors. Granulocyte precursors and monocytes are positive. On occasion, the number of peroxidase positive granules will be too scant for recognition by light microscopy, but the phospholipid envelope of the granule will be stained by the Sudan Black B reaction.

V. CYTOCHEMICAL CHARACTERISTICS OF LEUKEMIC CELLS

A. The AML, AMML, and AMoL Cell

With the employment of several cytochemical stains, in particular the peroxidase reaction and the NASDA/NASDA-F esterase reaction, it has become possible to subclassify the nonlymphocytic leukemias into three groups: acute myeloblastic leukemia (AML), acute myelomonocytic

leukemia (AMML), and acute monocytic leukemia (AMoL).

The peroxidase reaction will permit the separation of undifferentiated leukemia from poorly differentiated myeloblastic leukemia, the presence of 3% or more positive cells justifying removal from the undifferentiated leukemia category (Figure A). The fact that positivity may be seen in the cytoplasm of primitive cells devoid of granules probably represents staining of myeloperoxidase in the endoplasmic reticulum and the Golgi apparatus or reflects nuclear-cytoplasmic asynchrony. As expected, Auer rods are strongly peroxidase positive. It has been our experience[6] that all cases of AMML show peroxidase positivity, although the reaction is quite variable. In approximately 50% of cases of AMoL, the peroxidase reaction has been negative.

The chloroacetate esterase is usually positive in myeloblastic leukemia when the peroxidase is also positive. Its use is restricted to the identification of tissue deposits of leukemic cells (chloromas).

Using naphthol AS-D acetate esterase (NASDA), cases of AMoL invariably give a score of 3+ (Figure B). The addition of sodium fluoride results in a score of at least two full degrees lower, 0 to 0 to 1+ (Figure C). In AML cells the positivity is unaffected by sodium fluoride. Cases of AMML frequently reveal partial inhibition. This may mean that there is a population of both myeloblasts and monoblasts or a population of mixed myelomonoblasts (see Table 4).

The PAS reaction has been used routinely by many laboratories to aid in distinguishing acute lymphocytic leukemia (ALL) from non-ALL. Although many cases of acute granulocytic leukemia are PAS negative, careful review shows that approximately one third of cases of acute myeloblastic leukemia are PAS positive, some with coarse granules (Figure D). Close to 60% of cases of AMML are PAS positive, the reaction varying

TABLE 4

Stains	AML	AMML	AMoL	ALL
Peroxidase	1−3+	1−3+	0−2+	0
NASDA	2+	2−3+	3+	0−1+
NASDA-F	2+	1−2+	0−1+	0−1+
PAS	0−3+	0−3+	0−3+	0−3+

from a single glycogen granule to a fine-to-globular pattern. Almost 80% of cases of AMoL show PAS positivity, frequently with typical aggregated blocks or rings of PAS. Half of the AMoL cases are peroxidase negative, PAS positive, a type of cytochemical pattern which has heretofore been stated to be characteristic of ALL. Thus, it is worth emphasizing that in the absence of peroxidase the discovery of PAS-positive granules cannot be interpreted as a "lymphoid" characteristic.

The reaction pattern of N-acetyl-β-glucosaminidase in a series of acute nonlymphocytic leukemia cases reveals that reactivity correlates with an increasing monocytic component.[24]

The peroxidase, NASDA, NASDA-F, and PAS activity in AML, AMML, and AMoL are summarized in Table 4. The activity in ALL is included for comparison.

B. The CML Cell

A low leukocyte alkaline phosphatase (LAP) score is found in the vast majority of patients with chronic myelogenous leukemia (CML), but rarely is necessary for diagnosis. Occasionally the score is helpful in differentiating CML from polycythemia vera, some cases of myelosclerosis, and leukemoid reactions, where a high LAP score may be noted. Decreased enzyme activity is not unique to the CML cell, and the LAP score may be low in some cases of agnogenic myeloid metaplasia, megaloblastic anemia, infectious mononucleosis, infectious hepatitis, sarcoidosis, congenital hypophosphatasia, and paroxysmal nocturnal hemoglobinuria.

Successful treatment of CML has an inconstant association with an increase in previously depressed LAP scores, although the score may still be subnormal. The increased LAP score is not associated with a greatly increased proportion of neutrophils with 3+ or 4+ activity, but rather with selective removal of cells which lack alkaline phosphatase. It has been hypothesized[27] that the low LAP score in CML patients is due to the predominantly elderly neutrophils resulting from

accumulation of the expanded mass of neutrophils in storage pools (marrow, spleen, etc.), a subsequent delay before becoming circulating cells, and in many instances an extended life span in the peripheral blood. Reduction of the total granulocytic pool by drug treatment or removal of an important extramedullary site for storage (such as splenectomy) allows the earlier release into the circulation of younger neutrophils which possess LAP activity.

C. The ALL Cell

The peroxidase, NASDA, NASDA-F, and PAS reactions of the acute lymphocytic leukemia (ALL) cell are listed in Table 4. It is stated that in most cases of ALL at least a few and commonly many of the blast cells give positive PAS reactions. When present, PAS positivity is not diffuse, but is seen as coarse granules or blocks against a negative cytoplasmic background, and it is this pattern of reactivity rather than the percentage of positive blast cells that is said to be of diagnostic importance (Figure E). However, as was previously discussed, since blocks of PAS-positive material may be found in cases of non-ALL, the PAS stain is of limited value.

In one series of cases of acute lymphocytic leukemia stained with Oil Red O, 82% of the cases were found to contain positive pink cytoplasmic globules. This was in striking contrast to the rare positivity noted in the myeloid cells of AML.[28] However, the work of Shaw and Klemp[29] indicates that Oil Red O is of little diagnostic use in differentiating ALL from non-ALL. Although globular positivity was noted in six of 30 (20%) cases of ALL and in two of 21 (9%) cases of non-ALL, granular positivity was present in 11 of 30 (37%) cases of ALL and in 13 of 21 (62%) cases of non-ALL. It was suggested that aged alcoholic solutions of Oil Red O increase the staining of leukocyte granules.

It has recently been reported[30-32] that the majority of blast cells of T-lymphoblastic leukemia have strong acid phosphatase activity characteristically localized by electron microscopy in the membranes of the Golgi apparatus and in lysosomal granules in its vicinity (Figure F). The high acid phosphatase content of the T lymphoblasts may reflect a general property of the thymus-derived lymphocytes or may reflect differences in the proliferation kinetics of the T and non-T blasts, the release of lysosomal enzymes perhaps playing a role in the process of blast transformation and mitosis. In cases of ALL with negative surface markers or in cells of more differentiated B-cell leukemias, only a small proportion of cells react positively (less than 30%), and the reaction is never more than weak or moderate. Approximately 25% of cases of childhood ALL have been found to have T-cell characteristics and accompanying distinct clinical pathological features. The use of acid phosphatase may facilitate the recognition of T-ALL.

D. The CLL Cell

Beta-glucuronidase has been reported to be consistently low in patients with chronic lymphocytic leukemia (CLL)[23,33,34] in accord with its B-cell origin. Flandrin[34] reported that 18 of 20 untreated CLL patients examined had β-glucuronidase values below the normal range (control range 101 to 181). Up to 99% of the lymphocytes had no β-glucuronidase activity (mean 88%), and most of the cells were grade 0, 1, and 2. Comparison of β-glucuronidase activity with acid phosphatase activity showed close correlation between these two enzyme activities.[34] In 16 CLL cases with B-cell markers, Catovsky reported low (always <25%) or absent acid phosphatase activity.[32]

In 11 patients with CLL of T-cell origin, which is considered to be a rare disorder, all patients had a high content of β-glucuronidase and acid phosphatase in more than 90% of the peripheral blood lymphocytes.[35] Of the 11 patients, 9 had an atypical clinical course, and it may be that identification of this subset of CLL patients will have important prognostic and therapeutic considerations.

E. The Hairy Cell

The leukemic reticuloendothelial cell (hairy cell) is characterized by having strong acid phosphatase activity, although the intensity varies from patient to patient and from cell to cell. The enzymatic activity of these cells is characterized by resistance to inhibition by L(+) tartaric acid, corresponding to the high content of isoenzyme 5.[36] It has been our experience that not all morphologically identified hairy cells show tartrate resistance. However, any percentage of resistant cells is significant. Catovsky reported that tartrate resistance was evident only in hairy cells with strong acid phosphatase activity.[37] The weak

or moderate reaction found in lymphocytes and the strong one of monocytes are both completely inhibited by simultaneous incubation with L(+) tartaric acid.

The cytochemical reactions characteristic of granulocytic cells (peroxidase, Sudan Black B, chloroacetate esterase) are always negative in hairy cells. Nonspecific esterase reactions are negative or only moderately positive without sodium fluoride inhibition. The PAS reaction varies from case to case but is usually weakly positive in the form of fine small granules.[36,37]

F. The Mast Cell ("Leukemic")

Mast cell leukemia is a very rare disorder. There are no accurate figures as to the incidence, and only a few cases have been published. Most of the cases describe "tissue" mast cells, resembling the normal counterpart, or well-differentiated cells 15 to 30 μm in diameter with dense uniform basophilic granules that often obscure the nucleus. The nucleus is spherical to oval with dense chromatin. Both histamine[38] and heparin[39] are contained within the granules. Phagocytosis of latex particles is variable.

Rarely, a less differentiated form of mast cell leukemia has been noted and can be separated from other acute leukemias by cytochemical studies (Figure H). The two most important stains are the toluidine blue and peroxidase reaction. The former is positive in the majority of the cells, and the latter is always negative. These two reactions become even more critical in poorly differentiated mast cell leukemia where the cells may resemble promyelocytes (peroxidase positive; toluidine blue negative). Other cytochemical stains, including PAS and naphthol AS-D chloroacetate, have been studied with variable results. Nonspecific esterase (NASDA) reaction is strongly positive (2 to 3+).

APPENDIX:
TABLE OF CONTENTS

7. Histochemical Demonstration of Leukocyte Esterase Activity
8. Leukocyte Alkaline Phosphatase Determination (Using Naphthol AS Phosphate and Fast Blue BBN)
9. The Identification of Monocytes and Monoblasts Using Naphthol AS.D Acetate and Inhibition with Sodium Fluoride
10. A Method for Staining β-glucuronidase Activity in Leukocytes
11. A Method for Staining N-Acetyl-β-glucosaminidase

1. AN IMPROVED METHOD OF STAINING LEUKOCYTE GRANULES WITH SUDAN BLACK*[4] [1]

Method

1. Fix air-dried smears in formalin vapor for 10 min.
2. Immerse slides for 30 min in Sudan Black B solution.
3. Wash thoroughly for several minutes in absolute ethyl alcohol. (Gently wave the slide back and forth in a coplin jar.)
4. Counterstain in dilute Giemsa for 40 min (1 ml stock Giemsa to 49 ml distilled H_2O.
5. Air dry and coverslip. Permount® may be used.

Interpretation: lymphocytes and lymphoblasts are negative; normal granulocyte precursors are positive as well as myeloblasts, myelomonoblasts, and monocytes (also, on occasion, monoblasts).

Reagents

1. Sudan Black B Solution: add 0.3 g of Sudan Black B to 100 ml absolute ethyl alcohol; shake vigorously and frequently for 1 or 2 days or until all dye is dissolved; filter.
2. Buffer: mix a solution of 16 mg pure phenol crystals in 30 ml absolute ethyl alcohol with a solution of 0.3 g $Na_2HPO_4 \cdot 12 H_2O$ or 0.119 g Na_2HPO_4 in 100 ml H_2O.
3. Sudan Black Staining Solution: mix 30 ml of Sudan Black B solution with 20 ml of the buffer, filter under suction or double filter paper. Mixture should be neutral or slightly alkaline. Do not keep for use for more than a few weeks.
4. Dilute Giemsa stain: 1 ml Giemsa in 49 ml distilled H_2O.**
5. Fixative: 40% formalin (full strength).

2. METHOD FOR DEMONSTRATION OF LEUKOCYTE ACID PHOSPHATASE WITH TARTARIC ACID INHIBITOR[4] [2]

Reagents

Fixative solution		10% formalin with 1% $CaCl_2$	
40% formalin	25 ml		
distilled H_2O	75 ml	10% formalin with 1% $CaCl_2$	
	100 ml	Adjust weekly to pH 7.0 (± 0.1) with NaOH	
$CaCl_2$	1.0 g		

The working solution is freshly prepared from four stock solutions.

1. Michaelis veronal acetate buffer
   9.75 g sodium acetate. $3H_2O$.
   14.71 g sodium barbital dissolved in distilled water, make up to final volume of 500 ml.
   For 200 ml buffer: 3.90 g sodium acetate, 5.884 g sodium barbital; q.s. to 200 ml with distilled H_2O).
2. Substrate stock solution (make fresh each time)
   Naphthol, AS-BI phosphoric acid (sodium salt) (Sigma Chemicals) dissolved in N-N-dimethylformamide in 10 mg/ml concentration.
   For 1 test: 20 mg Naphthol AS-BI phosphoric acid (Na salt), 2 ml N-N-dimethylformamide.

*In particular phospholipids (membranes).
**Some prefer a more concentrated Giemsa stain. Various proportions may be tried.

3. 4% $NaNO_2$ in distilled water (make fresh each time)

4 g $NaNO_2$ in 100 ml H_2O.

For 1 test: 0.2 g $NaNO_2$ in 5 ml H_2O.

4. Pararosanilin hydrochloride (Sigma Chemicals)

2 g added to 50 ml 2N NCl; Heat gently without boiling; cool to room temperature; filter.

HCl (37% specific gravity 1.18); 16.7 ml HCl, q.s. to 100 ml with $H_2O \rightarrow$ 2N HCl,

2 g pararosanilin in 50 ml 2N HCl, or 0.5 g in 12.5 ml 2N HCl.

The fixative, Michaelis Veronal Buffer, and the pararosanilin hydrochloride may be made up and stored at 4°C.

Working Solution

10 ml of Solution 1 buffer
2 ml Solution 2 substrate
26 ml distilled water
3.2 ml Hexasonium pararosanilin

1.6 ml Solution 3, 1.6 ml Solution 4; mix, let stand 2 min, add to working solution

------

41.2 ml, for 1 Coplin jar

Adjust to pH 5.0 (± 0.1) with HCl or NaOH. Solution should be clear yellow. If not, filter

Procedure

1. Blood or bone marrow films are dried at room temperature.

2. Fix films for 10 min at 4°C in neutral formalin with 1% $CaCl_2$.

3. Rinse well with distilled water. Air dry or gently blot. Fixed films can be stored up to 1 week at −20°C, before reaction stain is done.

4. Incubate slides in working solution for 1 to ½ hr at 37°V.

5. Rinse well in distilled water.

6. Counterstain with hematoxylin for 15 min.

7. Rinse in distilled water.

Bright red granules are seen in the cytoplasm at the sites of acid phosphatase enzyme activity.

Tartaric Acid Step

To carry out the tartaric acid step, double the amounts in the working solution; to 40 ml of this add 300 mg L(+) tartaric acid. Perform the reaction on two similar slides in parallel (one slide in normal working solution, one slide in solution with tartaric acid). A large number of the "hairy cells" will be equally positive in both solutions; other positive leukocytes will be negative in the solution containing the tartaric acid.

2 X Working Solution

20 ml Solution 1 buffer
4 ml Solution 2 substrate
52 ml distilled water
6.4 ml hexazonium pararosanilin

3.2 ml Solution 3, 3.2 ml Solution 4; mix, let stand 2 min, add to working solution.

82.4 ml, for 2 Coplin jars

3. PEROXIDASE STAINING METHOD*

Principle

The peroxidase enzyme in the granules of the cells liberates the oxygen in the H_2O_2. This O_2 then oxidizes the benzidine and causes its disposition as a black compound at the site of activity. Sodium nitroprusside serves as a catalyst for this reaction.

---

*Dr. M. L. Ingram's modification of Goodposture's method; method used at the University of Rochester Medical Center.

Procedure

    1. Cut filter paper to about ½ in. longer than slide size and place over film.

    2. Drop Solution 1 onto filter paper until it is just wet (approx. 8 to 10 drops). Let stand ½ min.

    3. Add Solution 2 until it thoroughly floods the slide (like buffer on Wright's preparation). Gently blow to mix solutions. Let stand 1½ min.

    4. Peel off filter paper. Smears should be a definite red color. To remove excess stain, hold coverslip or slide with forceps and wash with running water.

    5. Counterstain with Wright's or Giemsa in the usual manner.

Solutions

1. Solution 1
   2 g benzidine base*
   1.2 g basic fuchsin
   4 ml sodium nitroprusside (saturated aqueous solution). To 10 ml distilled water add the sodium nitroprusside powder until the solution is definitely saturated.
   400 ml ethyl alcohol (95%)
   Rub the 2 g benzidine base in a mortar with small amount of alcohol, then add rest of alcohol, mixing well in mortar. Filter this solution. To filtered solution add basic fuchsin, then add 4 ml of the saturated sodium nitroprusside solution. Age for 2 to 4 days before using. It keeps indefinitely in a dark dropping bottle at room temperature, although it may be necessary to add additional nitroprusside if staining becomes less distinct.
2. Solution 2
   Make fresh each time.
   25 ml distilled H_2O
   4 drops of 3% hydrogen peroxide solution (if refrigerated, 3% stock hydrogen peroxide solution is good for 1 month).

Sources of Reagents

Benzidine — 25 g #71102 Hartman Leddon Co., Philadelphia

Sodium nitroprusside — 100 g Cat #P-2394 Distillion Products — Eastman Kodak Co., Rochester, N.Y.

*Benzidine may not be available because of associated toxicity.

Basic fuchsin — 10 g Cat #434. Certified; Allied Chemical, Morristown, N.J.; National Aniline, Charlotte, N.C.

95% Ethyl alcohol — 1 gal — pharmacy.

4. OIL RED O STAIN

Method

    1. Fix (thin) smears in formalin vapor for 15 min.

    2. Rinse in tap water by gently waving slide back and forth in a coplin jar.

    3. Prepare staining solution by mixing 30 cc Oil Red O and 20 cc distilled H_2O and allow to stand for 30 min.

    4. Filter through two thicknesses of Whatman #1 filter paper into a coplin jar and keep covered.

    5. Rinse slides briefly in 50% isopropyl alcohol, then transfer directly to staining solution (3 to 4) for 30 min.

    6. Rinse slides briefly in 50% isopropyl alcohol to remove excess stain, then in distilled H_2O by the same technique as in 2.

    7. Counterstain in Harris Hematoxylin® (filtered before use) for 10 min.

    8. Rinse in dilute ammonia water, then rinse in tap water for a few minutes by gently waving slide back and forth in a coplin jar. Blot dry carefully. Cover slip using Permount.

Reagents

    1. 40% Formalin
    2. Isopropyl alcohol (propanol)
    3. Oil Red O 0.2% in isopropyl alcohol
    4. Harris Hematoxylin

5. PERIODIC ACID SCHIFF METHOD

    1. Fix 10 to 15 min, in formal alcohol.[1]

    2. Was 4 to 5 times with running tap water.

    3. Incubate in 1% aqueous periodic acid[2] for 15 min at room temperature.

    4. Rinse 3 or 4 times in tap water.

    5. Incubate for 15 min in Schiff's Reagent[3] (Use Harleco Schiff Reagent®, Cat. #6073).

6. Wash in running tap water using 4 to 5 changes of water.

7. Counterstain in alum aqueous solution hematoxylin 10 to 15 min (Mallory's Formula Harleco Cat. #632 or Harris Hematoxylin Cat. #638).

8. Rinse in very dilute ammonia water (3 to 5 drops $NH_4 OH$ in 50 ml $H_2 O$).

9. Wash in tap water.

10. Dry and mount (Permount may be used).

Reagents

1. Formal alcohol: 10 ml 40% Formalin, 90 ml Absolute methanol. Keep refrigerated.

2. Periodic acid: 1 g Periodic Acid in 100 ml distilled $H_2 O$. Keep refrigerated. (Also available from Harleco.)

3. Schiff reagent: recommend purchase of this from Harleco.

6. TOLUIDINE BLUE STAIN FOR BASOPHILS AND MAST CELLS

Reagent

Saturated solution of Toluidine Blue in methanol (1 g Toluidine Blue in 100 ml methanol). The solution keeps indefinitely.

Method

Blood or bone marrow smears are air dried, covered with the Toluidine Blue solution for 10 min, washed with tap water, and air dried.

Results

The granules of basophils (or mast cells) stain a brilliant reddish violet. Remaining cells stain blue. Slight metachromatic staining may be noted with azurophilic granulation of promyelocytes and with platelets.

7. HISTOCHEMICAL DEMONSTRATION OF LEUKOCYTE ESTERASE ACTIVITY[43]

Method

1. Fix push smears in cold formalin-methanol for 30 sec. Wash in tap water for 30 sec.
2. Make incubation mixture as follows:
   a. Naphthol AS-D chloroacetate 50 mg.
   b. Dissolve in cold acetone (0.55 cc) in a 100-ml beaker.
   c. Add distilled $H_2 O$ (25 cc) — solution turns cloudy.
   d. Add 0.1 M Tris$^{®}$ buffer, pH 7.1 (25 cc).
   e. Add 50 mg Garnet GBC Diazo salt to mixture which should be mixing on a magnetic type mixer-stirrer. Allow to mix thoroughly (approx. 5 min)
3. Filter incubation mixture through a single sheet of filter paper into a coplin jar and incubate for 60 min at room temperature.
4. Wash in running tap water (4 to 5 changes of water).
5. Counterstain in Harris Hematoxylin for 15 min.
6. Rinse, dry, and mount with glycerin gelatin. Note: Never use Permount because the reaction will disappear in minutes.

Reagents

1. Formalin-methanol: 50 ml 40% formalin to 450 ml absolute methanol.

2. Naphthol AS-D chloroacetate and Garnet GBC Diazo salt are available from Sigma Chemical Co., St. Louis, Mo.

3. Hematoxylin (Harris formula) Harleco stains.

4. Tris buffer: 6.05 gm/500 ml distilled $H_2 O$. Adjust pH to 7.1.

Only granulocytes should show activity.

8. LEUKOCYTE ALKALINE PHOSPHATASE DETERMINATION (USING NAPHTHOL AS PHOSPHATE AND FAST BLUE BBN)[14,44]

Principle

The demonstration of the location of an enzyme depends on its action on a specific substrate, forming a product which will form an insoluble deposit at the site of the enzyme activity. This deposit is then stained so that its intensity may be graded.

Reagents

1. 10% formalin in absolute methanol
2. Stock substrate solution
3. 0.1% aqueous neutral red
4. Fast Blue (BBN)

Smear-making Procedure

If patient's white cell count (at least 40 to 50% neutrophils) is above 5000, make six capillary blood push smears, which should be somewhat thick. Wright's stain and label one of these smears with patient's name, source of blood (cap) and date. Label unstained smears with the same information on the back side with a red wax pencil.

If patient's white cell count is below 5000, obtain 5 cc of blood in EDTA and immediately make six buffy-coat push smears after spinning two macrohematocrit tubes of blood at 1800 rpm for 6 min. Wright's stain and label one of the smears with patient's name, source of blood (conc.) and date. Label unstained smears with the same information on the back side with a red wax pencil.

The smears may be stained immediately or kept for several weeks after fixation.

Staining Procedure

1. Select two smears from each patient; write the patient's name on each slide with a diamond-point pencil.

2. Fix smears in cold solution of 10% formalin in absolute methanol (0 to 4°C) for 30 sec in a coplin jar.

3. Pour off fixative and rinse slides 4 to 5 times with tap water (medium temperature). Air-dry slides.

4. Make incubating solution just before use by adding 100 mg of Fast Blue BBN to 100 ml of stock substrate solution which has quickly been brought to room temperature. Stir to dissolve the Fast Blue BBN diazonium salt. Filter mixture rapidly before use into coplin jar. Use glassware labeled LAP for this step. Clean glassware with detergent and hot water and rinse well with distilled water.

5. Always run a previously fixed control (example: smear from woman in third trimester of pregnancy).

6. Incubate smears for 15 min at room temperature, in coplin jars containing the freshly prepared incubating solution. Use incubating solution for only one set of smears.

7. Decant solution and wash smears with 4 to 5 changes of tap water. Air-dry smears.

8. Counterstain smears by immersion for 5 to 10 min in a coplin jar containing a 0.1% aqueous solution of safranin.

9. Pour off safranin stain and rinse smears very rapidly once in tap water. In order to preserve a brilliant reddish-orange nuclear stain, the shortest possible rinse is required.

10. Air-dry slides, label, and coverslip.

Interpretation

The Wright's stained smear is examined for the appropriate number of neutrophils per oilfield and also for the presence of immature myeloid and erythroid cells.

Examine smears under oil immersion. Sites of the LAP enzymatic activity are represented by discrete bright blue granules of varying size. Mature neutrophils are the usual cell in which this enzyme activity is noted, although earlier neutrophils may stain positively. One hundred consecutive neutrophils are graded visually from 0 to 4+ by the following criteria:

    0. No granules
    1. Extremely few blue granules
    2. Few to moderate number of blue granules
    3. Moderate to numerous granules
    4. Cytoplasm saturated by closely approximate granules

After grading 100 neutrophils, record in the LAP book in the corresponding columns of 0, 1+, 2+, 3+, 4+. Then multiply the number of 1+'s by 1, 2+'s by 2, 3+'s by 3, and 4+'s by 4. Add the four products for the final LAP index score.

- The normal score ranges from 40 to 100. It is unusual to find a 4+ cell in a normal smear.
- Chronic granulocytic leukemia (Ph[1] positive) is consistently low (below 15).
- Polycythemia vera, leukemoid reaction, infectious leukocytosis, and some myeloid metaplasia cases show elevated scores.
- Pregnancy from the third month on should be high as well as women on anovulatory pills.
- Cortisone treatment elevates the LAP score.
- Acute leukemias may be low, normal, or high.
- Secondary polycythemia should be normal.

Solutions for Leukocyte Alkaline Phosphatase Determination

1. 10% formalin in absolute methanol. Add 10 ml of absolute formalin (40%) to 90 ml methanol. Store in refrigerator at 0 to 4°C. Fix smears in fixative at this temperature.
2. Stock substrate solution:

   Dissolve 300 mg naphthol AS phosphate in 5 ml N, N-dimethyl formamide.

   Add 1000 ml of 0.2 M Tris buffer, pH 9.1.

   Stock solution must be stored in refrigerator at 2 to 4°C. It is stable for 2 to 3 months. Do not expose to higher temperatures since it will decompose.

   Naphthol AS phosphate solution will last indefinitely if added to Tris buffer just before use, i.e., 0.5 cc to 100 cc of Tris.

   0.2 M Tris buffer, pH 9.1.

$$\begin{array}{r} \text{Mol wt} = 121.14 \\ \underline{0.2} \\ 24.228 \text{ g/l } H_2O \end{array}$$

To have pH 9.1, add small volume of 6NHCL (usually less than 2 cc) using pH meter readings.

3. 0.1% aqueous safranin: 100 mg safranin per liter distilled H_2O

4. Fast Blue BBN 100 mg added to the substrate stock solution (100 cc)

   • Fast Blue BBN may be purchased from Sigma Chemicals, (Fast Blue BB salt, Catalogue #F0250)

   • Naphthol AS phosphate may be purchased from Cyclo Chemical Corporation, Los Angeles, Cal.

   • N,N-dimethyl formamide may be purchased from Fisher Scientific Co., Fair Lawn, N.J.

9. THE IDENTIFICATION OF MONOCYTES AND MONOBLASTS USING NAPHTHOL AS.D ACETATE AND INHIBITION WITH SODIUM FLUORIDE

Reagents

1. Formalin (40%).
2. Phosphate buffer 0.1 M Na_2HPO_4, 7.09 g/500 ml, use 60 ml; 0.1 M KH_2PO_4, 6.80 g/500 ml; use 40 ml.
3. Solution naphthol AS.D acetate (16 mg naphthol AS.D. acetate, 3 ml acetone, 2 ml propylene glycol).
4. Fast Blue BB Salt, 200 mg.
5. Sodium fluoride, 75 mg.

Method

1. Fix smears in Formalin vapor for 10 min, wash carefully, and air dry.
2. Incubation mixture consists of 100 ml phosphate buffer, 5 ml naphthol AS.D acetate solution and 200 mg Fast Blue BB salt. This is allowed to mix thoroughly in a magnetic stirrer for 3 to 4 min.
3. 50 ml of this is then filtered through one thickness of Whatman #1 filter paper into a coplin jar marked "Plain."
4. Immediately 75 mg of NaF is added to the remaining 50 ml in the mixing beaker and

allowed to dissolve. This is then filtered into a coplin jar as in 3 and marked NaF.

5. Formalin vapor fixed, washed, and air-dried smears are incubated in these two jars for 70 min at room temperature.
6. Following incubation the smears are removed from the mixture and washed in a coplin jar of tap water by waving the slide back and forth very gently in water so as not to dislodge the blood or bone marrow film. This gentle washing is especially important with bone marrow smears as they tend to peel off of the slide more rapidly than peripheral blood smears.
7. Counterstain in Harris hematoxylin for 10 min and wash as in 6.
8. Air dry or blot dry and examine with oil immersion lens.

Results

The reaction is manifested by the presence of blue granules in the nucleus and cytoplasm of both monocytes and granulocytes, but monocytes and monoblasts show the greatest degree of positivity before the addition of NaF. However, in the smears which have been exposed to NaF, the granulocytes remain positive, while in the monocytes the reaction is markedly or completely inhibited. It should be noted, however, that many monocytes retain a small degree of activity.

10. A METHOD FOR STAINING β-GLUCURONIDASE ACTIVITY IN LEUKOCYTES

Stock Substrate Solution

1. Dissolve 11 mg of naphthol (AS-BI-β-D-glucuronic acid in 1 ml of 0.05 M sodium bicarbonate (420 mg NaHCO$_3$ in 100 ml H$_2$O).
2. Bring to a final volume of 100 ml with acetate buffer.
3. This solution can be refrigerated, but should not stand for more than 2 weeks.

Acetate Buffer for Stock Substrate[4][5]
0.2 N sodium acetate-acetic acid, pH 5.0.

1. Sodium acetate: 8.2 g in 500 ml distilled H$_2$O.
2. Acetic acid: 6 ml in 494 ml distilled H$_2$O.
3. Add 118 ml acetic acid solution and 282 ml sodium acetate solution for buffer at pH 5.0.

Pararosanilin Solution[4][6]
Reagents: Pararosanilin hydrochloride, concentrated HCl.

1. Dissolve 1 g pararosanilin hydrochloride in 20 ml distilled H$_2$O and 5 ml concentrated HCl with gentle warming.
2. Filter after cooling and store at room temperature (solution may be stored indefinitely).

Sodium Nitrite Solution
Prepare a 4% solution by dissolving 4 g sodium nitrite in 100 ml H$_2$O (distilled). Prepare a fresh solution every 2 to 3 weeks.

Counterstaining Solution
Reagents: Harris Hematoxylin, Dilute ammonia water.

1. Prepare Hematoxylin by filtering through one thickness of Whatman #1 filter paper.
2. Prepare dilute ammonia water as follows: in 500 ml distilled water add about 40 to 50 drops of NH$_4$OH. Mix thoroughly.

Preparation of Working Solution
For a final volume of 41.2 ml:

1. 1.2 ml of hexazonium pararosanilin is prepared by mixing equal parts of pararosanilin solution and 4% sodium nitrite 0.6 ml pararosanilin and (0.6 ml 4% sodium nitrite). This should be prepared fresh each time.
2. After 1 min, 20 ml of the stock substrate solution is added.
3. Acetate buffer is added to a final volume of 41.2 ml.
4. The pH of the solution is adjusted to pH 5.2 to 5.4 using 1 N NaOH.
5. Filter solution through #1 Whatman filter paper into coplin jar.

The incubation solution should be pale yellow and clear.

Staining Procedure

1. Air dry smears at room temperature.
2. Keep unfixed smears in refrigerator at approx. 2°C. (This improves staining.)
3. Fix smears in 40% formalin vapor for 60 sec.
4. Rinse several times in a beaker filled with distilled water and allow to air dry.
5. Incubate the smears for 90 min at 37°C.
6. After incubation, rinse smears in distilled water and allow to stand until thoroughly dry.
7. Counterstain the smears in filtered Hematoxylin for 15 min, rinse briefly in dilute ammonia water in a coplin jar, and then rinse again in distilled water.
8. Allow to air dry and mount with Permount.

11. A METHOD FOR STAINING N-ACETYL-β-GLUCOSAMINIDASE

Citrate-citric Acid Buffer (0.1 M)
Solution A: 0.2 M solution of sodium citrate (granular), 5.882 g/100 ml.
Solution B: 0.2 M solution of citric acid, 3.842 g/100 ml.

pH	A	B
5.2	160 ml	90 ml

Dilute to 500 ml.

Fixative

40% formalin, 75 ml.
distilled water, 375 ml.
10% $CaCl_2$, 75 ml.
Mix and store in the refrigerator.

Working Solution

Dissolve 15 mg of naphthol AS-BI N-acetyl-β-glucosaminide in 2.5 ml of ethylene glycol monomethyl ether and add 47.5 ml of 0.*M* citrate-citric acid buffer, pH 5.2. Add 50 mg of fast garnet GBC to the magnetically stirring mixture. Filter through a #1 Whatman filter paper into a coplin jar. The working solution must be used immediately.

Staining Procedure

1. Treat slides in the formalin/$CaCl_2$ fixative for 15 min. Wash by waving in a coplin jar filled with distilled water.

2. Incubate in the working solution for 15 min.

3. Rinse by waving slides in distilled water.

4. Counterstain with neutral red for 10 min. Blot dry.

5. Do not mount in Permount (reaction fades) or glycerine jelly (removes the neutral red).

REFERENCES

1. **Stossel, T. P.,** Phagocytosis, *N. Engl. J. Med.,* 290, 774, 1974.
2. **Yam, L. T., Li, C. Y., and Crosby, W. H.,** Cytochemical identification of monocytes and granulocytes, *Am. J. Clin. Pathol.,* 55, 283, 1971.
3. **Bainton, D. F., Ullyot, J. L., and Farquhar, M. G.,** The development of neutrophilic polymorphonuclear leukocytes in human bone marrow, *J. Exp. Med.,* 134, 907, 1971.
4. **Nichols, B. A., Bainton, D. F., and Farquhar, M. G.,** Differentiation of monocytes — origin, nature, and fate of their azurophil granules, *J. Cell. Biol.,* 50, 498, 1971.
5. **Li, C. Y., Lam, K. W., and Yam, L. T.,** Esterases in human leukocytes, *J. Histochem. Cytochem.,* 21, 1, 1973.
6. **Bennett, J. M. and Reed, C. E.,** Acute leukemia cytochemical profile: diagnostic and clinical implications, *Blood Cells,* 1, 101, 1975.
7. **Wachstein, M. and Wolf, G.,** The histochemical demonstration of esterase activity in human blood and bone marrow smears, *J. Histochem. Cytochem.,* 6, 457, 1958.
8. **Fischer, R. and Schmalzl, F.,** Über die Hemmbarkeit der Esterase Aktivität in Blutmonocyten durch Natriumfluorid, *Klin. Wochenschr.,* 42, 751, 1964.
9. **Roche, J.,** Blood phosphatases, *Biochem. J.,* 25, 1724, 1931.
10. **Valentine, W. N. and Beck, W. S.,** Biochemical studies on leukocytes. I. Phosphatase activity in health, leukocytosis, and myelocytic leukemia, *J. Lab. Clin. Med.,* 38, 39, 1951.
11. **Wiltshaw, E. and Moloney, W. C.,** Histochemical and biochemical studies on leukocyte alkaline phosphatase activity, *Blood,* 10, 1120, 1955.
12. **Gomori, G.,** Microchemical determination of phosphatase in tissue sections, *Proc. Soc. Exp. Biol. Med.,* 42, 23, 1939.
13. **Kaplow, L. S.,** Cytochemistry of leukocyte alkaline phosphatases, *Am. J. Clin. Pathol.,* 39, 439, 1963.
14. **Rutenberg, A. M., Rosales, C. C., and Bennett, J. M.,** An improved histochemical method for the demonstration of leukocyte alkaline phosphatase activity: clinical application, *J. Lab. Clin. Med.,* 65, 698, 1963.
15. **Strauss, R. G., Bove, K. E., Jones, J. F., Mauer, A. M., and Fulginiti, V. A.,** An anomaly of neutrophil morphology with impaired function, *N. Engl. J. Med.,* 290, 478, 1974.
16. **Yam, L. T.,** Clinical significance of the human acid phosphatases, *Am. J. Med.,* 56, 604, 1974.
17. **Yam, L. T., Li, C. Y., and Lam, K. W.,** Tartrate-resistant acid phosphatase isoenzyme in the reticulum cells of leukemic reticuloendotheliosis, *N. Engl. J. Med.,* 284, 357, 1971.
18. **Bowling, M. C.,** *Histopathology Laboratory Procedures of the Pathologic Anatomy Branch of the National Cancer Institute,* U.S. Government Printing Office, Washington, D.C., 1967.
19. **Leder, L. D.,** The selective enzymocytochemical demonstration of neutrophil myeloid cells and tissue mast cells in paraffin sections, *Klin. Wochenschr.,* 42, 553, 1964.
20. **Tamaoki, N. and Essner, E.,** Distribution of acid-phosphatase, β-glucuronidase and N-acetyl-beta-glucosaminidase activities in lymphocytes of lymphatic tissues of man and rodents, *J. Histochem. Cytochem.,* 17, 238, 1969.
21. **Hayashi, M., Nakajima, Y., and Fishman, W. H.,** The cytologic demonstration of β-glucuronidase employing naphthol-AS-BI-glucuronide and hexazonium pararosanilin. A preliminary report, *J. Histochem. Cytochem.,* 12, 293, 1964.

22. Lorbacher, P., Yam, L. T., and Mitus, W. J., Cytochemical demonstration of beta-glucuronidase in blood and bone marrow smears, *J. Histochem. Cytochem.*, 15, 680, 1967.

23. Yam, L. T. and Mitus, W. J., The lymphocyte β-glucuronidase activity of lymphoproliferative disorders, *Blood,* 31, 480, 1968.

24. Reed, C. E. and Bennett, J. M., N-acetyl-β-glucosaminidase activity in normal and malignant leukocytes, *J. Histochem. Cytochem.*, in press.

25. Mitus, W. J., Berna, L. J., Mednicoff, I. B., and Dameshek, W., Cytochemical studies of glycogen content of lymphocytes and lymphocytic proliferations, *Blood*, 13, 748, 1958.

26. Gottfried, E. L., Lipids of human leukocytes. Relation to cell type, *J. Lipid Res.,* 8, 321, 1967.

27. Spiers, A. S. D., Liew, A., and Baike, A. G., Neutrophil alkaline phosphatase score in chronic granulocytic leukemia: effects of splenectomy and antileukemic drugs, *J. Clin. Pathol.*, 28, 517, 1975.

28. Bennett, J. M. and Dutcher, T. F., The cytochemistry of acute leukemia: observations of glycogen and neutral fat in bone marrow aspirates, *Blood*, 33, 341, 1969.

29. Shaw, M. T. and Klemp, V. A., Cytochemical staining with oil red O and for β-glucuronidase in the diagnosis of acute leukemia, *Am. J. Clin. Pathol.,* 61, 169, 1974.

30. Catovsky, D., Galetto, J., Okos, A., Miliani, E., and Galton, D. A. G., Cytochemical profile of B and T leukemic lymphocytes with special reference to acute lymphoblastic leukemia, *J. Clin. Pathol.*, 27, 767, 1974.

31. Catovsky, D., Frisch, B., and Van Noorden, S., B, T, and "null" cell leukemias. Electron cytochemistry and surface morphology, *Blood Cells,* 1, 115, 1975.

32. Catovsky, D., T-cell origin of acid phosphatase-positive lymphoblasts, *Lancet,* 1, 327, 1976.

33. Zittoun, R. Cadiow, M., Davo, C., Blanc, J. M., and Bowsser, J., Lymphocytic beta-glucuronidase in the lymphoproliferative syndromes, *Biomedicine,* 18, 415, 1973.

34. Flandrin, G. and Daniel, M. T., B-glucuronidase activity in Sezary cells, *Scand. J. Haematol.,* 12, 23, 1974.

35. Brouet, J. C., Flandrin, G., Sasportes, M., Preud'homme, J. L., and Seligmann, M., Chronic lymphocytic leukemia of T cell origin. An immunological and clinical evaluation in eleven patients, personal communication.

36. Yam, L. T., Li, C. Y., and Finkel, H. E., Leukemic reticuloendotheliosis. The role of tartrate acid phosphatase in diagnosis and splenectomy in treatment, *Arch. Int. Med.,* 130, 248, 1972.

37. Catovsky, D., Pettit, J. E., Galton, D. A. G., Spiers, A. S. D., and Harrison, C. V., Leukaemic reticuloendotheliosis ("Hairy" cell leukemia): a distinct clinico-pathological entity, *Br. J. Haematol.,* 26, 9, 1974.

38. Riley, J. F. and West, G. B., Presence of histamine in tissue mast cells, *J. Physiol.,* 120, 528, 1953.

39. Schiller, S. and Dorfman, A., Isolation of heparin from mast cells of the normal rat, *Biochim. Biophys. Acta,* 31, 278, 1959.

40. Wakem, C. J. and Bennett, J. M., Acute mast cell leukemia, *Clin. Res.,* 18, 687, 1970.

41. Sheehan, H. L. and Storey, G. W., An improved method of straining leukocyte granules with Sudan Black B, *J. Pathol. Bacteriol.,* 59, 336, 1947.

42. Goldberg, A. F. and Barka, T., Acid phosphatase activity in human blood cells, *Nature,* 195, 297, 1962.

43. Moloney, W. C., McPherson, K., and Fliegelman, L., Esterase activity in leukocytes demonstrated by the use of naphthol AS-D chloroacetate substrate, *J. Histochem. Cytochem.,* 8, 200, 1960.

44. Bennett, J. M., Nathanson, L., and Rutenberg, A., Significance of leukocyte alkaline phosphatase in Hodgkin's disease, *Arch. Int. Med.,* 121, 338, 1968.

45. Pearse, A. G., *Histochemistry,* Vol. 1, Little, Brown & Co., Boston, 1968, 583.

46. Barka, T. and Anderson, P. J., Histochemical methods for acid phosphatase using hexazonium pararosanilin as coupler, *J. Histochem. Cytochem.,* 10, 741, 1962.

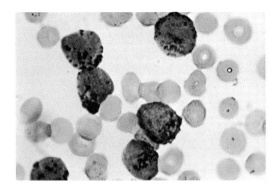

A. Peroxidase Reaction, Acute Myeloblastic Leukemia

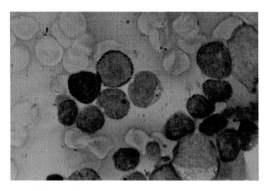

E. PAS Positive Reaction, Acute Lymphocytic Leukemia

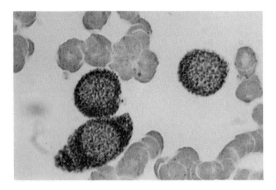

B. NASDA Reaction, Acute Monocytic Leukemia

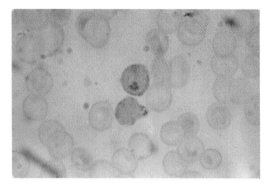

F. Acid Phosphatase Positive Reaction, Acute Lymphocytic Leukemia

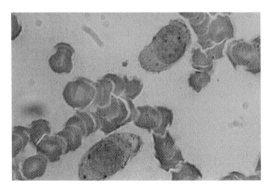

C. NASDA-F Reaction, Acute Monocytic Leukemia

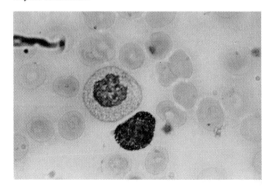

G. Toluidine Blue Reaction, Basophil (Positive) and Eosinophile (Negative Reaction)

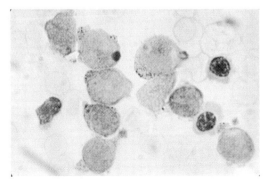

D. PAS Positive Reaction, Acute Myeloblastic Leukemia

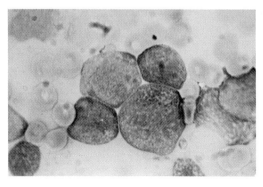

H. Toluidine Blue Reaction, Poorly Differentiated Mast Cell (1 Cell Positive)

Chapter 3
THE CYTOGENETICS OF LEUKEMIA AND SOME RELATED DISORDERS

Ernest Lieber and Lillian Y. F. Hsu

TABLE OF CONTENTS

I. INTRODUCTION

The concept that cancer is related to chromosomal abnormalities dates back to 1912 when Boveri hypothesized that chromosomal alterations are among the fundamental changes that result in malignancy.[1] In 1958 Ford et al.[2] studied mouse leukemia and found that, in general, neoplastic cells contained abnormal chromosomes. Individual neoplasms may show a certain degree of uniformity of their chromosomal complement. In 1960, Nowell and Hungerford were the first group to report a unique chromosomal aberration in patients with chronic myelogenous leukemia (CML),[3] which was designated as the Philadelphia chromosome (Ph[1]). Within the past two decades, numerous cytogenetic reports have further strengthened the relationship between chromosomes and leukemia.

In 1966, Baikie[4] wrote, "it seems likely that renewed progress must await either the development of *new methods* of study or the adoption, with or without modifications, of methods already developed in other fields of research but as yet unexploited in the study of leukemias." This statement presaged discoveries related to identification of specific chromosomes which were based on existing cytogenetic techniques. With the banding techniques predicted by Baikie, researchers reached their present vantage point in regard to the study of chromosomes and leukemia.

The development of a simple, direct bone marrow preparation for chromosome analysis by Tijo and Whang[5] in 1962 made it possible to study various granulocytic leukemias. The use of phytohemagglutinin in the cultures of peripheral blood leukocytes by Moorehead et al. (1960)[6] provided an easy method for the study of short-term lymphocyte chromosomes.

New staining techniques in the accurate identification of individual human chromosomes were introduced between 1968 and 1970.[7,8] With the new techniques, Caspersson et al.[9] were able to identify the Ph[1] chromosome as a partial deletion of the long arms of a No. 22 instead of a No. 21 which had been its previous designation.

In 1973, Rowley[10] was the first investigator to define the exact nature of the Ph[1] chromosome. Instead of a simple deletion of a No. 22

chromosome, she demonstrated a balanced reciprocal translocation between the long arm of a No. 22 and the long arm of a No. 9 chromosome, i.e., t(9q+;22q−). Furthermore, the new techniques showed evidence of nonrandom chromosomal abnormalities in various hematologic disorders.[11-41]

It is the purpose of this chapter to update cytogenetic studies using the new banding techniques in the leukemias and related disorders.

II. CHRONIC MYELOGENOUS LEUKEMIA

A. Prebanding

Since 1960, when Nowell and Hungerford[3] first described the Philadelphia chromosome as a consistent bone marrow finding in CML, there has been much speculation about its relevance to the leukemic state. It was originally thought to be a No. 21 chromosome with partial deletion of the long arm. It was found in the bone marrow but not in skin fibroblasts or lymphocytes of approximately 85% of patients with CML.[15-17] In a majority of cases, the Ph[1] chromosome persisted even during complete remission.[16,17] On occasion, the Ph[1] chromosome was duplicated and, in most of these cases, the double Ph[1] chromosomes were detected in the acute stage of the disease or shortly before the blastic crisis.[18] It was reported in only one set of monozygous twins.[19] Usually it was discordant for monozygous twins and, therefore, it was thought to be acquired.[19a] There are, however, several reports of the Ph[1] chromosomes present for some years before the onset of overt clinical disease. Canellos and Whang-Peng[20] reported an individual in whom the Ph[1] chromosome was present some 5 years before the disease became manifest. A similar case was reported by Baccarini et al.[21] Weiner[22] in 1965 reported a unique family in which several members had died with a diagnosis of leukemia; several other relatives were living with CML and had a Ph[1] chromosome in the bone marrow. Other family members were hematologically normal, but had a Ph[1] chromosome present in the bone marrow. These individuals subsequently developed clinical and hematologic signs of CML. Hirschhorn[23] has discussed the relationship of the presence of the Ph[1] chromosome in hematologically normal individuals and the subsequent development of overt disease in this unusual case. Muldal and Lajtha[24] have recently reviewed the implication of the Ph[1] chromosome. No other leukemic state is yet known to be associated with a specific and more or less constantly associated chromosomal finding.

With autoradiography, Prieto et al. in 1970[25] suggested that the Ph[1] chromosome is a No. 22 chromosome. Detailed discussion of CML prior to the use of banding techniques has been published in several comprehensive reviews.[24,26-30]

B. Origin of Ph[1] Chromosome

By using an X-linked enzyme, such as G6PD, Fialkow et al., in 1967,[31] were able to demonstrate a single enzyme pattern (G6PDA) in the erythroid and granulocyte cell population of a heterozygous female patient with Ph[1]-positive CML, while her skin fibroblasts showed both A and B types of G6PD. Evidently this can only be explained by the Lyon hypothesis and clonal origin of cells with Ph[1] chromosome. In other words, the cells with the Ph[1] chromosome were derived from a single cell which contained the active X chromosome carrying G6PDA.[31] The clonal origin of the Ph[1] chromosome was confirmed by Lawler and Sanger[32] using an X-linked blood group marker, Xg[a]. Further investigation on two interesting patients with mosaic 46, XY/47,XXY Klinefelter's syndrome, and Ph[1]-positive CML brought additional evidence of the clonal origin of the Ph[1] chromosome,[33,33a] since only cells with 46, XY showed the Ph[1] chromosome. Gahrton et al.[34] presented further evidence of the clonal origin of the Ph[1] chromosome by tracing its origin to either the maternal or paternal chromosome No. 22. By use of fluorescent staining techniques, they demonstrated morphologic similarities between their patient's No. 22 chromosome and the patient's mother's No. 22 chromosome. Using the same technique with their second patient, they similarly demonstrated the origin of the No. 22 chromosome to be paternal.[34]

In twin studies, several presumably monozygous pairs showed only one affected with positive CML, while the other one was unaffected and had no Ph[1] chromosome. This again implied the acquired nature of Ph[1] chromosome.[35]

C. Postbanding

In 1972, Caspersson et al.[9] and O'Riordan et al.,[36] using the newly introduced quinacrine fluorescent banding techniques, identified the Ph[1] chromosome to be a No. 22 and not a No. 21, as previously believed. Rowley, in 1973,[10] studied the bone marrow chromosomes of nine patients with Ph[1]-positive CML. In each case she further confirmed the 22q− nature of Ph[1] chromosome and, in addition, she found an unexpected extra piece of weakly fluorescent chromosomal material on the distal end of the long arm of a No. 9 chromosome, indicating a reciprocal translocation t(9q + ;22q−).[10] Her interpretation was further supported by other investigators.[37,37a,38] The exact chromosome break points are 9q34 and 22q11.

The accumulated cytogenetic data on CML have shown that, although the translocation involved the long arms of chromosomes 9 and 22 in approximately 93% or more of the Ph[1]-positive cases, various other recipient chromosomes for the 22q material have been reported. These included 2q, 3p, 6p, 10q, 11p, 12p, 13p, 16p, 17p, 17q, 19q, 21p, and 22q[38-41]

Additional cytogenetic findings in patients with Ph[1]-positive CML were also reported, such as absence of a Y chromosome.[42,43]

D. Ph[1]-negative CML

Other chromosomal abnormalities in Ph[1]-negative CML patients have been reported. These included missing Y,[44] trisomy 8,[45] and trisomy 13.[46] It is interesting to note that a few patients reported by Sandberg and Sakurai with Ph[1]-negative CML and a missing Y chromosome had rather long periods of survival and better response to therapy.[42]

It is possible that patients with Ph[1]-negative CML may represent a different type of disorder.[47] The clinical course is more rapidly fatal with a mean course of 18 months as opposed to 45 months in Ph[1]-positive CML patients. An age difference has also been noted; Ph[1]-negative patients tend to be older than Ph[1] patients. Males who are Ph[1]-negative also appear to respond poorly to treatment. In addition, the blood picture varies from typical Ph[1]-negative disease. As Ph[1]-negative patients may form a distinct subgroup of patients, Kenis and Koulischer[48] have suggested the term chronic myeloid leukemia for Ph[1]-negative patients. This clinical-cytogenetic picture seems to have remained constant even in the postbanding era.

E. Acute Phase of CML

In the acute phase of Ph[1] (+) CML, 70 to 80% of patients develop other chromosomal abnormalities.[39,49,50] The two most frequently seen karyotypic changes are the presence of an additional Ph[1] and trisomy 8.[39,51] Close to 30% of patients in the blastic phase developed an isochromosome for the long arm of 17 (17qi).[39,50-52]

In the cases of two Ph[1] chromosomes, only one 9q + chromosome has been observed.[39] This again indicated an initial single event in the formation of the reciprocal translocation involving t(9q + ;22q−), and the duplication of the Ph[1] chromosome is possibly a result of mitotic nondisjunction.

In general, alteration of the original karyotype observed in patients with CML is a grave sign; it usually indicates an imminent blastic crisis.[53,54] DeGrouchy and Turleau[55] proposed seven models of numerical and structural changes occurring in the acute phases of CML. These included: (1) duplication of the Philadelphia chromosome, isolated and associated with other abnormalities; (2) acquisition of an extra single supernumerary, probably a C group chromosome; (3) acquisition of several supernumerary chromosomes; (4) loss of one or more chromosomes G, Y, 17, 8; (5) loss and acquisition; (6) structural rearrangements i(17q) as well as others; (7) polyploidization. Although reported before banding, their analyses led to the conclusion that the sixth model was seen in over 50% of karyotypes from patients with CML in the acute blastic phase. These findings have been well corroborated with banding techniques.

F. Summary

A unique chromosomal abnormality, the Ph[1] (22q−), was found in 85% of patients with CML. It was not only demonstrated to be acquired, but also to be of clonal origin. The clonal origin of Ph[1] implies that malignancy in general arises as a consequence of mutation or chromosomal event in a single cell. The Ph[1] chromosome has been found in precursor cells of the erythroid-myeloid-megakary-ocytic series, again indicating that the initial mutation occurs in a common stem cell.

The new chromosome banding techniques have identified the nature of the balanced reciprocal translocation of the Ph[1] chromosome. In 93% or more cases of Ph[1]-positive CML, the translocation involves the long arms of a No. 9 and a No. 22 chromosome, i.e., t(9q + ;22q−) with break points at 9q34 and 22q11. However, 7% showed other recipient chromosomes for the 22qter regions. The fact that all translocations are balanced in nature and all involve a rearranged 22q11→22qter suggests a position effect due to a displaced 22q11→22qter rather than a rearranged recipient chromosome. This position effect possibly causes a specific myeloproliferative process, i.e., CML, which then predisposes the patient to be more susceptible to true leukemia.[55a]

In the blastic crisis of CML, other nonrandom chromosome aberrations such as double Ph[1], trisomy 8, and isochromosome of 17 (17qi) have been frequently found. In the cases with two Ph[1] chromosomes, only one 9q + chromosome has been detected, again implying a single chromosome mutation. In general, a change of karyotype in patients with CML suggests an imminent acute blastic crisis.

III. ACUTE MYELOGENOUS LEUKEMIA

A. Prebanding

Prior to the use of the current banding techniques, 35 to 50% of cases with acute myelogenous leukemia (AML) were found to have what appeared to be random chromosomal abnormalities.[27,29,39] Although no consistent chromosomal aberrations were recognizable, the C group chromosomes appeared to be involved more often, as expected, in both gain or loss of chromosomes. Perhaps due to the inadequate cytogenetic techniques, structural chromosomal aberrations were rarely seen. A change in ploidy in AML was noted by Cervenka and Koulischer in the distribution of the modal chromosome number.[28] Hypodiploid states accounted for 11%, pseudodiploid states for 6.3% and hyperdiploid states accounted for 29.5%. Sandberg et al.[56] suggested that a diploid or hypodiploid chromosomal complement is more frequently seen in patients with AML, whereas hyperdiploid states tend to be seen more often in patients with acute lymphocytic leukemia (ALL).

Hart et al.[57] suggested that patients with extra D and E chromosomes appeared to have a better prognosis, whereas shorter survival seemed to be associated with an extra C group chromosome. Fitzgerald[58] found that male patients missing a C group chromosome had survival times three times longer than those patients who had trisomy for a C group chromosome. However, Fitzgerald drew the conclusion that, in general, chromosomal aberration did not appear to influence the course of the disease.

B. Postbanding

With the new banding techniques, it has become clear that there is a nonrandom chromosomal involvement in patients with different types of AML. Chromosomal aberrations have been observed in 15 to 100 % of patients with AML in different studies.[12,39,50,59,60] Rowley found 50% of her 50 patients showed chromosomal abnormalities,[39] Mitelman et al.[12] first reported about 43% of their 30 patients with aneuploidy, then Levan and Mitelman[50] found only 15% with chromosomal aberrations in a larger series of 186 patients. Hsu[59] identified 14 cases with chromosomal aberrations (4 were trisomy 8) in 46 patients with a clinical diagnosis of AML between 1974 and 1977. Ford et al.,[60] however, reported that all 12 of their patients with AML showed chromosomal aberrations, and each included at least trisomy 9.

The combined data showed that about 30% of cases had chromosomal abnormalities and that the chromosomes affected most commonly in AML are 8, 21, 7, 9, 17, X, Y, and 5. Chromosome No. 8 is the most frequently involved chromosome of all. Chromosomes No. 8 and 9 are almost always trisomic or translocated, chromosomes No. 7 and 5 are more frequently seen with loss of material or monosomy, chromosome No. 21 exhibits trisomy and monosomy, chromosome No. 17 is frequently involved in isochromosome formation of the long arm, and both X and Y are frequently lost.

To reiterate, chromosome No. 8 is not only frequently involved in trisomy, but also in structural rearrangement. A reciprocal translocation t(8q−;21q+) or t(8; 21) (q22; q22) has been identified in at least five patients with AML.[39] In Rowley's collected series, 8% of patients with AML showed this specific site for

insertion or activation of a specific oncogenic virus.[11] The specific chromosome aberration may represent one step in a two-step system of carcinogenesis as postulated by Knudson.[61].

Rowley[39] also identified two cases of translocation involving chromosomes 6 and 9, i.e., t(6; 9) (p23; q34). In 1977, Rowley et al.[62] and Okada et al.[63] reported another type of translocation in four patients with acute promyelocytic leukemia, i.e., a reciprocal translocation of t(15; 17) (q22; q21). [62,63] Since each of these two structural rearrangements involved identical breakage points, i.e., 6p23 and 9q34 for the former translocation and 15q22 and 17q21 for the latter, it evidently indicates nonrandom involvements.

In one of the trisomy 8 patients observed by Hsu,[59] the trisomy 8 cells completely disappeared during the remission and reappeared before the relapse, this time accompanied by other additional chromosomal abnormalities.

As to the possible prognostic value of chromosomal aberration in the banded studies, Nilsson et al.,[64] in 1977, suggested that the karyotype could be an important prognostic indicator in acute non-lymphocytic leukemias (AL). They found that the prognosis was more favorable in patients with only normal karyotypes (mean survival time of 8 months). The patients who showed both normal and abnormal karyotypes had an average 2.5-month survival time, whereas patients with only abnormal karyotypes showed the least survival time averaging 1 month.

C. Summary

Chromosomal abnormalities have been demonstrated in the bone marrow in about 30% of patients with AML. The banding studies have definitely indicated nonrandom chromosomal involvement. The most frequently affected chromosome is No. 8 with trisomy in most instances and reciprocal translocation, i.e., t(8q−;21q+) in a significant percent. The other commonly involved chromosomes are 7, 21, 9, 17, X, Y, and 5. Chromosomes 7 and 5 are associated with deletion or monosomy. Chromosome 21 showed both gain and loss, chromosome 9 was associated with trisomy, chromosome 17 was involved in isochromosome formation, and the sex chromosomes were frequently lost. It is conceivable that with more studies and follow-up the relationship between the cytogenetic finding and the clinical course will be better correlated.

IV. CHRONIC LYMPHOCYTIC LEUKEMIA

A. Prebanding

Cytogenetic studies of the leukemic cells in chronic lymphocytic leukemia (CLL) have not revealed any consistent or even observable gross abnormalities.[26,28,29] Woodliff and Cohen[65] studied the PHA-stimulated peripheral blood lymphocytes from 40 patients with diagnosed CLL. Normal karyotypes were found in 10 patients, and 30 other patients showed an increased aneuploidy but no anueploid cell lines. In none of the karyotypes from the 40 patients was a persistent marker detectable. Differences in survival time could not be correlated with the aneuploid and normal karyotypes. Gunz et al.[66] reported a family with CLL in which several members had an apparent deletion of the short arms of a G-group chromosome and they designated this marker chromosome as the Christ Church (New Zealand) chromosome (or Ch[1] for its place of original observation). However, this finding has not been substantiated. Hence, it probably represented an isolated marker and possibly a balanced translocation state, although undetected without banding techniques.

A lower mitotic rate as well as decreased synthesis of protein has been observed in 72-hr PHA-stimulated lymphocytes from patients with CLL. However, after 5 to 7 days of PHA stimulation, a maximal response was achieved.[67,68]

B. Postbanding

Crossen[69] studied the lymphocytes of 20 patients with CLL using the new banding techniques. All the cultures were 72-hr PHA-stimulated peripheral blood lymphocytes. He concluded that the chromosomes in CLL have normal banding patterns. Since CLL could be either a T or B cell disorder[70,71] in Crossen's 69 studies, using PHA may have allowed the investigators to observe the chromosome complement of stimulated T cells. Therefore, it is difficult to know whether or not the karyotypes are representative of the leukemic cells.

If Dameshek's[72] conception of CLL is ac-

cepted, namely that the disease may be merely an accumulation of immunologically incompetent lymphocytes, then there may be no malignant cell at all. The rare karyotypic changes seen may be due to therapeutic measures.

V. ACUTE LYMPHOCYTIC LEUKEMIA

A. Prebanding

In more than 500 patients with acute lymphocytic leukemia (ALL) studied by Whang-Peng et al.,[73] Sandberg and Hossfeld,[27] and Oshimura and Sandberg,[74] chromosomal abnormality was found in about 50% of patients either prior to treatment or at some stage of the disease. Hyperdiploidy was the predominant finding. In the series of Whang-Peng et al.,[73] the most common chromosomal group involved in aneuploidy was the G group and the next most common was the B group. A Gq− chromosome which appeared to be a Ph[1] chromosome was observed in four patients, and two of these chromosomes were later proven to be 21q−. They noted disappearance of the aneuploid cells during remission and suggested that aneuploid cells appeared to have no prognostic significance, nevertheless they recommended eradication of aneuploid cells in order to achieve a long remission.

B. Postbanding

In the series of Oshimura and Sandberg,[74] banding studies were possible in 16 cases with chromosomal abnormalities. Of these 16, 4 patients were found to have a similar chromosomal abnormality in their bone marrow cells; all 4 patients had a partial deletion of the long arm of one of their No. 6 chromosomes, i.e., del(6) (pter→q21; q25→qter). In addition, two patients had only 6q−, and two had other chromosomal abnormalities as well. Evidently, this type of deletion indicates a nonrandom chromosomal involvement. This chromosomal abnormality may very well prove to be a specific abnormality for ALL, since such an abnormality has not been previously reported in AML.

Using T and B lymphocyte membrane markers it has been shown that 26% of ALL cases were T cell in type, 4% were B cell, and the 70% with no detectable membrane markers were null type.[75] Study of the surface antigens in the two cases with 6q− of Oshimura and Sandberg showed one to be a T cell ALL and one to be null cell ALL.

In at least six instances of ALL, a Ph[1]-like chromosome was detected in the bone marrow cells.[76-81]. In at least five of these cases, a Ph[1] chromosome was identified with banding techniques. However, as stated earlier, two Ph[1]-appearing chromosomes in Whang-Peng's series were verified as 21q−, instead. This would suggest an earlier stem cell involvement of the Ph[1] formation and the initial cell, with the chromosome mutation later giving rise to a predominantly lymphoid population.

VI. ERYTHROLEUKEMIA

Several investigators studied 28 patients with erythroleukemia (EL)[82-84] prior to banding. Besides these 28 cases, 24 more cases were reviewed by Cervenka and Koulischer.[28] Cytogenetically, differences between EL, erythremic myelosis and DiGuglielmo's disease are not clear. The cytogenetic findings in all 54 cases show hypodiploid states to predominate in the karyotypes. Random structural changes have also been observed. A ring chromosome has been demonstrated in three cases;[84-86] however, in each report the ring appeared to represent a different chromosomal group.

With banding techniques, Petit and Fondu[87] identified a monosomy 7 in a patient with erythroleukemia.

VII. DOWN SYNDROME AND LEUKEMIA

It is an established fact that children with Down syndrome have a significantly greater incidence of acute leukemia than normal children.[88-92] Apparently, different figures have been reported from studies in different geographic areas; a 12-fold increase of leukemia deaths above expectation was observed in California, while in Pennsylvania the increase was 61-fold.[93] In general, it is believed that there is an increase of 12- to 15-fold in the incidence of leukemia in patients with Down's syndrome.[91] The cytogenetic studies by Harnden and O'Riordan of 89 children with leukemia showed two patients with trisomy 21, one with a reciprocal balanced translocation, and 86 pa-

tients with normal karyotypes. They indicated that in children with leukemia any increase in constitutional chromosomal abnormalities other than trisomy 21 must be relatively small. It has been shown that children with Down's syndrome who develop leukemia have predominantly acute lymphocytic leukemia, as do normal children who become leukemic.[90,92] The identification of the Ph[1] chromosome as a 22q− has corrected the erroneous belief of a relationship between trisomy 21 and myelogenous leukemia.

As to the possible mechanisms which cause the increased susceptibility of Down's syndrome to leukemia, many studies have been carried out. In 1967 Todaro and Martin[94] found that cultured fibroblasts from patients with Down's syndrome showed an increased SV40 transformation rate in vitro. It was suggested that patients with Down's syndrome carry an intrinsic susceptibility of the trisomic cells to oncogenic agents. Gregory et al.[95] demonstrated a high frequency of partial leukocyte dysfunction against staphylococci in children with Down's syndrome and suggested that it could be one of the leukemogenic factors.

Higurashi et al.[96] observed increased chromosomal damage in patients with Down's syndrome who had chicken pox. A constitutional (genetic) change may lead to the patient with Down's syndrome being more susceptible to exogenous influences which may further affect the chromosomes. Lambert et al.[97] studied DNA repair mechanism in leukocytes from patients with Down's syndrome with UV and X-ray exposure. The results indicated that DNA repair mechanism is significantly impaired in leukocytes from such patients, which possibly is a contributing factor in causing increased susceptibility to leukemia in these children.

VIII. POLYCYTHEMIA VERA

A. Prebanding

Cervenka and Koulischer[28] reviewed 86 cases of polycythemia vera (PV) in the literature before the advent of banding. The majority (65% of karyotypes had diploid cell lines. Some of these patients were studied before and some after treatment. Occasionally, a chromosome resembling the Ph[1] chromosome was found.[29] Several groups of investigators reported a significant number of cases with partial deletion of an F group chromosome.[98-102] This morphologically aberrant F group chromosome deletion was not clarified until banding studies were employed.[103]

The recent report of the PV study group found a preponderance of C group chromosome abnormalities. This study demonstrated that 26% of patients studied before treatment had chromosome abnormalities. Hyperdiploidy appeared to be the most common type of aberration observed. The findings of hyperdiploidy as the commonest manifestation of cytogenetic alterations have been reported by others also.

B. Postbanding

Using the banding techniques, nonrandom chromosomal involvements have also been demonstrated in patients with PV.[11] The most common chromosomal aberrations are trisomy 8,[11,45,104] trisomy 9,[11] partial trisomy 1q,[104,105] and 20q−.[103] The latter chromosomal aberration has been observed mostly in patients who had received P32 and/or chemotherapy. The 7q− chromosome has been reported in a few instances.[11,106,107] Thus far, no large series has been studied with banding techniques. Shiraishi et al.[108] analyzed 13 patients and found definite karyotypic abnormalities in 5 patients, including 3 with Fq− (one was proven to be 20q−;) one with both 11q− and 13q−, and 1 with a missing Y. They believe that cytogenetic changes do not play a crucial role in the genesis of PV. It also seems that aberrant clones most likely do not indicate that clinical leukemia is imminent.[109]

C. Summary

Chromosomal aberrations were found in about 26% of patients with untreated PV. Hyperdiploidy was the most frequent finding. The banding techniques again showed nonrandom chromosomal involvement with the most common abnormalities being trisomy 8, trisomy 9, partial trisomy 1q, and a partial deletion of the long arm of a No. 20 chromosome 20q−. Most of the patients with 20q− had received either P32 or chemotherapy or both. Thus far, the relationship between the cytogenetic findings and the clinical course is not clear.

IX. MULTIPLE MYELOMA

Woodliff[26] and Cervenka and Koulischer[28] have reviewed the cytogenetic changes associated with multiple myeloma (MM). A marker chromosome has been identified in perhaps as many as 50% of cases prior to banding.[28] The marker appears to be in both bone marrow and peripheral blood. At times it appeared to be a submetacentric chromosome or a large acrocentric chromosome,[28] but these markers are not demonstrated consistently. Of 51 patients reported by several investigators,[28] 4 were hypodiploid, 11 were pseudodiploid, 23 were diploid, 13 cases were hyperdiploid, and 23 markers were seen in the aneuploid lines.

Using G banding in 1973, Wurster-Hill et al.[110] found a 14q+ marker with two extra terminal bands in the bone marrow cells of two patients with MM and plasma cell leukemia. One of the patients had a bimodal number of cells 42 and 46; the abnormal chromosome was seen only in the cells with 42 chromosomes, which has been the case in those patients studied prior to banding as well. In both cases the abnormal 14 replaced a normal one. In 1975, Philip [111] demonstrated this marker in one patient with MM. In a series of 22 patients with myelomatosis, Weitze and Rowley,[112] using quinacrine fluorescence, observed this 14q+ marker chromosome in the blood and bone marrow cells of three patients with MM and in the peripheral blood lymphocytes of one patient with plasma cell leukemia. In the patient with plasma cell leukemia, both No. 14 chromosomes were replaced by the 14q+ marker chromosome. Thus, it appears that the 14q+ marker is seen to occur in a nonrandom fashion in this disorder. The high incidence of this marker seen in several related disorders has led to the assumption that genes regulating lymphoid cell proliferation may be located on the No. 14 chromosome.[112a] Further studies are needed to determine the significance of this interesting relationship.

X. MACROGLOBULINEMIA OF WALDENSTRÖM

Chromosomal changes were first reported in

this entity in 1961. Bottura et al.[113] first described a large supernumerary chromosome appearing rather like a large No. 2 or B group chromosome. Since then, German et al.[114] and Benirschke et al.[115] have described chromosomes having the appearance of a large metacentric No. 1 chromosome. This extra chromosome has been found in peripheral blood lymphocytes and bone marrow. The size of the marker has not been identical in all reports. The percentage of cells in reported cases showing the marker chromosome varied from 2 to 51%.[28] DeNava[29] reported nine cases of MGW, all with normal metaphase chromosomes. Therefore, the question of a marker chromosome, although established in some cases, cannot be said to be uniquely associated with MGW. The discrepancy may be accounted for by different stages of the disease or even some heterogeneity of the disease process and pathology as reflected in the cells studied. Verification of such findings awaits further banding studies.

XI. HODGKIN'S DISEASE AND NON-HODGKIN'S LYMPHOMAS

Several reviews dealing with the cytogenetics of malignant lymphomas and Hodgkin's Disease (HD) have appeared before banding techniques were consistently used.[26,28,29,116] In 1970, Spiers and Baikie[117] raised the possibility of a connection between the E group chromosomes No. 17 and/or No. 18 and the malignant lymphomas including HD. They analyzed the previously reported cases up to 1970 (all unbanded) and found five cases of HD with a constant loss of an E group chromosome. They also found a number of structural rearrangements involving the E group chromosomes including an isochromosome for a No. 17 or No. 18.

Reeves,[118] with banding, studied ten cases of malignant lymphomas, including three cases of HD. The cells studied were obtained either from the tumors (lymph nodes or spleen) or from peripheral blood stimulated with phytohemagglutinin. Hyperdiploidy with a rare diploid complement was seen in the cultured cells from these three patients. Each patient's cells contained a number of random rearrangements or markers. In the first case a 14q + was seen in all analyzed cells. Many complex rearrangements were also seen in the two other cases. The non-Hodgkin's lymphomas also showed a variety of numerical and structural chromosomal alterations. An isochromosome i(18q) was also seen in a non-Hodgkin's lymphoma. Most interesting was the observation that all the break points appeared to involve either the light staining bands or the centromeres.

Reeves[118] claimed that he could differentiate HD from other malignant lymphomas on the basis of numerical chromosomal changes. Approximately half of the HD cases had 57 to 80 chromosomes as the modal number, whereas other lymphomas had 54 to 56 in the chromosomal complement.

Fleischmann et al.[119] studied nine cases of HD (banded) among other lymphomas and found E group chromosomal involvement in four cases and C group chromosomal involvement in two cases. Four cases were found to have normal karyotypes.

XII. BURKITT'S LYMPHOMA

Prior to the use of banding techniques, tumor preparation from patients with Burkitt's lymphoma (BL) demonstrated hyperdiploid and tetraploid cell lines along with normal karyotypes. A marker chromosome, resembling a No. 2 chromosome, was occasionally observed by several investigators.[26,28]

In 1972, Manolov and Manolova[120] identified a similar chromosomal abnormality involving one No. 14 chromosome, i.e., 14q + with an extra band of medium staining intensity in biopsies and cell cultures in all 12 patients with BL. Their findings were subsequently confirmed by Jarvis[121] and Jarvis et al.[122] in 1974 in the lymphoblastoid cell lines of additional patients. The 14q + marker was not observed in cell lines obtained from patients with infectious mononucleosis nor from 18 lines infected with EB virus derived from fetal cord blood. Jarvis et al. suggested that this represented an in vivo type of transformation leading to the formation of the marker No. 14 chromosome. However, Prigogina and Fleischman[123] have demonstrated a similar 14q + marker in two patients with non-Burkitt's lymphomas. Zech et al.[124] not only further confirmed the 14q + marker chromosomes in patients with BL, but also demonstrated that the 14q + was a recipient chromosome of a balanced reciprocal trans-location, i.e., t(8q−;14q+), in at least 12 patients studied with banding techniques.

McCaw et al.[125] have found the t(8q−;14q+) in biopsied material from two African and three North American BLs. Further, they found the 14q+ translocation in both Ebstein Barr virus (EBV) negative and positive specimens. They feel that nonrandom translocation is related to lymphocytic neoplasia rather than to EBV. The recent evidence of Fukuhara et al.[126] that a large acrocentric 14q+ chromosome marker was found in several cases of non-Burkitt's lymphomatous disease seems to support the assumption of McCaw et al.[112a,125] The marker chromosome in the report of Fukuhara et al. appeared to be a 14:14 tandem long arm translocation.

XIII. CONCLUDING REMARKS

The relationship of chromosomal abnormalities and the susceptibility to develop neoplasia has been the subject of much investigation and speculation.[1,23,127-135] An increased susceptibility to leukemia and other malignancies has been clearly demonstrated in patients irradiated for ankylosing spondylitis [136] and individuals exposed to atomic bomb radiation.[137] This increased risk may be related to the long term chromosome damage caused by irradiation. Children with Down syndrome also have been shown to have a higher incidence of acute leukemia and begin life with a constitutional chromosomal abnormality. Four recessively inherited disorders associated with chromosomal breakage and rearrangement, Fanconi's anemia,[128,129,134-138] ataxia telangiectasia,[128,129,134,139-142] Bloom's syndrome,[126,129,134,143,144] and xeroderma pigmentosum (no spontaneous breakage is seen — the defect is in defective DNA repair after UV exposure) may serve as models in attempting to bridge the two events, i.e., chromosomal damage — fragility and instability — and the increased risk of developing neoplasia.

In 1966, Todaro[145] and co-workers showed that cultured fibroblasts derived from individuals with Fanconi's anemia and Down's syndrome[94] had a greater tendency to undergo an in vitro transformation. Following exposure to an oncogenic virus, SV40, the cultured fibro-

blasts lost their orderly monolayer pattern and developed characteristics associated with malignancy, namely the loss of contact inhibition. Thus, this model provided further evidence that preexistent chromosomal aberrations or instability might lead to increased susceptibility to malignancy in vivo. Furthermore, by using somatic cell hybridization, it has been shown that specific mammalian chromosomes play a role in neoplastic transformation and even neoplastic suppression.[146] In 1971, Klein[147] and his co-workers, by fusing normal mouse cells and malignant mouse cells, produced a hybrid initially showing no malignant potential. However, when certain chromosomes of the normal parent were eliminated, the hybrid regained its malignant potential. Fusion of two malignant cell types results in a malignant cell if there is no chromosome loss, but if specific chromosomes are lost, the cells may lose their malignant potential.

Yamamoto et al.[148] have proposed a model for the genetic control of neoplasia, possibly determined by the balance of genes for expression (E) and suppression (S) of malignancy. A chromosomal change brought about by a carcinogenic agent might alter the balance between (E) and (S) genes.

The banding techniques have demonstrated nonrandom chromosome involvement in various leukemias and related disorders. It has also become clear that chromosomal break points (either induced or spontaneous) are nonrandom in nature. von Koskull and Aula[149] demonstrated that the break points in five patients with Fanconi's anemia occur exclusively in the lightly stained regions of the chromosomes corresponding to the R bands. They further found statistically significant involvement of chromosomes 1, 2, 3, 6, and 13 with little breakage in the X and Y chromosomes. There is also evidence that even X-rays do not damage chromosomes in a random fashion.[150,151]

Recently, a new technique has been described by Latt[152] that can accurately define sister chromatid exchange (SCE). Sister chromatid exchange involves the homologous exchange of regions of two sister chromatids, which does not lead to a cytological alteration of chromosome morphology. It has been shown that several chromosome breaking agents induce increased SCE, which was also shown to be dose dependent. Thus, SCE determination may serve as a potent indicator of the presence of a mutagen, but is also of potential importance as a means of detecting subtle chromosome instability or fragility.[153] An increased SCE has been demonstrated in Bloom's disease, but is not seen in Fanconi's anemia.[154]

Rowley[155] has postulated that for each nonrandom chromosomal event a possibly specific etiologic agent may be active, so that this exogenous (environmental) agent acts in some manner to alter the genetically susceptible genome and induce or trigger a subsequent neoplastic change. There is evidence that in some mice the leukemogenic susceptibility may be genetically controlled at the H2 locus.[156] Thus, a virus may act as an inducer to produce leukemia in a genetically susceptible host. [157,159,160]

Such associations of leukemia and HLA are not yet established in man. Finally, Mitelman et al.[160] found that they could induce some tumors in mice (indistinguishable histologically one from the other) with different oncogenic agents, Rous sarcoma virus (RSV) and 7,12-dimethylbenz(a) anthracene (DMBA) In each instance, although the tumor was the same, the karyotype was distinct and apparently of a nonrandom character.

The development of the various techniques, such as banding which demonstrates involvement of specific chromosomes, examination of sister chromatid exchange, and somatic cell hybridization, along with advances in immunology, will further our understanding of the role of chromosomes in leukemia and other neoplastic conditions.

REFERENCES

1. Boveri, T., *Zur Frage der Enstening Maligner Tumoren*, Gustav Fischer, Jena, 1914.
2. Ford, C. E., Hamerton, J. L., and Mole, R. H., Chromosomal changes in primary and transplanted reticular neoplasms of the mouse, *J. Cell. Physiol.*, 52 (Suppl. 1), 235, 1958.
3. Nowell, P. C. and Hungerford, D. A., A minute chromosome in human chronic granulocytic leukemia, *Science*, 132, 1497, 1960.
4. Baikie, A. G., Chromosomes and leukemia, *Acta Haematol.*, 36, 157, 1966.
5. Tijo, J. H. and Whang, J., Chromosomal preparation of bone marrow cells without prior *in vitro* or *in vivo* colchicine administration, *Stain Technol.*, 37, 17, 1962.
6. Moorehead, P. S., Nowell, P. C., Mellman, W. J., Battips, D. M. J. and Hungerford, D. A., Chromosome preparations of leukocytes cultured from human peripheral blood, *Exp. Cell. Res.*, 20, 613, 1960.
7. Paris Conference (1971), Standardization in Human Cytogenetic Birth Defects, *Original Article Series VIII*, The National Foundation, New York, 1972.
8. Shaw, M. W. and Chen, T. R., The application of banding techniques to tumor chromosomes, in *Chromosomes and Cancer*, German, J., Ed., John Wiley & Sons, New York, 1974, 135.
9. Caspersson, T., Gahrton, G., Lindsten, J., and Zech, L., Identification of the Philadelphia chromosome as a No. 22 by quinacrine mustard fluorescence analysis, *Exp. Cell. Res.*, 63, 238, 1970.
10. Rowley, J., A new consistent chromosomal abnormality in chronic myelogenous leukemia identified by quinacrine fluorescence and Giemsa staining, *Nature* (London), 243, 290, 1973.
11. Rowley, J. D., Nonrandom chromosomal abnormalities in hematological disorders of man, *Proc. Natl. Acad. Sci. U.S.A.*, 72, 152, 1975.
12. Mitelman, F., Nilsson, P. G., Levan, G., and Brandt, L., Nonrandom chromosomal changes in acute myeloid leukemia: chromosomal banding examination of 30 cases at diagnosis, *Int. J. Cancer*, 18, 31, 1976.
13. Mitelman, F. and Levan, G., Clustering of aberrations to specific chromosomes in human neoplasms. II. A survey of 287 neoplasms, *Hereditas*, 82, 167, 1976.
14. Rowley, J. D., Golomb, H. M., Vardiman, J., Fukuhara, S., Doughterty, C. J., and Porter, D., Further evidence for a nonrandom chromosomal abnormality in acute promyelocytic leukemia, *Int. J. Cancer*, 20, 869, 1977.
15. Ezdinli, E. Z., Sokal, J. E., Crosswhite, B. S., and Sandberg, A. A., Philadelphia chromosome positive and negative in chronic myelocytic leukemia, *Ann. Intern. Med.*, 72, 175, 1970.

16. **Frei, E., Tijo, J. H., Wang, J., and Carbone, P. P.**, Studies of the Philadelphia chromosome in patients with chronic myelogenous leukemia, *Ann. N.Y. Acad. Sci.*, 113, 1973. 1964.

17. **Canellos, G. P., Devita, V. T., Whang-peng, J., and Carbone, P. P.**, Hematologic and cytogenetic remission of blastic transformation in chronic granulocytic leukemia, *Blood*, 38, 671, 1971.

18. **Kamada, N. and Uchino, H.**, Double Ph[1] chromosome in leukemia, *Lancet*, 1, 1107, 1967.

19. **Goh, K. and Swisher, S. N.**, Identical twins and chronic myelocytic leukemia: chromosomal studies of a patient with myelocytic leukemia and his normal identical twin, *Arch. Intern. Med.*, 114, 439, 1964.

19a. **Dougan, L., Scott, I. D., and Woodliff, H. J.**, A pair of twins one of whom has chronic granulocytic leukemia, *J. Med. Genet.*, 3, 217, 1966.

20. **Canellos, G. P. and Whang-Peng, J.**, Philadelphia chromosome positive preleukemic state, *Lancet*, 1, 1227, 1972.

21. **Baccarini, M., Zaccaria, A., and Tura, S.**, Philadelphia chromosome positive preleukemic state, *Lancet*, 2, 1094, 1973.

22. **Weiner, L.**, A family with high incidence leukemia and unique Ph[1] chromosome findings, *Blood* 26 (Abstr.), 871, 1965.

23. **Hirschhorn, K.**, Cytogenetic alterations in leukemia, in *Perspectives in Leukemia*, Damesheck, W. and Dutscher, R., Eds., Grune & Stratton, New York, 1968, 113.

24. **Muldal, S. and Lajtha, L. G.**, Chromosomes and leukemia, in *Chromosomes and Cancer*, German, J., Ed., John Wiley & Sons, New York, 1974.

25. **Prieto, F., Egozcue, J., Forteza, G., and Marco, F.**, Identification of the Philadelphia (Ph[1]) chromosome, *Blood*, 35, 23, 1970.

26. **Woodliff, H. J.**, *Leukemia Cytogenetics*, Year Book Medical Publishing, Chicago, 1971.

27. **Sandberg, A. and Hossfeld, D. K.**, Chromosomal abnormalities in human neoplasia, *Annu. Rev. Med.*, 21, 379, 1970.

28. **Cervenka, J. and Koulischer, L.**, Chronic myeloid granulocytic leukemia, in *Chromosomes in Human Cancer*, Gorlin, R. J., Ed., Charles C Thomas, Springfield, Ill., 1973, 55

29. **DeNava, C. M. C.**, Les anomalies chromosomiques au cour des hemopathies malignes et non malignes, *Monogr. Ann. Genet. (Paris) L'expansion*, 1, Editorial, 1969.

30. **Stryckmans, P. A.**, Current concepts in chronic myelogenous leukemia, *Semin. Hematol.*, 11, 101, 1974.

31. **Fialkow, P. J., Gartler, S. M., and Yoshida, A.**, Clonal origin of chronic myelocytic leukemia in man, *Proc. Natl. Acad. Sci. U.S.A.*, 58, 1468, 1967.

32. **Lawler, S. D. and Sanger, R.**, X_g blood groups and clonal origin theory of chronic myeloid leukemia, *Lancet*, 1, 584, 1970.

33. **Fitzgerald, P. H., Pickering, A. F., and Eiby, J. R.**, Clonal origin of the Philadelphia chromosome and chronic myeloid leukemia: evidence from a sex chromosome mosaic, *Br. J. Haematol.*, 21, 473, 1971.

33a. **Moore, M. A. S., Ekert, A., Fitzgerald, M. G., and Carmichael, A.**, Evidence for the clonal origin of chronic myeloid leukemia from a set chromosome mosaic: clinical, cytogenetic and marrow culture studies, *Blood*, 43, 15, 1974.

34. **Gahrton, G., Lindsten, J., and Zech, L.**, Clonal origin of the Philadelphia chromosome from either the paternal or the maternal chromosome No. 22, *Blood*, 43, 837, 1974.

35. **Goh, K. and Swisher, S. N.**, Identical twins and chronic myelocytic leukemia, *Arch. Intern. Med.*, 115, 475, 1965.

36. **O'Riordan, M. L., Robinson, J. A., Buckton, K. E., and Evans, H. J.**, Distinguishing between chromosomes involved in Downs Syndrome (trisomy 21) and chronic myeloid leukemia (Ph[1]) by fluorescence, *Nature* (London), 230, 167, 1971.

37. **Lawler, S. D., O'Malley, F., and Lobb, D. S.**, Chromosome banding studies in Philadelphia chromosome positive myeloid leukemia, *Scand. J Haematol.*, 17, 17, 1976

37a. **Prigogina, E. L. and Fleischman, E. W.**, Certain patterns of karyotype evolution in chronic myelogenous leukemia, *Humangenetik*, 30, 113, 1975.

37b. **Gahrton, J., Lindstein, J., and Zech, L.**, Involvement of chromosomes 8, 9, 19 and 22 in Ph[1] positive and Ph[1] negative chronic myelocytic leukemia in the chronic and blastic stages, *Acta. Med. Scand.*, 196, 355, 1974.

38. **Gahrton, G., Zech, L., and Lindsten, J.**, A new variant translocation (19q + ,22q−) in chronic myelocytic leukemia, *Exp. Cell. Res.*, 86, 214, 1974.

39. **Rowley, J. D.**, Population cytogenetics of leukemia, in *Population Cytogenetics: Studies in Humans*, Hook, E. B. and Porter, I., Eds., Academic Press, New York, 1977, 189.

40. **Van Den Blij-Philipsen, M., Breed, W. P. M., and Hustnix, T. W. J.** A case of chronic myeloid leukemia with a translocation t(12;22) (p13; g11), *Humangenetik*, 39, 229, 1977.

41. **Fleischman, E. W., Prigogina, E. L., Volkova, M. A., and Petkovitch, I.**, Unusual translocation t(10:22) in chronic myelogenous leukemia, *Humangenetik*, 39, 127, 1977.

42. Sandberg, A. P. and Sakurai, M., The missing Y chromosome and human leukemia, *Lancet*, 1, 375, 1973.

43. Lawler, S. D., Lobb, D. S., and Wiltshaw, E., Philadelphia chromosome positive bone marrow cells showing loss of the Y in males with chronic myeloid leukemia, *Br. J. Haematol.*, 27, 247, 1974.

44. Hossfeld, D. K. and Wendhorst, E., Ph[1] negative chronic myelocytic leukemia with a missing Y chromosome, *Acta Haematol.*, 52, 232, 1974.

45. Hsu, L. Y. F., Aiter, A. and Hirschhorn, K., Trisomy 8 in bone marrow cells of parents with polycythemia vera and myelogenous leukemia, *Clin. Genet.*, 6, 258, 1974.

46. Hsu, L. Y. F., Papenhausen, P., Greenberg, M. L., and Hirschhorn, K., Trisomy D in bone marrow cells in a patient with chronic myelogenous leukemia, *Acta Haematol.*, 52, 61, 1974.

47. Tijo, J. H., Carbone, P. O., Whang, J. , and Frei, E., The Philadelphia chromosome and chronic myelogenous leukemia, *J. Natl. Cancer Inst.*, 36, 587, 1966.

48. Kenis, Y., and Koulischer, L., Étude clinique et cytogénétique de 21 patients atteunts de leucémie myéloide chronique, *Eur. J. Cancer*, 3, 83, 1967.

49. Hossfeld, D. K., Identification of chromosome anomalies in the blastic phase of chronic myelocytic leukemia (CML) by Giemsa and quinacrine banding techniques, *Humangenetik*, 23, 111, 1974.

50. Levan, G. and Mitelman, F., Chromosomes and the etiology of cancer, in *Chromosomes Today*, Proc. 6th Int. Chromosome Conference, De la Chappelle, A. and Sorsa, M., Eds., Helsinki, August 1977, Elsevier-North Holland, Amsterdam, 1977, 363.

51. Goh, K., Additional Philadelphia chromosomes in acute blastic crisis of chronic myelocytic leukemia: possible mechanism of producing additional chromosomal abnormalities, *Am. J. Med. Sci.*, 267, 229, 1974.

52. Sharp, J. C., Potter, A. M., and Guyer, R. J., Karyotypic abnormalities in transformed chronic granulocytic leukemia, *Br. J. Haematol.*, 29, 587, 1975.

53. Whang-peng, J., Canellos, G. P., Carbone, P. O., and Tijo, J. H., Clinical implications of cytogenetic variants in chronic myelocytic leukemia (CML), *Blood*, 32, 755, 1968.

54. Sandberg, A. A., Hossfeld, D. K., Ezdinli, E. E., and Crosswhite, L. H., Chromosomes and causation of human cancer and leukemia VI blastic phase, cellular origin and the Ph[1] in CML, *Cancer*, 27, 176, 1971.

55. DeGrouchy, J. and Turleau, C., Clonal evolution in the meyloid leukemias, in *Chromosomes and Cancer*, German, J., Ed., John Wiley & Sons, 1974.

55a. Borgaonkor, D. S., Philadelphia chromosome translocations and chronic myeloid leukemia, *Lancet*, 1, 1250, 1973.

56. Sandberg, A. A., Takagi, N., Sofuni, T., and Crosswhite, L. H , Chromosomes and causation of human cancer and leukemia, *Cancer*, 22, 1268, 1968.

57. Hart, J. S., Trujillo, J. U., Freireich, E. J., George, S. L., and Frei, E., Cytogenetic studies and their clinical correlates in adults with acute leukemia, *Ann. Intern. Med.*, 75, 353, 1971.

58. Fitzgerald, P. H., Crossen, P. E., and Hamer, J . W.,Abnormal karyotypic clones in human acute leukemia: their nature and clinical significance, *Cancer*, 31, 1069, 1973.

59. Hsu, L. Y. F., unpublished data.

60. Ford, J. H., Pittman, S. M., Singh, S., Wass, E. J., Vincent, P. C., and Gunz, F. W., Cytogenetic basis of acute myeloid leukemia, *J. Natl. Cancer Inst.*, 55, 761, 1975.

61. Knudson, A. G., Mutation and cancer: statistical study of retinoblastoma, *Proc. Natl. Acad. Sci. U.S.A.*, 68, 820, 1971.

62. Rowley, J. D., Golomb, H. M., Vardiman, J., Fukuhara, S., Dougherty, C., and Potter, D., Further evidence for a nonrandom chromosomal abnormality in acute promyelocytic leukemia, *Int. J. Cancer*, 20, 869, 1977.

63. Okada, M., Miyazaki, T., and Kumota, K., 15/17 translocation in acute promyelocytic leukemia, *Lancet*, 1, 961, 1977.

64. Nilsson, P. G., Brandt, L., and Mitelman, F., Prognostic implications of chromosome analysis in acute non-lymphocytic leukemia, *Leukemia Res.*, 1, 31, 1977.

65. Woodliff, H. J. and Cohen, G., Cytogenetic studies in chronic lymphocytic leukemia, *Med. J. Aust.*, 1, 970, 1972.

66. Gunz, F. W., Fitzgerald, P. H., and Adams, A., An abnormal chromosome in chronic lymphocytic leukemia, *Br. Med. J.*, 2, 1097, 1962.

67. Goh, K. O., Pseudodiploid chromosomal pattern in chronic lymphocytic leukemia, *J. Lab. Clin. Med.*, 69, 938, 1967.

68. Havermann, K. and Rubin, A. D., The delayed response of chronic lymphocytic leukemia lymphocytes to phytohemagglutinin *in vitro*, *Proc. Soc. Exp. Biol. Med.*, 127, 668, 1968.

69. Crossen, P., Giemsa banding patterns in CLL, *Humangenetik*, 27, 151, 1975.

70. Catovsky, D. and Holt, P. J. L., T or B lymphocytes in chronic lymphocytic leukemia, *Lancet*, 1, 976, 1971.

71. Wilson, J. D. and Nossal, G. J. V., The T or B cell nature of chronic lymphocytic leukemia lymphocytes, *Lancet*, 1, 1153, 1971.

72. Damashek, W., Chronic lympocytic leukemia an accumulative disease of immunologically incompetent lymphocytes, *Blood,* 29, 566, 1967.
73. Whang-peng, J., Freireich, E. J., Oppenheim, J. J., Frei, E., and Tijo, J. H., Cytogenetic studies in 45 patients with acute lymphocytic leukemia, *J. Natl. Cancer Inst.,* 42, 881, 1969.
74. Oshimura, M. and Sandberg, A. A., Chromosomal 6q- anomaly in acute lymphoblastic leukemia, *Lancet,* 2, 1405, 1976.
75. Belpomme, D., Mathe, G., and Davis, A. J. S., Clinical significance and prognostic value of the T-B immunological classification of human primary acute lymphoid leukemias, *Lancet,* 1, 555, 1977.
76. Propp, S. and Lizzi, F. A., Philadelphia chromosome in acute lymphoblastic leukemia, *Blood,* 36, 353, 1970.
77. Schmidt, R., Dar, H., Santorineou, M., and Sekine, I. Ph[1] chromosome and loss and reappearance of the Y chromosome in acute lymphoblastic leukemia, *Lancet,* 1, 1145, 1975.
78. Secker Walker, L. M., and Hardy, J. D., Philadelphia chromosome in acute leukemia, *Cancer,* 38, 1619, 1976.
79. Rausen, A. R., Kim, H. J., Burstein, Y., Rand, S., McCaffrey, R. M., and Kung, P. C., Philadelphia chromosome in acute lymphocytic leukemia of childhood, *Lancet,* 1, 432, 1977.
80. Van Biervliet, J. P., Van Hemel, J., Geurts, K., Punt, K., and DeBoer-Van Wering, E., Philadelphia chromosome in acute lymphocytic leukemia, *Lancet,* 2, 617, 1975.
81. Mandel, E. M., Shabtai, F., Gafter, U., Klein, B. L., Halbrecht, I., and Djaldetti, M., Ph[1]- positive acute lymphocytic leukemia with chromosome 7 abnormalities, *Blood,* 49, 281, 1977.
82. Klossoglou, K. A., Mitus, W. J., and Damashek, W., Chromosomal aberrations in acute leukemia, *Blood,* 26, 611, 1965.
83. Castoldi, G., Yam, L. T., Mitus, W. J., and Crosby, W. H., Chromosomal studies in erythroleukemia and chronic erythremic myelosis, *Blood,* 31, 202, 1968.
84. Krogh-Jensen, M., *Chromosome Studies in Acute Leukemia,* Munksgaard, Copenhagen, 1969, 1.
85. DiGrado, F., Mendes, F. T., and Schroeder, E., Ring chromosome in a case of DiGuglielmo syndrome, *Lancet,* 2, 1243, 1964.
86. Crossen, P. E., Fitzgerlad, P. H., Menzies, R. C., and Brehaul, L. A., Chromosomal abnormality megaloblastosis and arrested DNA synthesis in erythroleukemia, *J. Med. Genet.,* 6, 95, 1969.
87. Petit, P., Alexander, M., and Fondu, P., Monosomy F in erythroleukemia, *Lancet,* 2, 1326, 1973.
88. Warkany, J., Schubert, W. K., and Thompson, J. N., Chromosome analyses in mongolism (Langdon-Down Syndrome) associated with leukemia, *N. Engl. J. Med.,* 268, 1, 1963.
89. Buchanan, J. G., and Becroft, D. M. O., Down's syndrome and acute leukemia: a cytogenetic study, *J. Med. Genet.,* 7, 67, 1970.
90. Rosner, F. and Lee, L. L., Down's Syndrome and acute leukemia, *Lancet,* 1, 110, 1973.
91. Harnden, D. G. and O'Riordan, M. L., Down's Syndrome and leukemia, *Lancet,* 1, 260, 1973.
92. Down's syndrome and acute leukemia, (editorial), *Lancet,* 2, 1187, 1972.
93. Jackson, E. W., Turner, J. H., Klauber, M. R., and Morris, F. D., Down's Syndrome: variation of leukemia occurrence in institutionalized populations, *J. Chronic Dis.,* 21, 247, 1968.
94. Todaro, G. J. and Martin, G. M., Increased susceptibility of Down's Syndrome fibroblasts to transformation by SV 40, *Proc. Soc. Exp. Biol. Med.,* 124, 1232, 1967.
95. Gregory, L., Williams, R., and Thompson, E., Leucocyte function in Down's Syndrome and acute leukemia, *Lancet,* 1, 1359, 1972.
96. Higurashi, M., Tamura, T., and Nakatake, T., Cytogenetic observations in cultured lymphocytes from patients with Down's Syndrome and measles, *Pediatr. Res.,* 7, 582, 1973.
97. Lambert, B., Hansson, K., Bui, T. H., Funes-Cranioto, F., Lindsten, J., Holmberg, M., and Strausmanis, R., DNA repair and frequency of X-ray and u.v. light induced chromosome aberrations in leukocytes from patients with Down's Syndrome, *Ann. Hum. Genet.,* 39, 293, 1976.
98. Kay, H. E. M., Lawler, S. D., and Millard, R., The chromosomes in polycythemia vera, *Br. J. Haematol.,* 12, 507, 1966.
99. Millard, R. E., Lawler, S. D., Kay, H. E. M., and Cameron, C. B., Further observations in patients with a chromosomal abnormality associated with polycythemia vera, *Br. J. Haematol.,* 14, 363, 1968.
100. Lawler, S. D., Millard, R. E., and Kay, H. E. M., Further cytogenetic investigations in polycythemia vera, *Eur. J. Cancer,* 6, 223, 1970.
101. Visfeldt, J., Primary polycythemia, *Acta Pathol. Microbiol. Scand. Sect.* 79, 513, 1971.
102. Hirschhorn, K. and Bloch-Shtacher, N., Transformation of genetically abnormal cells, in *Genetic Concepts and Neoplasia,* Anderson, W., Ed., Williams & Wilkins, Baltimore, 1970, 191.
103. Reeves, B. R., Lobb, D. S., and Lawler, S. D., Identity of the abnormal F group chromosome associated with polycythemia vera, *Humangenetik,* 14, 159, 1972.
104. Wurster-Hill, D., Whang-Peng, J., McIntyre, R. O., Hsu, L. Y. F., Hirschhorn, K., Modan, B., Pisciotta, A. V., Pierre, R., Balcerzak, S. P., Weinfeld, A., and Murphy, S., Cytogenetic studies in polycythemia vera, *Semin. Hematol.,* 13, 13, 1976.

105. Hsu, L. Y. F., Pinchiaroli, D., Gilbert, H. S., Wittman, R., and Hirschhorn, K., Partial trisomy of the long arm of chromosome 1 in myelofibrosis and polycythemia vera, *Am. J. Hematol.,* 2, 375, 1977.

106. Rowley, J. D., Deletions of chromosome 7 in hematological disorders, *Lancet.* 2, 1385, 1973.

107. Tsuchimoto, T., Bühler, E. M., Stadler, G. R., Mayer, A. C., and Obrecht, J. P., Deletion of chromosome 7 in polycythemia vera, *Lancet,* 1, 566, 1974.

108. Shiraishi, Y., Hayata, I., Sakurai, M., and Sandberg, A. A., Chromosomes and causation of human cancer and leukemia. XII. Banding analysis of abnormal chromosomes in polycythemia vera, *Cancer,* 36, 199, 1975.

109. Nowell, P., Jensen, J., Gardner, F., Murphy, S., Chaganti, R. S. K., and German, J., Chromosome studies in "preleukemic" III myelofibrosis, *Cancer,* 38, 873, 1976.

110. Wurster-Hill, D. H., McIntyre, O. R., Cornwell, G. G., and Maurer, L. H., Marker chromosome 14 in multiple myeloma and plasma cell leukemia, *Lancet,* 2, 1031, 1973.

111. Philip, P., Marker chromosome 14q+ in multiple myeloma, *Hereditas,* 80, 155, 1975.

112. Weitze, L. and Rowley, J. P., 14q+ marker chromosomes in multiple myeloma and plasma cell leukemia, *Lancet,* 1, 96, 1978.

112a. McCaw, B. K., Hecht, F., Hamden, D., and Teplitz, R. L., Somatic rearrangement of chromosome 14 in human lymphocytes, *Proc. Natl. Acad. Sci. U.S.A.,* 72, 2071, 1975.

113. Bottura, C., Ferrari, J. , and Veiga, A. A., Chromosome aberrations in Waldenström's Macroglobulinemia, *Lancet,,* 1, 1170, 1961.

114. German, J. L., Bird, C. E., and Bearn, A. G., Chromosomal abnormalities in Waldenström's Macroglobulinemia, *Lancet,* 2, 48, 1961.

115. Benirschke, K., Brownhill, L., and Ebàugh, F. G., Chromosomal abnormalities in Waldenström's Macroglobulinemia, *Lancet,* 1, 594, 1962.

116. Miles, C. P. Geller, W., and O'Neill, F., Chromosomes in Hodgkin's disease and other malignant lymphomas, *Cancer,* 19, 1103, 1966.

117. Spiers, A. S. D. and Baikie, A. G., A special role of the group 17-18 chromosomes in reticulo endothelial neoplasia, *Br. J. Cancer,* 24, 77, 1970.

118. Reeves, B. R., Cytogenetics of malignant lymphomas, *Humangenetik,* 20, 231, 1973.

119. Fleischmann, T., Hakansson, C. H., and Levan, A., Chromosomes of malignant lymphomas: studies in short term cultures from lymph nodes of twenty cases, *Hereditas,* 83, 47, 1976.

120. Manolov, G. and Manolova, Y., Marker band in one chromosome 14 from Burkitt's lymphoma, *Nature* (London), 237, 33, 1972.

121. Jarvis, J. E., Herpes virus and oncogenesis, *Nature* (London), 252, 348, 1974.

122. Jarvis, J. E., Bay, G., Rickinson, A. B., and Epstein, M. A., Cytogenetic studies on human lymphoblastoid cell lines from Burkitt's lymphoma and other sources, *Int. J. Cancer,* 14, 716, 1974.

123. Prigogina, E. L. and Fleischman, E. W., Marker chromosome 14q+ in two non-Burkitt lymphomas, *Humangenetik,* 30, 109, 1975.

124. Zech, L., Haglund, U., Nilsson, K., and Klein, G., Characteristic chromosomal abnormalities in biopsies and lymphoid cell lines from patients with Burkitt and non-Burkitt lymphomas, *Int. J. Cancer,* 17, 47, 1976.

125. McCaw, B. K., Epstein, A. L., Kaplan, H. S., and Hecht, F., Chromosome 14 translocation in African and North American Burkitt's lymphomas, *Int. J. Cancer,* 19, 482, 1977.

126. Fukuhara, S., Shivakawa, S., and Uchino, H., Specific marker chromosome 14 in malignant lymphomas, *Nature* (London), 259, 210, 1976.

127. DeGrouchy, J. and DeNava, C., A chromosomal theory of carcinogenics, *Ann. Intern. Med.,* 69, 381, 1968.

128. Schroeder, T. M. and Kurth, R., Spontaneous chromosomal breakage and high incidence of leukemia in inherited disease, *Blood,* 37, 96, 1971.

129. German, J., Genes which increase chromosomal instability in somatic cells and predispose to cancer, in *Progress in Medical Genetics,* Vol. 8, Steinberg, A. G. and Bearn, A. G., Eds., Grune & Stratton, New York, 1972.

130. German, J., Ed., *Chromosomes and Cancer,* John Wiley & Sons, New York, 1974.

131. Nowell, P. C., The clonal evolution of tumor cell population, *Science,* 194, 23, 1976.

132. DiPaolo, J. A. and Popescu, N. C., Relationship of chromosome changes to neoplastic cell transformation, *Am. J. Pathol.,* 65, 711, 1976.

133. Hirschhorn, K., Chromosomes and cancer, in *Cancer and Genetics,* Bergsma, D., Ed., A. Liss, New York, 1976, 113.

134. Hecht, F. and McCaw, B. K., Chromosome instability syndromes, in *Genetics of Human Cancer,* Mulvihill, J. J., Miller, R. W., and Fraumeni, J. F., Jr., Eds., Raven Press, New York, 1977, 105.

135. Chromosomes and cancer, *Lancet,* 2, 277, 1977.

136. Buckton, K. E., Jacobs, P. A., Court Brown, W. M., and Doll, R., A study of the chromosome damage persisting after X-ray therapy for ankylosing spondylitis, *Lancet,* 2, 676, 1962.

137. **Bloom, A. D.**, Induced chromosomal aberrations in man, in *Advances in Human Genetics,* Vol. 3, Harris, H. and Hirschhorn, K., Eds., Plenum Press, New York, 1972, 99.

138. **Swift, M. R. and Hirschhorn, K.,** Fanconi's anemia: inherited susceptibility to chromosomal breakage in various tissues, *Ann. Intern. Med.,* 65, 496, 1966.

139. **Hecht, F., McCaw, B. K., and Koler, R.,** Ataxia - telangiectasia - clonal growth of translocation lymphocytes, *N. Engl. J. Med. ,* 289, 286, 1973.

140. **Bochkov, N. P., Lopukhin, Y. M., Kuleshov, N. P., and Kovalchuk, L. V.,** Cytogenetic study of patients with ataxia telangiectasia, *Humangenetik,* 24, 115, 1974.

141. **Harnden, D. G.,** Ataxia telangiectasia syndrome: cytogenetic and cancer aspects, in *Chromosomes and Cancer,* German, J., Ed., John Wiley & Sons, 1974, 619.

142. **Oxford, J. M., Harnden, D. G., Parrington, J. M., and Delhanty, J. D. A.** Specific chromosome aberrations in ataxia telangiectasia, *J. Med. Genet.,* 12, 251, 1975.

143. **Sawitsky, A., Bloom, D., and German J.,** Chromosomal breakage and acute leukemia in congenital telangiectatic erythema and stunted growth, *Ann. Intern. Med.,* 65, 487, 1966.

144. **German, J.,** Bloom's syndrome. II. The prototype of human genetic disorders predisposing to chromosome instability and cancer, in *Chromosomes and Cancer,* German, J., Ed., John Wiley & Sons, New York, 1974, 601.

145. **Todaro, G. J., Green, H., and Swift, M. R.,** Susceptibility of human diploid fibroblast staining to transformation by SV40 virus, *Science,* 153, 1252, 1966.

146. **Miller, O. J.,** Cell hybridization in the study of the malignant process, including cytogenetic aspects, in *Chromosomes and Cancer,* German, J., Ed., John Wiley & Sons, New York, 1974, 521.

147. **Klein, G., Bregula, U., Wiener, F., and Harris, F.,** The analysis of malignancy by cell fusion. I. Hybrids between tumor cells and L cell derivatives, *J. Cell. Sci.,* 8, 659, 1971.

148. **Yamamoto, T , Rabinowitz, Z., and Sachs, L.,** Identification of the chromosomes that control malignancy, *Nature* (London) New Biol., 243, 247, 1973.

149. **von Koskull, H. and Aula, P.,** Non-random distribution of chromosome breaks in Fanconi's anemia, *Cytogenet. Cell Genet.,* 12, 423, 1973.

150. **Caspersson, T., Haglund, U., Lindell, B., and Zech, L.,** Radiation induced non-random chromosome breakage, *Exp. Cell. Res.,* 75, 541, 1972.

151. **Seabright, M.,** High resolution studies on the pattern of induced exchanges in the human karyotype, *Chromosoma,* 40, 333, 1973.

152. **Latt, S. A.,** Microfluorometric detection of deoxyribonuclease acid replication in human metaphase chromosomes, *Proc. Natl. Acad. Sci. U.S.A.,* 70, 3395, 1973.

153. **Kato, H.,** Induction of sister chromatid exchanges by chemical mutagen and its possible relevance to DNA repair, *Exp. Cell. Res.,* 85, 239, 1974.

154. **Chaganti, R. S. K., Schonberg, S., and German, J.,** A many fold increase in sister chromatid exchanges in Bloom's Syndrome lymphocytes, *Proc. Natl. Acad. Sci.,* U.S.A., 71, 4508, 1974.

155. **Rowley, J. D.,** Do human tumors show a chromosome pattern specific for each etiologic agent, *J. Natl. Cancer Inst.,* 52, 315, 1974.

156. **Lilly, F., Boyse, E. A., and Old, L. J.,** Genetic basis of susceptibility to viral leukemogenesis, *Lancet,* 2, 1207, 1964.

157. **Snell, G. D.,** The H_2 locus of the mouse: observations and speculations concerning its comparative genetics and its polymorphism, *Folia Biol.* (Prague), 14, 335, 1968.

158. **McDevitt, H. O. and Bodmer, W. F.,** Histocompatibility antigens, immune responsiveness and susceptibility to disease, *Am. J. Med.,* 52, 1, 1972.

159. **Gatti, R. A.,** Role of immunological factors in cancer susceptibility, in *Genetics of Human Cancer,* Mulvihill, J. J., Miller, R. W., and Fraumeni, J. F., Jr., Eds., Raven Press, New York, 1977, 329.

160. **Mitelman, F., Mark, J., Levan, G., and Levan, A.,** Tumor etiology and chromosome pattern, *Science,* 176, 1340, 1972.

Chapter 4

THE ROLE OF VIRUSES IN INDUCING NEOPLASIA IN BLOOD CELLS WITH SPECIAL REFERENCE TO THE ISOLATION OF PUTATIVE HUMAN LEUKEMIA VIRUS

William G. Baxt

TABLE OF CONTENTS

I. INTRODUCTION

Over 200 years ago, Peyrilhe[1] proposed the viral theory of cancer — postulating that cancer was caused by a contagious virus. It was not until 1908 that Ellerman and Bang[2,3] discovered the first virus that could actually induce cancer. They reported the transmission of erythromyeloblastic leukemia of chickens by cell-free filtrates of leukemic cells. Two years later, in 1911, Rous discovered the transmission of solid tumors in chickens by cell-free filtrates.[4,5] These discoveries eventually led to the isolation and characterization of the first RNA tumor viruses — avian leukemia and Rous sarcoma virus.

During the ensuing two decades, the diseases caused by avian leukemia virus and Rous sarcoma virus were further characterized. Concurrently, several investigators began to inbreed strains of mice, enabling Bittner, Andervont, and Bryan[6–8] to isolate an agent that caused murine mammary tumors, and enabling Gross[9] to successfully induce leukemia in C3H mice by the inoculation of extracts of AK-leukemic cells. In the following years, numerous strains of murine leukemia viruses were identified. In 1964, Harvey[10] isolated a virus from a stock of Moloney murine leukemia virus, which induced pleomorphic sarcomas in mice. Moloney[11] later reported the induction of rhabdomyosarcomas in mice using similar methods, and

Kirsten and Mayer[12] isolated a murine sarcoma virus from stocks of murine leukemia virus passaged in rats. In 1966, Finkel et al.[13] reported the first isolation of a virus from a naturally occurring osteosarcoma.

A number of strains of RNA tumor viruses have been isolated and shown capable of inducing true neoplastic processes in a wide spectrum of animals: leukemia and sarcoma RNA tumor viruses have been isolated from snakes, frogs, hamsters, guinea pigs, rats, cows, cats, dogs, marmosets, and monkeys, and mammary RNA tumor viruses from mice and monkeys. Since this time, a great deal has been learned about RNA tumor viruses which has been amply reviewed elsewhere.[14,15]

In the late 1950s, Dmochowski reported the first studies that implicated RNA tumor viruses in human leukemia.[16–18] In these studies, sections of human leukemic lymph nodes and plasma pellets were examined by electron microscopy, and viral-like particles were identified. However, studies done by other laboratories failed to verify these data.[19–21] Electron micrographic studies done in the early and mid 1960s purported to demonstrate RNA tumor viruses in human leukemic plasma,[22–27] but negative staining did not reveal the internal structures of these particles. It was concluded by other investigators that these structures were probably mycoplasma.[28–31] Interest in the RNA tumor viruses waned until 1960 when

Baltimore and Temin independently discovered that RNA tumor viruses contained a new enzyme — RNA-dependent DNA polymerase (reverse transcriptase).[32,33] With this discovery, investigators began to look for biochemical evidence implicating the RNA tumor viruses in human leukemia.

The first biochemical work implicating the RNA tumor viruses in human leukemia was that of Gallo et al.,[34,35] who reported the finding of reverse transcriptase activity in extracts made from human leukemic cells. Penner et al.[36] and Kiessling et al.[37] also reported finding reverse transcriptase-like activity in extracts made from human leukemic cells. Spiegelman detected reverse transcriptase-like activity in extracts made from cells from patients with a broad spectrum of leukemias.[38]

Gallo[40] and Sarngadharan et al.[39] then went on to purify reverse transcriptase from large quantities of human leukemic lymphoblasts. It was later demonstrated that the human leukemic RNA-dependent DNA polymerase was inhibited by an antibody made against the RNA-dependent DNA polymerase of simian sarcoma virus (SSV).[41-43]

The first genetic experimental data implicating the RNA tumor viruses in human leukemia were carried out with RNA extracted from human leukemic white blood cells (WBC). This RNA was annealed to ^{3}H-DNA (cDNA) probes generated endogenously by Rauscher leukemia virus (RLV), an agent known to cause leukemia and sarcoma in mice.[44] In each case, greater than 65% of the RNAs tested hybridized to the RLV probe but failed to hybridize to probes generated by murine mammary tumor virus or avian myeloblastosis virus. However, the data of these experiments were very weak.

A particulate fraction was then isolated from leukemic WBC which had three known characteristics of RNA tumor viruses: a density of 1.16 g/cc, 70S RNA, and RNA-dependent DNA polymerase.[45-47] These particulate fractions were used to generate radiolabeled cDNA probes which were shown to have a high degree of complementarity to the RNA of several known RNA tumor viruses.[44,45] Approximately 40% of these human probes were homologous to the RNA of RLV, and 65% of the probe was homologous to the RNA of SSV.

These probes were further used in DNA:DNA hybridization experiments to detect complementary sequences in human normal and leukemic WBC nuclear DNA. Although it was found that both normal and leukemic WBC nuclear DNA contained sequences homologous to the human particulate fraction-directed cDNA, the leukemic WBC nuclear DNA appeared to have qualitatively more information complementary to the leukemic cDNA.[48] The complementary sequences present in both normal and leukemic WBC DNA were removed by exhaustive hybridization of the probe to normal WBC DNA. The remaining single-stranded probe was reisolated and shown to be unable to react with normal WBC DNA and then challenged with the nuclear DNA from the same leukemic patient. In every case, more than 25% of the residue probe reacted with host leukemic DNA, implying the presence of DNA sequences in the leukemic genome not detectable in the normal genome[48] and possibly complementary to a potential human leukemogenic virus.

These observations were extended by performing similar experiments on two sets of identical twins. Since identical twins derive their genomes from the same fertilized egg, any vertically transmitted information must be present in both. The data obtained revealed that if particulate fractions are isolated from the leukemic twin's WBC and used to generate probes (cDNA) which are then extensively annealed to normal WBC DNA, when the nonannealing fraction is reisolated and rechallenged with the DNA extracted from both the normal and leukemic twin, the remaining fraction unable to anneal to normal WBC DNA will anneal to the leukemic twin's DNA but not to the normal twin's DNA.[49]

Further studies of the leukemic specific sequences reisolated after exhaustive hybridization to normal WBC nuclear DNA which were done by rechallenging probe with the DNA from patients with different types of leukemia have revealed that these sequences are the same in similar types of leukemia. Additional studies done by rechallenging such recycled probes with the DNA extracted from different organs of the same patient suggested that these sequences were not present in all the cells of leukemic patients.[50] Additional work done by polysomal messenger RNA analyses have shown that the information contained in the unique sequences may be expressed in the RNA of leukemic WBC in a 350S polysomal fraction containing a messenger RNA of about 20S in size.[51]

These experiments were extended even further

by the isolation of a subfraction of the human cDNA complementary to RLV-70S RNA by hybridization techniques. cDNA made from a particulate fraction extracted from human leukemic WBC was annealed with RLV-70S RNA. The duplexes were reisolated by hydroxyapatite chromatography. The human leukemic cDNA isolated was then shown to be 100% homologous to RLV-70S RNA. This cDNA was then annealed to normal and RLV-infected BALB/c mice splenic DNA. The RLV-specific cDNA annealed to the RLV-infected splenic DNA but failed to anneal to the normal mouse spleen DNA, suggesting the presence of murine leukemic specific nuclear DNA sequences homologous to part of the informational content of the RLV genome. This was further verified by the hybridization of the RLV-specific cDNA to human normal and leukemic WBC nuclear DNA. The RLV-specific cDNA annealed completely to the human WBC leukemic cDNA but failed to anneal to the human normal WBC DNA.[52] All of these data supported the possibility that the nuclear DNA of human leukemic WBC may contain sequences which are not present in the nuclear DNA of nonleukemic WBC and which may be complementary to part of the genetic information encoded in the RNA of a known leukemogenic virus. The implication of this could be that the leukemic WBC had been infected by such a virus with the consequent integration of viral-specific information into the normal host genome.

Since these studies, a number of laboratories have confirmed the existence of viral-specific sequences in lower mammals that are only detectable in cells after they are infected by a given RNA tumor virus.[53-61]

These data also suggested the possibility of the relationship between mouse leukemogenic RNA tumor viruses and the putative leukemogenic human agent. Hybridization experiments done with the human leukemic particulate fraction cDNA have revealed that the informational content of these probes has a much greater similarity to the mouse genome than to the genome of higher mammals.[62]

Miller et al. have made similar observations[47] and shown that the primate genome of sarcoma-producing RNA tumor viruses is more closely related to the rodent genome than to higher mammals. Benveniste and Todaro have shown that the genome of SSV is also more closely related to

the genome of murine RNA tumor viruses than to the genome of higher mammalian RNA tumor viruses.[63]

These data may all point to the fact that the human leukemogenic virus may be of murine origin — infecting higher primate hosts directly rather than moving up the evolutionary ladder.

II. GROWTH OF POTENTIAL HUMAN LEUKEMOGENIC VIRUS

Several laboratories have attempted to grow RNA tumor viruses in tissue cultures derived from human leukemic white cells. These attempts were fruitless until recently when two laboratories were able to first show the release of reverse transcriptase-containing particles from human leukemic WBC in short-term tissue cultures.[64-66] One of these groups then isolated a particle from the supernatant of such cultures which possessed a density of 1.16 g/cc, the electron micrographs of which resembled immature introcytoplasmic RNA tumor viruses.[67] This group has recently gone on to demonstrate that these particles possess 70S RNA and can endogenously generate cDNA which is 45% complementary to the RNA of murine leukemia virus and 65% complementary to the RNA of SSV.[68]

Gallagher et al.[69] have been successful in growing an RNA tumor virus from *one* patient with acute myelogenous leukemia. This particle possesses a density of 1.16 g/cc and has an enzymatic activity that is similar to that of RNA-dependent DNA polymerase and which was inhibited by an antibody made against the RNA-dependent DNA polymerase of SSV. This particle may also have an antigen which is partially related to the P^{30} antigen of SSV and the woolly monkey tumor virus.[70] Hybridization studies reveal that the genome of this agent(s) is homologous with the genome of both SSV and the woolly monkey virus.[38] The electron micrographs of this particle reveal that it has morphological characteristics virtually identical to that of known RNA tumor viruses.[69] However, the virus has not been successfully isolated from a large number of other leukemic marrows.

Even more recently, two other laboratories have reported studies further supporting the growth of RNA tumor viruses from short-term tissue culture of human leukemic WBC. Vosika et al.[71] reported detecting reverse transcriptase activity in high-speed pellets harvested from short-term tissue cultures of two patients with preleukemic stages. However, a more vigorous characterization of these particles was not reported.

Zurcher et al.[72] reported the growth of a particle that resembles an RNA tumor virus on electron microscopy from a short-term tissue culture derived from a patient with leukosarcoma. Preliminary antigenic screening of this particle revealed that it was not grossly related to Moloney leukemia virus, RLV, or SSV.

III. DIRECT PURIFICATION OF A POTENTIAL HUMAN LEUKEMOGENIC VIRUS

At the same time, a third laboratory was avoiding the risks and artifacts of tissue culture and purifying a particulate fraction from large quantities of human leukemic material.[73]

The purification procedure used took advantage of a number of the characteristics of RNA tumor viruses: density (isopycnic steps), size (sedimentation velocity step), and resistance to nuclease and protease treatment.

The ability of detergent-treated particulate fractions to generate RNase-sensitive ^{3}H-DNA bound to a 35 to 70S RNA has been used as an assay for C-type particles,[74] based on the fact that such a complex would represent an RNA-dependent DNA polymerase DNA product bound to its viral 70S RNA template. This assay was used as a method to follow the purification of C-type particles. The feasibility of this approach was confirmed by results obtained using either added known quantities of RLV to normal murine splenic tissue or RLV-infected BALB/c spleens in the purification procedure. Viral purification could be followed at each step in the procedure by comparing the number of counts per minute migrating as a 70S element per milligram of protein. The results indicated that about a 7500-fold purification can be accomplished. These results also confirmed that a known RNA tumor virus is resistant to both micrococcal nuclease and to trypsin, steps which were added to the procedure to further degrade any residual host nucleic acids and proteins. By comparing final viral recovery to the known initial input of virus, about 20% of the total viral input is recovered on the basis of net yield of 35 to 70S RNA; 10% of the total initial ability to generate 35 to 70S migrating radioactivity is recovered.

This method was used to follow the purification of human particles from human leukemic spleens. Figure 1 is a gross illustration of the RNase-sensitive radioactivity migrating in the 35 to 70S region of glycerol sedimentation gradients generated from particulate fractions from each of the six major steps in the purification procedure of a human leukemic spleen. Counts per minute are expressed as a function of protein concentration. As can be seen from the figure, approximately a 4000 to 5000-fold purification was accomplished in this manner; 8% of the ability to endogenously generate 35 to 70S radioactivity was recovered.

The purification of six leukemic spleens yielded results within the same range as that noted above. Four fresh normal spleens and 500 g of pooled post-mortem normal spleens were taken through the procedure, and all fractions obtained during this purification were unable to generate 35 to 70S migrating radioactivity.

As a further control, a known quantity of RLV (14 mg) was added to 500 g of pooled post-mortem normal human spleens and also taken through the procedure. Each fraction at each step of the purification procedure had the ability to generate 70S migrating radioactivity. The extent of purification as calculated above was approximately 5500-fold; 10% of the ability to generate 35 to 70S radioactivity was recovered.

High molecular weight RNA was extracted from the isolated final viral fractions by detergent treatment and purification of a 10 to 30% glycerol-TNE (a Tris® -saline EDTA buffer) sedimentation velocity gradient. The RNA so purified on the sedimentation velocity gradients was followed by OD_{260}. Figure 2 illustrates the RNA OD_{260} profile and the endogenous reaction product generated by the final pellet obtained from the purification of RLV added to pooled normal human spleens. As can be seen from the figure, OD_{260} absorbing material sedimented in the 70S and 55S regions of the gradient. These were the identical regions where the RNase-sensitive high molecular weight products of the endogenous reaction migrated. This is consistent with the previous observations that the early endogenous reaction products of C-type particles are bound to viral high molecular weight RNA. These data also demonstrate the ability of the purification procedure used here to purify known

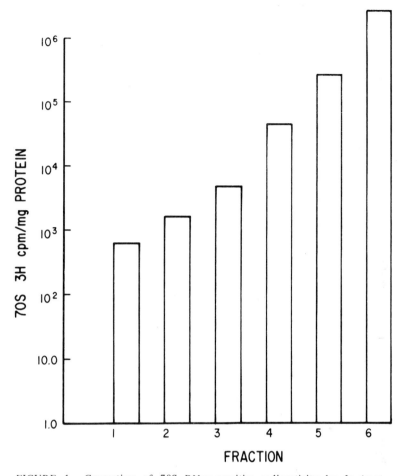

FIGURE 1. Generation of 70S RNase-sensitive radioactivity by Je (acute myelogenous leukemia) spleen fractions. The assay for the generation of 70S migrating radioactivity was performed as outlined. The numbers on the abscissa correspond to the steps of the C-particle purification procedure. Ribonuclease-sensitive radioactivity migrating in the 70S region of the sedimentation gradients was summarized and expressed as counts per minute per milligram of each fraction on the ordinate. The background radioactivity of 15 to 20 cpm was subtracted, and the protein concentration was determined by the method of Lowry.[77]

C-type particles from large quantities of human spleen and excludes the possibility that the normal tissue possesses factors which may inhibit or degrade viral particles. Figure 2B illustrates profiles of the OD_{260} profile and the endogenous reaction product generated by the final pellet isolated from a human leukemic spleen. Both the high molecular weight RNA and the endogenous reaction product sedimented in the 70S and 55S regions of the gradient. These profiles of sedimentation are indistinguishable from the sedimentation profiles obtained with added RLV (Figure 2A).

The 70S RNA was reisolated by ethanol precipitation. All six leukemic spleens so purified yielded RNA with sedimentation patterns similar to the one illustrated. The total yield of RNA (measured by OD_{260}) was between 5 and 21 μg. The high molecular weight RNA was resistant to DNase and degraded by RNase. DNA was undetectable by the diaminobenzoic acid method. No detectable nucleic acids were extracted from the final pellets of normal spleens.

Electron micrographs were made from aliquots taken from each of the six major steps of the

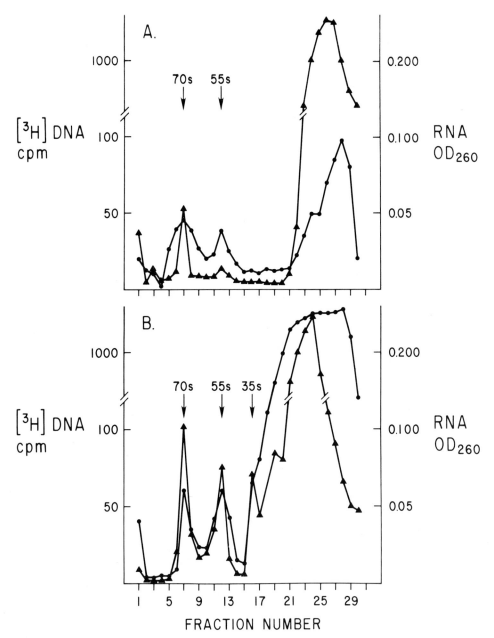

FIGURE 2.   Sedimentation profile of purified RLV and human particulate fraction high molecular weight RNA. (A) RLV added to 500 g of pooled normal post-mortem spleens. ▲ represents the sedimentation velocity profile of the endogenous reaction of the final viral pellet (generation of 70S migrating radioactivity) as followed by radioactivity. ● represents the sedimentation velocity profile of the RNA extracted from the final viral pellet as followed by OD_{260}. (B) Human leukemic spleen (acute myelogenous leukemia). ▲ represents the sedimentation velocity profile of the endogenous reaction of final viral pellet as followed by radioactivity. ● represents the sedimentation velocity profile of the RNA extracted from the final viral pellet as followed by OD_{260}.

The background radioactivity of 15 to 20 cpm was subtracted. The background OD_{260} absorbing material of 0.025 OD_{260}/ml was subtracted.

particle purification. The photoelectron micrographs of the early fraction reveal little other than host cell elements, but the photoelectron micrographs of the last two fractions reveal the presence by negative staining of particles virtually identical to those demonstrated by Mak et al.[68] These particles do not resemble typical RNA tumor viruses but do resemble photoelectron micrographs of known RNA tumor viruses published elsewhere.[75,76]

This is the first example of the direct purification of oncornavirus-like particles from human leukemic tissue. The obvious advantage of this approach is that it was accomplished without the need to resort to the use of tissue culture. Work is presently under way to further characterize the particle's nucleic acids and proteins.*

IV. CONCLUSION

Clearly, all of the work done to date investigating the role of RNA tumor viruses in human leukemia implies nothing about their possible etiologic role in this disease. Although the data seem to be mounting supporting their presence in human leukemic tissue, it will take a great deal of work to prove that they are etiologic in this disease, since it will be impossible to fulfill Koch's postulates with a leukemogenic agent. Studies are presently under way to elucidate the genetic changes that take place after leukemogenic RNA tumor viruses infect cells. Hopefully, the results of these studies will provide the necessary tools to detect such changes in human cells potentially transformed by such affinity, and will come closer to proving that leukoviruses are etiologic in human leukemia.

*Supported by NIH research grant no. CA 15376 from the National Cancer Institute and a Leukemia Society of America Scholarship.

REFERENCES

1. **Peyrilhe, B.,** Dissertation Academique sur le Cancer qui a Remporté le Prix Double de l'Academie des Sciences, Arts et Belles Lettres de Lyon, le 8 Decembre, 1773, Chez Ruault, Paris, 1773, 135.
2. **Ellerman, V. and Bang, O.,** Experimentelle leukämie bei hühnern, *Zentralbl. Bakteriol. Parasitenkd. Infektionskr. Hyg. Abt. 1 Orig.,* 46, 595, 1908.
3. **Ellerman, V. and Bang, O.,** Experimentelle leukämie bei hühnern, *Z. Hyg. Infektionskr.,* 63, 231, 1909.
4. **Rous, P. A.,** Transmissable avian neoplasm (sarcoma of the common fowl), *J. Exp. Med.,* 13, 696, 1910.
5. **Rous, P. A.,** Sarcoma of the fowl transmissable by an agent from the tumor cells, *J. Exp. Med.,* 13, 397, 1911.
6. **Bittner, J. J.,** Some possible effects of nursing on the mammary gland tumor incidence in mice, *Science,* 84, 162, 1936.
7. **Bittner, J. J.,** Milk influence of breast tumors in mice, *Science,* 95, 462, 1942.
8. **Andervont, H. B. and Bryan, W. R.,** Properties of the mouse mammary tumor agent, *J. Natl. Cancer Inst.,* 5, 143, 1944.
9. **Gross, L.,** "Spontaneous" leukemia developing in C3H mice following inoculation in infancy with AK-leukemic extracts or AK-embryos, *Proc. Soc. Exp. Biol. Med.,* 76, 27, 1951.
10. **Harvey, J. J.,** An unidentified virus which causes the rapid production of tumors in mice, *Nature,* 204, 1104, 1964.
11. **Moloney, J. B.,** A virus-induced rhabdomyosarcoma of mice, *Natl. Cancer Inst. Monogr.,* 22, 139, 1966.
12. **Kirsten, W. H. and Mayer, L. A.,** Morphologic responses to a murine erythroblastosis virus, *J. Natl. Cancer Inst.,* 39, 311, 1967.
13. **Finkel, M. P., Biskis, B. O., and Jenkins, P. B.,** Virus induction of osteosarcomas in mice, *Science,* 151, 698, 1966.
14. **Gross, L.,** *Oncogenic Viruses,* 2nd ed., Pergamon Press, Oxford and New York, 1970.
15. **Tooze, J.,** *The Molecular Biology of Tumor Viruses,* Cold Spring Harbor Laboratory, Cold Spring Harbor, New York, 1973.
16. **Dmochowski, L. and Grey, C. E.,** Subcellular structures of possible viral origin in some mammalian tumors, *Ann. N. Y. Acad. Sci.,* 68, 559, 1957.
17. **Dmochowski, L., Grey, C. E., Dreyer, D. A., Sykes, J. A., Shullenberger, C. C., and Howe, C. D.,** Studies in human leukemia, *Proc. Soc. Exp. Biol. Med.,* 101, 686, 1959.
18. **Dmochowski, L., Taylor, H. G., Grey, C. E., Dreyer, D. A., Sykes, J. A., Langford, P. L., Rogers, T., Shullenberger, C. C., and Howe, C. D.,** Viruses and mycoplasma (PSLO) in human leukemia, *Cancer Bull.,* 18, 1345, 1965.
19. **Bessis, M. and Thiéry, J. P.,** Études au microscope électronique sur les leucémies humaines. II. Les leucémies lymphocytaires. Comparison avec la leucémie de la souris de souche AK, *Nouv. Rev. Fr. Hematol.,* 2, 387, 1962.

20. Braunsteiner, H., Fellinger, K., and Pakesch, G., On the occurrence of virus-like bodies in human leukemia, *Blood,* 115, 476, 1960.
21. Leplus, R., Debray, J., Pinet, J., and Bernhard, W., Lésions nucléaires décélécs au microscope électronique dans des cellules de "lymphomes malins" chez l'homme, *C. R. Acad. Sci.,* 253, 2788, 1961.
22. Almeida, J. D., Hasselback, R. C., and Ham, A. W., Virus-like particles in blood of two acute leukemia patients, *Science,* 142, 1487, 1963.
23. Benyesh-Melnick, M., Smith, K. O., and Fernbach, D. J., Association of mycovirus-like particles with acute leukaemia of childhood, *Nature,* 202, 1129, 1964.
24. Benyesh-Melnick, M., Smith, K. O., and Fernbach, D. J., Studies on human leukemia. III. Electron microscopic findings in children with acute leukemia and in children with infectious mononucleosis, *J. Natl. Cancer Inst.,* 33, 571, 1964.
25. Burger, C. L., Harris, W. W., Anderson, N. G., Bartlett, T. W., and Kinseley, R. M., Virus-like particles in human leukemic plasma, *Proc. Soc. Exp. Biol. Med.,* 115, 151, 1964.
26. Murphy, W. H., Eriel, I. J., and Zaraionitis, C. J. D., Virus studies of human leukemia, *Cancer,* 18, 1329, 1965.
27. Murphy, W. H., Furtado, D., and Plata, E., Possible association between leukemia in children and virus-like agents, *JAMA,* 191, 110, 1965.
28. Smith, K. O., Benyesh-Melnick, M., and Fernbach, D. J., Studies on human leukemia. II. Structure and quantitation of mycovirus-like particles associated with human leukemia, *J. Natl. Cancer Inst.,* 33, 557, 1964.
29. Dmochowski, L., Grey, C. E., Dreyer, D. A., Sykes, J. A., Langford, P. L., and Taylor, H. G., Mycoplasma (pleuropneumonia-like organisms PPLO) and human leukemia, *Med. Rec. Annu.,* 57, 563, 1964.
30. Dulbecco, R., Viruses in carcinogenesis, *Ann. Int. Med.,* 70, 1019, 1969.
31. Prince, A. M. and Adams, W. R., Virus-like particles in human plasma and serum. Role of platelet lysosomes, *J. Natl. Cancer Inst.,* 37, 153, 1966.
32. Baltimore, D., Virus RNA-dependent DNA polymerase, *Nature,* 226, 1209, 1970.
33. Temin, H. M. and Mizutami, S., RNA-dependent DNA polymerase in virions of Rous sarcoma virus, *Nature,* 226, 1211, 1970.
34. Gallo, R. C., Yang, S. S., and Ting, R. C., RNA-dependent DNA polymerase of human acute leukaemic cells, *Nature,* 228, 927, 1970.
35. Gallo, R. C., Reverse transcriptase. The DNA polymerase of oncogenic RNA viruses, *Nature,* 234, 194, 1971.
36. Penner, P. E., Cohen, L. H., and Loeb, L. A., RNA-dependent DNA polymerase in human lymphocytes during gene activation by phytohemagglutinin, *Nature (London) New Biol.,* 232, 58, 1971.
37. Kiessling, A. A., Weber, G. H., Deeney, A. O., Possehl, E. A., and Beaudreau, G. S., Deoxyribonucleic acid polymerase activity associated with a plasma particulate fraction from patients with chronic lymphocytic leukemia, *J. Virol.,* 7, 221, 1971.
38. Spiegelman, S., unpublished data.
39. Sarngadharan, M. G., Sarin, P. S., Reitz, M. S., and Gallo, R. C., Reverse transcriptase activity of human acute leukaemic cells: purification of the enzyme response to AMV 70S RNA and characterization of the DNA product, *Nature (London) New Biol.,* 240, 67, 1972.
40. Gallo, R. C., Sarin, P. S., Smith, R. G., Bobrow, S., Sarngadharan, M. G., Reitz, M. S., and Abrell, J., RNA-directed and primed DNA polymerase activities in tumor viruses and human lymphocytes in *DNA Synthesis In Vitro,* (Proc. 2nd Annual Steenbock Symp.), Wells, R. and Inman, R., Eds., University Park Press, Baltimore, Md., 1973, 251.
41. Todaro, G. J. and Gallo, R. C., Immunological relationship of DNA polymerase from human acute leukaemia cells and primate and mouse leukaemia virus transcriptase, *Nature,* 244, 206, 1973.
42. Gallagher, R. E., Todaro, G. J., Smith, R. G., Livingston, D. M., and Gallo, R. C., Relationship between RNA-directed DNA polymerase (reverse transcriptase) from human acute leukemic blood cells and primate type-C viruses, *Proc. Natl. Acad. Sci. U.S.A.,* 71, 1309, 1974.
43. Gallo, R. C., Gallagher, R. E., Miller, N. R., Mondal, H., Saxinger, W. C., Mayer, R. J., Smith, R. G., and Gillespie, D. H., Relationships between components in primate RNA tumor viruses and in the cytoplasm of human leukemic cells: implications to leukemogenesis, *Cold Spring Harbor Symp. Quant. Biol.,* 39, 933, 1974.
44. Hehlmann, R., Kufe, D., and Spiegelman, S., RNA in human leukemic cells related to the RNA of a mouse leukemia virus, *Proc. Natl. Acad. Sci. U.S.A.,* 69, 435, 1972.
45. Baxt, W. G., Hehlmann, R., and Spiegelman, S., Human leukemic cells containing reverse transcriptase associated with a high molecular weight viral-related RNA, *Nature (London) New Biol.,* 240, 72, 1972.
46. Gallo, R. C., Miller, H. R., Saxinger, W. C., and Gillespie, D., DNA related to a primate RNA tumor virus genome which is synthesized endogenously by reverse transcriptase in virus-like particles from fresh human acute leukemic blood cells, *Proc. Natl. Acad. Sci. U.S.A.,* 70, 3219, 1973.
47. Miller, N. R., Saxinger, W. C., Reitz, M. S., Gallagher, R. E., Wu, A. M., Gallo, R. C., and Gillespie, D. H., Systematics of RNA tumor viruses and virus-like particles of human origin, *Proc. Natl. Acad. Sci. U.S.A.,* 71, 3177, 1974.
48. Baxt, W. G. and Spiegelman, S., Nuclear DNA sequences present in human leukemic cells and absent in normal white blood cells, *Proc. Natl. Acad. Sci. U.S.A.,* 69, 3737, 1972.

49. Baxt, W. G., Yates, J. W., Wallace, J. W., Holland, J. F., and Spiegelman, S., Leukemia-specific DNA sequences in leukocytes of the leukemic member of identical twins, *Proc. Natl. Acad. Sci. U.S.A.*, 70, 2629, 1973.
50. Baxt, W. G., unpublished data.
51. Baxt, W. G., unpublished data.
52. Baxt, W. G., Sequences present in both human leukemic cell nuclear DNA and Rauscher leukemia virus, *Proc. Natl. Acad. Sci. U.S.A.*, 71, 2853, 1974.
53. Viola, M. V. and White, L. R., Differences in murine leukaemia virus-specific DNA sequences in normal and malignant cells, *Nature*, 246, 485, 1973.
54. Sweet, R. W., Goodman, H. C., Cho, J. R., Ruprecht, R. M., Redfield, R. R., and Spiegelman, S., The presence of unique DNA sequences after viral induction of leukemia in mice, *Proc. Natl. Acad. Sci. U.S.A.*, 71, 1705, 1974.
55. Evans, R. M., Baluda, M. A., and Shoyab, M., Differences between the integration of avian myeloblastosis virus DNA in leukemic cells and of endogenous viral DNA in normal chicken cells, *Proc. Natl. Acad. Sci. U.S.A.*, 71, 3152, 1974.
56. Markham, P. D. and Baluda, M. A., Integrated state of oncornavirus DNA in normal chicken cells and in cells transformed by avian myeloblastosis virus, *J. Virol.*, 12, 721, 1974.
57. Varmus, H. E., Vogt, P. K., and Bishop, J. M., Integration of deoxyribonucleic acid specific for Rous sarcoma virus after infection of permissive and nonpermissive hosts, *Proc. Natl. Acad. Sci. U.S.A.*, 70, 3067, 1973.
58. Shoyab, M., Baluda, M. A., and Evans, R., Acquisition of new DNA sequences after infection of chicken cells with avian myeloblastosis virus, *J. Virol.*, 13, 331, 1974.
59. Neiman, P. E., Rous sarcoma virus nucleotide sequences in cellular DNA: measurement by RNA-DNA hybridization, *Science*, 178, 750, 1972.
60. Shoyab, M., Evans, R. M., and Baluda, M. A., Presence of leukemic cells of avian myeloblastosis virus-specific DNA sequences absent in normal chicken cells, *J. Virol.*, 14, 47, 1974.
61. Varmus, H. E., Guntaka, R. V., Fan, W. J. W., Heasley, S., and Bishop, J. M., Synthesis of viral DNA in the cytoplasm of duck embryo fibroblasts and in enucleated cells after infection by avian sarcoma virus, *Proc. Natl. Acad. Sci. U.S.A.*, 71, 3874, 1974.
62. Baxt, W. G., unpublished data.
63. Benveniste, R. E. and Todaro, G. J., Homology between type-C viruses of various species as determined by molecular hybridization, *Proc. Natl. Acad. Sci. U.S.A.*, 70, 3316, 1973.
64. Kotler, M., Weinberg, E., Haspel, O., Olshevsky, U., and Becker, Y., Particles released from arginine deprived human leukaemic cells, *Nature (London) New Biol.*, 244, 197, 1973.
65. Kotler, M., Balabanova, H., Weinberg, E., Friedmann, A., and Becker, Y., Oncornavirus-like particles released from arginine-deprived human lymphoblastoid cell lines, *Proc. Natl. Acad. Sci. U.S.A.*, 72, 4592, 1975.
66. Mak, T. W., Aye, M. T., Messner, H., Sheinin, R., Till, J. E., and McCulloch, E. A., Reverse transcriptase activity: increase in marrow cultures from leukaemic patients in relapse and remission, *Br. J. Cancer*, 29, 433, 1974.
67. Mak, T. W., Manaster, J., Howatson, A. F., McCulloch, E. A., and Till, J. E., Particles with characteristics of leukoviruses in cultures of marrow cells from leukemic patients in remission and relapse, *Proc. Natl. Acad. Sci. U.S.A.*, 71, 4336, 1974.
68. Mak, T. W., Kurtz, S., Manaster, J., and Housman, D., Viral-related information in oncornavirus-like particles isolated from cultures of marrow cells from leukemic patients in relapse and remission, *Proc. Natl. Acad. Sci. U.S.A.*, 72, 623, 1975.
69. Gallagher, R. E. and Gallo, R. C., Type C RNA tumor viruses isolated from cultured human acute myelogenous leukemia cells, *Science*, 187, 350, 1975.
70. Sherr, C. J. and Todaro, G. S., Type C viral antigens in man. I. Antigens related to endogenous primate virus in human tumors, *Proc. Natl. Acad. Sci. U.S.A.*, 71, 4703, 1974.
71. Vosika, G. J., Krivit, W., Gerrard, J. M., Coccia, P. F., Nesbit, M. E., Coalson, J. J., and Kennedy, B. J., Oncornavirus-like particles from cultured bone marrow cells preceding leukemia and malignant histiocytosis, *Proc. Natl. Acad. Sci. U.S.A.*, 72, 2804, 1975.
72. Zurcher, C., Brinkhof, J., Bentvelzen, P., and deMan, J. C. H., C-type virus antigens detected by immuno-fluorescence in human bone tumour cultures, *Nature*, 254, 457, 1975.
73. Baxt, W. G., The purification of particles resembling oncornaviruses from human acute leukemic spleens, in preparation.
74. Schlom, J. and Spiegelman, S., Simultaneous detection of reverse transcriptase and high molecular weight RNA unique to oncogenic RNA viruses, *Science*, 174, 840, 1971.
75. Moenig, V., Frank, H., Gunsmann, G., Ohms, P., Schwarz, H., Schafer, W., and Strandstrom, H., C-type particles produced by a permanent cell line from a leukemic pig. II. Physical, chemical and serological characterization of the particles, *Virology*, 57, 179, 1974.
76. Nermut, M. V., Frank, H., and Schafer, W., Properties of mouse leukemia viruses. III. Electron microscopic appearance as revealed after conventional preparation techniques as well as freeze-drying and freeze-etching, *Virology*, 49, 345, 1972.
77. Lowry, O. H., Rosebrough, N. J., Farr, A. L., and Randall, R. J., Protein measurement with the Folin phenol reagent, *J. Biol. Chem.*, 193, 265, 1951.

Chapter 5
HUMAN LEUKEMIA-ASSOCIATED ONCORNAVIRUSES

N. Gabelman

TABLE OF CONTENTS

I. INTRODUCTION

Leukemia is thought to stem from the inability of some hematopoietic precursor cells to mature.[1] The factors contributing to this block in maturation are not understood. It has been hypothesized, however, that at least some RNA viruses, all belonging to a single group with common morphological, biophysical, and biochemical characteristics, can induce leukemia, probably by transforming hematopoietic "stem cell" populations.[2]

These viruses are variously designated RNA tumor viruses,[3] oncornaviruses,[4] retraviruses,[5] leukoviruses,[6] and deoxyriboviruses.[7] These viruses have been isolated from a number of mammalian,[8] avian,[9] reptilian,[10] and osteichthyan[11] species.

The ability of oncornaviruses to cause cancer and leukemia in animals has been recognized for more than six decades. Ellerman and Bang[12] reported the transmission of an avian leukemia by cell free filtrates in 1908. This finding was followed by the discovery of an avian sarcoma virus by Peyton Rous in 1911,[13] a murine mammary tumor virus by Bittner in 1939,[14] and a murine leukemia virus by Gross in 1951.[15] Since 1951, oncornaviruses have been isolated from a number of higher vertebrates. The literature has been reviewed extensively by Temin,[16] Green,[17] Duesberg,[18] and Tooze.[19]

Initial studies which attempted to establish an etiologic role for oncornaviruses in the leukemias of mammals were conducted in laboratory mice bred for a high incidence of leukemia and were thus open to questions concerning the role of the host in the observed leukemogenesis. More recent studies have established that some naturally occurring leukemias, notably those of feral mice,[20] outbred cats,[21] and cows,[22] are the result of oncornavirus infection, but the ability of oncorna- viruses to induce leukemia appears to be under the genetic control of the host.[23] The feline and bovine leukemias are transmitted from animal to animal by classical (horizontal) infection,[24] and in each of the well-studied mammalian leukemias of viral origin, protection against the disease can be conferred by vaccination.[25]

An extension of the data demonstrating an etiologic role for the oncornaviruses in mammals to man would lead one to predict that some leukemias have oncornaviruses as their etiologic agents. However, since viremia does not appear to accompany human leukemia and the shedding of oncornavirus particles from human tumor cells is equally infrequent, support for this hypothesis by isolation of an unequivocally human oncornavirus has not been possible. This situation has been further complicated by the impossibility of ap- plying Koch's postulates to any putative "human" isolate. Notwithstanding all of these difficulties, there is a growing body of virologic, serologic, molecular biologic, and epidemiologic evidence which suggests that oncornaviruses play some role in human leukemias. What follows is a review of the pertinent literature with special emphasis on the virological and immunological data involved with the search for a human tumor virus.[26]

II. CHARACTERISTICS OF ONCORNAVIRUSES

A. Morphology

The oncornaviruses share several properties in common. They are all roughly spherical particles about 100 nm in diameter, with a nucleoprotein core (nucleoid) surrounded by one or more outer membranes made up of unit membrane, from the outer surfaces of which spikes project.[27,28] These spikes are made up of glycoproteins and are much more obvious in avian than in mammalian on- cornaviruses.[29]

When the nucleoid is electron-dense, spherical, and centrally located, the particle is designated as type C.[30] Those oncornaviruses which have cen- trally located but electron-luscent annular nucle- oids are designated type A and are thought by some investigators to represent immature type C particles.[31] The relationship between the A and C forms is not clear. In type B particles, the

electron-dense nucleoid is eccentrically located with respect to the envelope and often surrounded by an inner membrane.[32] None of these type B viruses appears to be involved in the etiology of leukemia in any of the species studied,[30] and all of the data reviewed will refer to type C oncorna- viruses.

B. Biochemical and Biophysical Characteristics

Most type C oncornaviruses have a buoyant density in isopycnic sucrose gradients of 1.15 to 1.19 g/ml.[16-19] The oncornavirus nucleoprotein core (nucleoid) contains a high molecular weight RNA of about 10^7 daltons (ca. 70S).[33] The 70S RNA is thought to be the viral genome, however, there is no direct evidence to support this supposi- tion since the RNA itself is not infectious.[34]

Under denaturing conditions, the 70S RNA dissociates into subunits with an apparent molecu- lar weight of 2.5×10^6 daltons (ca. 35S) and a number of 4 to 7S RNAs.[35] Each of the subunits is thought to contain at least four genetic loci. These loci are designated sarc, which regulates expression of the transformed phenotype in in- fected cells;[36] pol, which specifies the RNA dependent DNA polymerase; env, which specifies the major envelope glycoprotein (p67/71); and gag, which specifies the other major structural proteins. Each of the subunits of the viral genome can code for about 300,000 daltons of proteins, most of which have been identified.[37] The num- ber of structural and enzymic proteins which have been identified varies slightly from species to species, but in general, six or seven structural proteins can be identified.[38,39] According to the present nomenclature, such proteins are designated by a lower case p, while those proteins which are glycosylated are designated by a lower case gp placed before the number indicating the molecular weight in thousands of daltons. Thus, for example, there are two structural proteins which are identi- fied as residing in the envelope, a gp 67/71 and a p15(E), and four internal structural proteins, the p10, p12, p15, and p30. It should be understood that these values are not in complete agreement for all species or even among multiple isolates of the same virus and are offered for the sake of clarity and uniformity of nomenclature. Each of the structural proteins appears to have multiple antigenic determinants, and according to the sys- tem described above, are designated as type, group, or interspecies. The interspecies determinant of the major structural protein of a murine virus is then designated p30interspec.[40]

The best-studied of the enzymic proteins is the RNA dependent DNA polymerase (reverse transcriptase). This enzyme appears to be present in the core of all oncornaviruses, whether they are transforming or not.[41] Expression of enzymic activity requires that the surrounding viral envelope be disrupted, usually by detergent. This enzyme appears to be primer dependent and, except when copying synthetic polyribonucleotides templates, requires all four deoxynucleoside triphosphates, the divalent cation Mn^{++} or Mg^{++} and a reducing agent (type C oncornaviruses exhibit a preference for Mn^{++}).[42] The products of the reverse transcriptase mediated reaction are single and double stranded DNAs.[43] The enzyme itself has been purified from a number of different oncornaviruses, and its properties have been extensively studied in a number of different laboratories.[44,45] The best present estimates are that the virus contains about 10 molecules of RT protein per virion. The purified enzyme of the murine oncornaviruses has a molecular weight of about 70,000 daltons.[46] In addition to DNA polymerizing activity, the purified enzyme has a ribonuclease H activity which degrades the RNA moiety from DNA:RNA hybrids.[47]

The virion RNA dependent DNA polymerase carries an antigenic activity which is distinct from all other antigens of the virus particle and its polypeptides. Its polypeptide constitution does not correspond to any of the major viral structural polypeptides as would be expected from the minute quantities of enzyme (ca. 10 molecules) present in each virus particle. The mammalian enzymes are immunologically distinct from one another, although there is some cross reactivity between the enzymes isolated from different mammalian type A viruses. There is no cross reactivity between the enzymes isolated from type A and type B mouse viruses.[48]

C. Oncornavirus Replication

Based on the present status of our knowledge of the system, the replicative cycle of the oncornaviruses is the same for all of the known species. The cycle can, for conceptual purposes, be divided into two parts. In the first part of the replicative cycle, the virion attaches to the cell and, by mechanisms which are not understood, allows its RNA along with the reverse transcriptase to enter the cell's cytoplasm.[49] There, the reverse transcriptase causes the synthesis of a DNA copy of the viral RNA (provirus). Present evidence indicates that a fraction of the proviral DNA can be recovered as closed circular DNA, and it is presumably that form which integrates into the cellular DNA.[50] Once the proviral DNA is integrated into the cellular DNA, the second part of the life cycle of the virus begins. During this period, the integrated DNA is expressed by the normal processes of transcription.[51] The two types of product that have been characterized are new virion RNA and mRNA. Much of the mRNA that specifies the sequence of viral protein is of the same length as the virion RNA, but there may also be shorter RNAs.[52] The virus-specific proteins have two known functions: one is the transformation of cells that occurs when a sarcoma virus infects a fibroblast; the second is to provide the protein for new virion production.

Thus, the life cycle of the oncornaviruses appears to involve the invasion of the cell by the viral RNA accompanied by the viral reverse transcriptase, which then synthesizes a DNA copy(s) of the viral genome which is integrated into the host cell genome and which thereafter functions as a cellular gene.

What appears to be implied by this stable association of the provirus with the DNA of the cell is the possibility that cellular repressor mechanisms of one sort or another may participate in regulating the expression of viral as well as cellular genes and may inhibit viral expression for one or many generations. Thus, an initial infection involving horizontal transmission need not result in immediate expression of overt virus.[53] Subsequent transmission may then be either vertical or horizontal, and since the viral genome is multicistronic, viral expression might be incomplete and result in the synthesis of a variety of virally ordered gene products as well as whole virus.[54,55]

III. DETECTION OF ONCORNAVIRUS-RELATED MACROMOLECULES IN HUMAN LEUKEMIC CELLS

A. Isolation of Leukemic Cell-associated Oncornaviruses

Since oncornaviruses are associated with the neoplastic diseases of animals belonging to a number of genera, similar viruses ought to be associated with and perhaps involved in the neoplastic process in humans. Although viremia has not been detected in human leukemia, it remains possible that oncornaviruses are present in the latent state in leukemic cells. Virally ordered macromolecules have been detected in a variety of leukemic tissues. These include cellular nucleic acid sequences homologous to viral RNAs,[56] RNA directed DNA polymerases of viral origin,[57,58] the presence of intracellular proteins that cross react with antibodies to virus specific proteins,[59-62] and infrequently electron microscopic identification of virus-like particles.[63] In many of the preliminary reports, the virus-like components were shown to be closely related to similar components from previously isolated primate type C oncornaviruses.

The relevant oncornaviruses are the simian sarcoma virus (SSV-1),[64] the gibbon ape leukemia virus (GaLV),[65] and the baboon endogenous virus (BEV).[66] SSV-1 is typical class II exogenous type C oncornavirus which was recently isolated from a spontaneous fibrosarcoma of a woolly monkey.[64] The virus is oncogenic when inoculated into some primates and transforms fibroblasts in tissue culture.[67] The SSV-1 is associated with a non-transforming helper virus designated simian sarcoma associated virus (SSAV).[68] GaLV is also a class II, type C oncornavirus originally isolated from a lymphosarcoma in a gibbon ape.[65] GaLV is leukemogenic when injected into primates.[69] GaLV and the SSV-1/SSAV complex are immunologically cross reactive[70] and genetically related.[71]

The BEV was isolated from "virus negative" baboon tissues and cell lines and can be distinguished from other previously isolated oncornaviruses.[72] Some normal baboon tissues have been shown to express low levels of virus specific RNA and p30, the major structural protein of oncornaviruses.[73] Nucleic acid sequences homologous with those of BEV can be detected in noninfected baboon cells.[74] The evidence indicates that the virus is transmitted genetically and does not appear to induce neoplasia in permissive hosts.[72] BEV appears to be a typical class I (endogenous) virus.

B. Isolation of Oncornaviruses from Human Tumor Cells

In view of the increasingly suggestive evidence for the presence of oncornavirus information in human tumor cells, a number of laboratories attempted to isolate oncornaviruses from human tissues. Several laboratories have reported spontaneous budding of type C particles from human leukemic leukocytes.[75-77]

Activation of oncornavirus expression was attempted using the deoxyuridine analogues 2-bromo 5-deoxyuridine (BrdU) and 5-iodo-5-deoxyuridine (IdU). These halogenated pyrimidines have been shown to activate oncornavirus expression in virus-negative murine cells.[78,79] The mechanism of induction is not understood, but, apparently, the incorporation of IdU and BrdU into cellular DNA plays a vital role in the activation of murine class I viruses.[80]

Another method employed for the activation of oncornavirus synthesis is cocultivation. Initial studies by Rubin and Temin showed that class II oncornaviruses defective for replication in a particular cell line may be induced to replicate by cocultivation of the restrictive cell line carrying unexpressed virus information with a permissive one.[81] It is also true that certain xenotropic oncornaviruses, not capable of replication in their own host cells, will replicate after cocultivation with an appropriate cell line.[82]

Finally, it has been shown that virus expression can be achieved when nonreplicating cells such as peripheral leukocytes are exposed to mitogens such as phytohemaglutinin, and in one case, to growth stimulatory factor isolated from a particular strain of whole human embryo cells.[83]

IV. CANDIDATE HUMAN LEUKEMIA-ASSOCIATED ONCORNAVIRUSES

Despite extensive research efforts and increases in the sophistication of the isolation techniques employed, the identification and isolation of type C oncornaviruses and their components in human solid tumors and leukemias continues to remain a rare event. Type C particles have been detected in short-term cultures of human leukemic cells,[84] lymphoma cells,[85] and human liposarcomas.[86] Subsequent isolation and characterization of these particles has not been reported, and their significance in the etiology of leukemias and solid tumors has not been assessed.

A relatively few candidate human tumor or leukemia-associated viruses have to date been isolated and extensively characterized. Among these are the ESP-1 virus isolated from a serially cultured line derived from a child with Burkitt's lymphoma.[87] The line was reported to contain a group-specific antigen and reverse transcriptase not related to any of the known oncornaviruses.[88] The isolate created great excitement in the scientific community, but the data reported by Priori et al. were not confirmed. Subsequent studies by Gilden revealed a mouse-related antigen in the ESP-1 isolate.[89] Scolnick and co-workers[90] provided evidence that the reverse transcriptase of the virus was also mouse-related. While the possibility exists that the ESP-1 isolate is in fact a human virus and that all or at least some human viruses are mouse-related, it is most probable that the ESP-1 isolate represents a contamination of the Burkitt cells with a murine virus.

Another putative human tumor-related virus was the RD114 isolate reported by McAllister et al.[91] Initially, the virus was induced by inoculating kittens *in utero* with cells of the RD line of human rhabdomyosarcoma cells.[92] The investigators reported here again that the virus isolate (RD114) was probably not rescued from the cat, but rather from the human component of the in vivo cocultivation. The particle isolated from the cocultivation was a typical type C particle which originated in a cell with typical human karyotype. The RD114 isolate was immunologically characterized as a mammalian virus unrelated to feline oncornaviruses or to any of the well-studied mammalian or avian oncornaviruses.

Subsequent reports by Sarma et al.[93] and Baluda and Roy-Burman[94] indicated that the RD114 isolate is a highly repressed endogenous virus of cats which was apparently "activated" by cocultivation with a human cell line and which is immunologically and biochemically distinct from conventional feline leukemia-sarcoma viruses.

More recently, Gallagher and Gallo[95] reported the isolation of a typical, budding type C oncornavirus from several cultures of leukemic leukocytes from a patient with acute myelogenous leukemia (AML). The virus was reported to contain a reverse transcriptase and p30 antigens related to those of the SSV-1/SSAV/GaLV group of primate oncornaviruses.[64,65] The host range of the virus has apparently not been completely characterized, but the virus (HL23V) can productively infect human rhabdomyosarcoma (A204 cells), Kirsten Sarcoma Virus-infected, nonproducer rat cells (K-NRK), and dog thymus cells.[96] The virus has thus far been isolated twice. The first two isolates were obtained from the cultured leukocytes of one patient, and the third isolate from the same patient's marrow 14 months later.[97]

Release of these particles from the leukemic leukocytes in culture required the addition to the culture medium of a factor isolated from whole human embryo cells designated WHE-1,[97] which supported exponential growth and myeloid differentiation of human AML leukocytes. The virus was shown by electron microscopy to bud from the surface of the AML leukocytes in characteristic fashion. The virus banded in isopycnic neutral sucrose gradients at 1.16 g/ml. Electron micrographs made from material pelleted from fractions at this density showed typical type C particles.[95] An antiserum to the reverse transcriptase protein isolated from SSV-1/SSAV marked inhibited the polymerizing activity of the HL23v-1 reverse transcriptase.[98] In addition, three of the secondary isolates from various kinds of cells infected with HL23V appear to contain baboon related proteins as well as 70S RNA. These findings are of interest in that they indicate that HL23V may be a mixture of SSV-1 and BEV, or alternatively, that HL23v-1 and other class II viruses may induce class I viruses (e.g., BEV) after infection.[99]

Another type C oncornavirus was isolated recently from the bone marrow cells of a 41-year-old patient with a lymphoblastic leukemia.[100] In this case, the bone marrow cells were cultured in liquid suspension in the presence of PHA, and the virus was isolated from the tissue culture supernatant using the Millipore® filter technique after 3 days of culture in the presence of PHA. In other experiments, the authors seeded bone marrow cells from the same patient on top of 24-hr culture of XC cells and several days later observed the presence of syncytia. The pattern was typical of that found when the XC cells are infected with a murine leukemia virus.[101]

When fresh leukemic bone marrow cells were cocultivated with XC cells, syncytia were also produced. Cocultivation of XC cells with bone marrows from patients with other leukemias, polycythemia vera, aplasia, and normal marrows did not produce syncytia.

The particles released from the XC cocultivations were typical type C particles which would apparently grow in human embryonic kidney cells in serial culture and in rat cells. Examination by electronmicroscopy confirmed that the particles budded from the cultures and were of typical type C morphology.[100]

Studies of the immunological relationships of the virus isolate to well-studied oncornaviruses of various species by immunofluorescence suggest that the virus has affinities for both the SSV-1 and the FMR group of murine leukemia viruses.[100]

An oncornavirus-like particle was recently isolated from a human breast carcinoma cell line (MC7).[102] The virus was designated 734B and does not appear to be immunologically related to the murine leukemia viruses or to SSV-1/SSAV/GaLV group of viruses, but does appear to have immunological relatedness to the murine mammary tumor virus group. The authors suggest that the virus may in fact be related to an agent present in human breast carcinoma cells. No further information confirming this hypothesis has been supplied either by the investigators or another independent laboratory.

Panem et al.[103] have also reported the isolation of a type C oncornavirus (HEL12) spontaneously released from cultures of a diploid human cell strain. The virions were reported to have the properties of known oncornaviruses and to share antigenic determinants with the major interspecies specific antigen (p30) of SSV-1. The authors also report that antiserum to the reverse transcriptase of GaLV inhibits the reverse transcriptase of the HEL12 virus isolate and that of SSV-1 but had no effect on the corresponding enzymes of avian or murine RNA tumor viruses. In addition, the authors once again reported the presence of detectable BEV.[99]

Mak et al.[104] also reported the isolation of an oncornavirus-like particle from cultures of marrow cells obtained from leukemic patients. The particles were reported to contain RNA molecules similar to those isolated from well-studied murine leukemia viruses. The oncornavirus isolate appeared to be related to both the murine leukemia viruses and the SSV-1 as judged by sequence homology of a DNA complementary to the viral 70S RNA synthesized during and endogenous reaction with the viral genomic RNAs extracted from several well-characterized type C oncornaviruses. The cDNA demonstrated no homology with avian oncornaviruses. There are no data, however, which describe the infectivity or host range of the isolate, nor do the authors indicate in their published work whether viral information

contained in the 70S RNA isolated was homologous with the marrow cell DNA.

Gabelman and co-workers also described a human tumor associated oncornavirus.[105-107] The investigators attempted to isolate oncornaviruses from human lung tumor cells placed in serial culture. Standard electron microscopic and biochemical assays for the presence of virus revealed no virus-like particles budding from the cytoplasmic membranes of these cells or in the cytoplasmic vacuoles or present in the tissue culture medium. Biologic assays for type C particles involving the cocultivation of these tumor lines with XC cells also yielded negative results. Attempts to induce virus synthesis in a number of these lines with bromodeoxyuridine or iododeoxyuridine were also unsuccessful.

However, since the possibility existed that human tumor cell associated virus might be defective for replication in the cell of origin, the investigators attempted the cocultivation of these tumor lines with a number of other mammalian cells in tissue culture as a method of inducing virus expression. Cocultivation of two of the serially passaged human tumor cell lines with XC cells did result in the isolation of overt virus (S-XC[107] and L 104),[105-107] and the remainder of their work to date has been concerned with the characterization of one of these isolates, v-L 104, and the cell line from which it was derived (L104).

The L 104 cell line resulted from the cocultivation of rat (XC) and human cells and appears karyotypically to be rat derived. The majority of the chromosomes appeared to be of rat origin, and further examination of the banded material confirmed their original supposition. There are 10 to 12 marker chromosomes present in the karyotype, many of which could readily be identified as rat; however, the origin of some segments of the marker chromosomes examined could not be established.

The possibility that some of those unidentified chromosome segments might be of human origin was supported by the finding that the cell membrane carried human HL-A antigens and that the cytoplasmic extracts of L 104 cells contained glucose-6-phosphate dehydrogenase (G-6-P) and lactate dehydrogenase (LDH) molecules which migrated on starch gels in the same fashion as do human G-6-PD and LDH.[111] The HL-A antigens composed about 5% of HL-A antigen present on the cell surface, and the human cytoplasmic enzymes observed constituted about 5% of that enzyme present in the cytoplasm. All of this evidence is suggestive of the presence of human genetic information within the L-104 genome; however, the presence of human elements in the rat cell genome has not yet been unequivocally established.

The virus particle isolated from the L-104, designated v-L-104, was a typical type C oncornavirus, which sedimented at about 1.16 to 1.19 g/ml in isopycnic sucrose gradients, contained a high molecular weight RNA (ca. 70S) and a DNA polymerase capable of transcribing an RNA template. The polymerase had similar characteristics to those of other well-studied RNA dependent DNA polymerases and was shown to be immunologically related to the viral polymerases of the simian sarcoma/gibbon ape leukemia group (SSV-1/GaLV) of viruses.

The structural proteins of the virus were recognized by antisera to whole disrupted virions of p30 proteins of the SSV-1/GaLV group of viruses. Immunofluorescence and tissue culture studies have since shown that the virus isolate is also related to the baboon endogenous virus (BEV) (unpublished data). The data thus far gathered appear to indicate that L-104 bears a striking similarity to HL23v,[95] HEL12,[103] and the virus reported by Nooter and co-workers,[100] as well as the BaEV and the SSV-1/SSAV/GaLV group of viruses.

All of these viruses appear to demonstrate differences in infectivity for cells of different species. Most notably, HL23v appears to infect some human and lower primate cell types, whereas v-L104 does not.[107] In addition, preliminary data indicate that HL23v promotes the formation of syncytia in XC, whereas in contrast, v-L-104 promotes syncytium formation in KC cells but not in XC cells. This difference is reminiscent of the differences in the abilities of SSV-1/SSAV/GaLV group to induce syncytium formation in XC but not in KC cells and indicates that there are detectable differences between HL23v, the virus isolated by Nooter and co-workers, and v-L-104. Unfortunately, no similar data has been reported for the other isolates described above.

V. EXPERIMENTAL INDUCTION OF NEOPLASIA IN ANIMALS WITH HUMAN TUMOR RELATED ONCORNAVIRUSES

While there is good experimental evidence for the ability of viruses of the SSV-1/SSAV/GaLV group to induce neoplasia in monkeys and gibbon apes,[108] there is, however, only one report of the induction of solid tumors and/or leukemia in nonprimate experimental animals by one of the human tumor-associated virus isolates. This report by Gabelman et al.[104] indicates that v-L-104 was capable of inducing tumors with the histologic characteristics of malignant lymphoma, reticulum cell type, and in one case, stem cell leukemia in Wistar rats. The disease became evident only after long periods of incubation (greater than 120 days). In contrast, the inoculation of L-104 cells into neonatal rats resulted in the rapid production of tumors (about 10 days) with the histologic characteristics of sarcomas.

VI. SEROLOGIC STUDIES OF HUMAN TUMOR-RELATED ONCORNAVIRUS EXPRESSION IN HUMANS

The reports of isolations of SSV and BEV related viruses from several laboratories as reviewed above have stimulated considerable debate over the origin of these viruses and their role in human neoplastic disease.[110] In the absence of a reference human oncornavirus with which to compare these isolates and since it is manifestly impossible to satisfy Koch's postulates, it has not been possible to establish the human origin of the isolates thus far characterized or to identify a role for them in human cancer directly.

An approach to this problem which might satisfy Koch's postulates indirectly would rest on the ability of the investigator to show virus related information in cancer cells not present in normal cells. Using the techniques of molecular hybridization, Speigelman and co-workers[111,112] demonstrated the presence of murine mammary tumor virus related information in the DNAs of human breast tumor cells, but not in the DNAs of sarcoma, leukemia, or lymphoma cells. Conversely, DNAs from human sarcoma, leukemia, or lymphoma cells demonstrated sequence homology with Rauscher murine leukemia virus RNAs. None of these human tumor cell DNAs shared sequences in common with any of the avian oncornaviruses or normal cellular DNAs.

Attempts to demonstrate the presence of primate oncornavirus related information in human DNAs have been somewhat less successful. Most of the human tumor or leukemia related virus isolates have recently been shown to contain a BEV related component and an SSV-1(SSAV) related component. Gallo and co-workers have been able to demonstrate homology between BEV component of HL23v and human DNA. They have not succeeded in identifying SSV-1(SSAV) related sequences in human leukemic or normal tissues.[113]

The failure to identify SSV-1(SSAV) related sequences in the DNA of leukocytes from patient HL23 may result from their being absent from the DNAs examined. However, such a situation is most unlikely and would require an alternative mechanism for oncornavirus replication from the one currently accepted by the scientific community. The alternative possibility is that SSV(SSAV) sequences are present in the cellular DNA but at levels below the sensitivity of the molecular hybridization systems.

In view of that possibility, other workers have attempted to detect viral information at the translational level, looking for viral proteins within the cell by immunological methods. The rationale for this approach to the detection of oncornavirus information in human cells rests upon earlier work in animal systems. For example, expression of the endogenous (genetically transmitted) viruses of mice[114] or infection with the exogenous (horizontally infecting) viruses of cats[115] and nonhuman primates[116] are known to result in the synthesis of humoral antibody. Similarly, inoculation of killed Rauscher leukemia virus into human patients was shown to result in the production of humoral antibody against the viral antigens.[117] Immunologically based systems should therefore be expected to detect minimal amounts of information because protein synthesis involves multiple rounds of translation and the resultant amplification of the sought after information. The immunological approach therefore offers the possibility of detecting both horizontally and vertically transmitted viruses in situations where hybridization techniques fail.

Initial data published by Strand and August,[118] using competitive radioimmunoassays

(RIA) in a heterologous system with anti RD114 antibody and ^{125}I-labeled Rauscher murine leukemia virus p30 or gp67/71, detected interspecies determinants for murine feline and primate antigens. They reported the presence of such antigens in all human tissues including tumor tissues, but found especially high titers of competitive antigens in systemic lupus erythematosus.

Sherr and Todaro detected antigens related to the major structural proteins of type C oncornaviruses of the SSV/SSAV/GaLV group in the peripheral leukocytes of five patients with acute leukemia. The data were obtained by using a homologous antibody and iodinated antigen in a competitive RIA.[119]

Charman et al.[120] look for interspecies antigens with an RIA using an antiserum prepared in goats by sequential immunization with feline leukemia virus (FeLV), RD114, and SSV-1. The antiserum inhibited all mammalian oncornaviruses but did not recognize human tumor tissue antigen.

Concurrent with attempts to find antigens cross reactive with known viral antigens in human normal and tumor cells were efforts to identify humoral antibody synthesized in response to such antigens in human sera. Prowchownik and Kirsten[121] reported the inhibition of reverse transcriptase activity of an SSV-BEV related complex of viruses isolated from human embryonic lung, designated HEL12, by the sera of two of ten patients with acute myelocytic leukemia. They also reported that the sera inhibited the related HL23v, BEV, and SSV polymerases, but not the polymerases of Gross, Kirsten, or avian myeloblastosis viruses.

Similarly, Snyder et al. showed cross reactivity between type C simian, murine, and feline (but not avian) oncornavirus proteins and human sera when assessed with RIA and radioimmunoprecipitation techniques.[122]

The authors, however, found no clear-cut differences in the reactivity of sera from normal or neoplastic individuals. The authors conclude that their work neither confirms nor denies the possibility that oncornaviruses are associated with human cancer.

Stephenson and Aaronson[123] looked for the presence of antibody cross reactive to SSV and BEV p30 and gp71 by RIA and were unable to find such cross reactivity in over 200 samples examined.

Gabelman et al., however, using immunofluorescence techniques, were able to find antibodies which cross reacted with v-L-104 antigens in 6 of 100 sera obtained from cancer patients, while finding no such cross reactivity with v-L104 antigens in 100 sera obtained from hospital staff or medical students employed as controls.[124]

The immunologic data reviewed above are contradictory and the contradictions will not be resolved without further study. Particular emphasis should be placed on efforts to understand the basis for the differences between the data of Stephenson and Aaronson, who find no cross reactivity with SSV-1(SSAV) related antigens in any of the human sera they tested, and the other investigators discussed above who report some cross reactivity to SSV(SSAV) related antigens in human sera obtained both in cancer patients and normal controls. What appears to be required here is an evaluation of the test systems with special regard to the characteristics of the reagents employed.

VII. SUMMARY

The present state of knowledge of the role of oncornaviruses in human cancer is obviously not satisfactory. The findings reviewed above suggest the presence in man and primates of primate-related oncornavirus information. The mode of transmission of this viral information is not understood. Neither the infectious nor the genetic mode of transmission is exclusively supported by the data, and it may well be that both horizontal (infectious) and genetic (vertical) transmission play a role in leukemogenesis, since oncornavirus expression in other mammals, and probably in man, is controlled by multiple genetic restrictive mechanisms[125] which make it possible for many generations to elapse between the initial infection and expression of the viral information as overt virus and/or leukemogenesis. Thus, information initially introduced into the cell or organism by infection might express itself many generations later in patterns characteristic of genetic, rather than infectious, transmission. Indeed, both hori-

zontal and vertical transmission of viral information may, and probably do, play a role in the leukemogenic process.

The role of oncornavirus information in the leukemogenic process, after its introduction into the organism, is equally unclear. It has been proposed, for example, that horizontal infection may result in depression of genetically transmitted viral information with a resultant alteration in the cell surface, which can be recognized as "nonself" by the immune surveillance system and destroyed.[126] Gabelman and co-workers suggest that infection of some cells with class II viruses results in the expression of class I virus information. This hypothesis is supported by the finding that v-L104 isolates, which did not contain BEV related information after initial isolation, did contain a BEV-related component after passage in non-human cells (Gabelman et al., unpublished data). It is not clear whether these isolates contained a BEV component at levels below the ability of the assay to detect it or whether the BEV component was induced after passage in cells containing unexpressed BEV-like information.

Alternate possibilities suggested by various investigators include some role in chemical carcinogenesis. Chemical carcinogens do not appear to transform by activating oncornavirus genomes; however, there is evidence that suggests a role for oncornaviruses, however peripheral, in chemical carcinogenesis. For example, immunization against oncornaviruses has been reported to protect against the effects of chemical carcinogens.[127] Long-term interferon therapy is reported to reduce the incidence of chemically-induced tumors.[128] The incidence of chemically-induced tumors is also reduced with neutralizing antibodies.[129]

Needless to say, a proven role for oncornaviruses in human cancer would represent a major breakthrough in our efforts to control the disease in the human population since it would then be possible to vaccinate the population and consequently send our major threat to life in this country down the road traveled by poliomyelitis, diphtheria, and measles.

REFERENCES

1. Friend, C., Preisler, H. D., and Scher, W., Studies on the control of differentiation of murine virus-induced erythroleukemia cells, *Curr. Top. Dev. Biol.,* 8, 81, 1974.
2. Brommer, E. J. P., *The Role of the Stem Cell in Rauscher Murine Leukemia,* Radiobiological Institute, Org. Health Res. TNH, Rijswijk, Z. H., Netherlands, 1972, 127.
3. Gross, L., Attempts at the classification of mouse leukemia viruses, *Acta Haematol.,* 32, 81, 1964.
4. Nowinski, R. C., Old, L. J., Sarkar, N. H., and Moore, D. H., Common properties of the oncogenic RNA viruses (oncornaviruses), *Virology,* 42, 1152, 1970.
5. Temin, H. M. and Baltimore, D., RNA directed DNA synthesis and RNA tumor viruses, *Adv. Virus Res.,* 17, 129, 1972.
6. Fenner, F., *The Biology of Animal Viruses,* Academic Press, New York, 1968.
7. Temin, H. M., The cellular and molecular biology of RNA tumor viruses especially avian leukosis-sarcoma viruses and their relatives, *Adv. Cancer Res.,* 19, 47, 1974.
8. Friend, C., Cell-free transmission in adult Swiss mice of diseases having the character of a leukemia, *J. Exp. Med.,* 105, 307, 1957.
9. Fujinami, A. and Inamoto, J., Ueber Geschwulste bie Japonischen haushuhnen inbesondere uber einen transplantablen tumor, *Z. Krebsforsch.,* 14, 94, 1914.
10. Zeigel, R. F. and Clark, H. F., Electron microscopic observations on a "C-type" virus in cell cultures derived from a tumor bearing viper, *J. Natl. Cancer Inst.,* 43, 1097, 1969.
11. Sonstegard, R. A. and Papas, T. S., Descriptive and comparative studies of type C virus DNA polymerase of fish (northern pike, *Esox lucius*), *Proc. Am. Assoc. Cancer Res.,* 18, 202, 1977.
12. Ellerman, V. and Bang, O., Experimentelle Leukemie bie Huhnen, *Zentralbl. Bakteriol. 1. Abt. Orig.,* 46, 595, 1908.
13. Rous, P., A sarcoma of the fowl transmissible by an agent separable from tumor cells, *J. Exp. Med.,* 13, 397, 1911.
14. Bittner, J. J., Breast cancer in mice, *Am. J. Cancer,* 35, 90, 1939.
15. Gross, L., Is leukemia caused by a transmissible virus? A working hypothesis, *Blood,* 9, 557, 1954.
16. Temin, H. M., Mechanism of cell transformation by RNA tumor viruses, *Annu. Rev. Microbiol.,* 25, 609, 1971.
17. Green, M., Oncogenic viruses, *Annu. Rev. Biochem.,* 39, 701, 1970.
18. Duesberg, P. H., On the structure of RNA tumor viruses, *Curr. Top. Microbiol. Immunol.,* 51, 79, 1970.
19. Tooze, J., Ed., *The Molecular Biology of RNA Tumor Viruses,* Cold Spring Harbor Laboratory, New York, 1973.
20. Gardner, M. B., Klement, V., Henderson, B. F., Meier, H., Estes, J. D., and Huebner, R. J., Genetic control of type C virus of wild mice, *Nature,* 259, 143, 1976.
21. Jarrett, W. F. H., Martin, W. B., Crighton, G. W., Dalton, R. G., and Stewart, M. F., Leukemia in the cat: transmission experiments with leukemia (lymphosarcoma), *Nature,* 202, 566, 1964.
22. Miller, J. M., Miller, L. D., and Olson, C., Inoculation of calves with particles resembling C-type virus from cultures of bovine lymphosarcoma, *J. Natl. Cancer Inst.,* 48, 423, 1972.
23. Lilly, F. and Pincus, T., Genetic control of murine viral leukemogenesis, *Adv. Cancer Res.,* 17, 231, 1973.
24. Hardy, W. D., Jr., Old, L. J., Hess, P. W., Essex, M., and Cotter, S. M., Horizontal transmission of feline leukemia virus. A field study, *Nature,* 244, 266, 1973.
25. Ferrer, J. F., Stock, N. D., and Lin, P., Detection of replicating C-type viruses in continuous cell cultures established from cows with leukemia, effect of culture medium, *J. Natl. Cancer Inst.,* 47, 613, 1971.
26. Spiegelman, S., Axel, R., Baxt, W., Kufe, D., and Scholm, J., Human cancer and animal viral oncology, *Cancer,* 34, 1406, 1974.
27. Bernhard, W., The detection and study of tumor viruses with the electron microscope, *Cancer Res.,* 20, 712, 1960.
28. De Harven, E., Morphology of murine leukemia viruses, in *Experimental Leukemia,* Rich, M., Ed., Appleton-Century-Crofts, New York, 1968, 97.
29. Rifkind, D. B. and Compans, R. W., Identification of spiked proteins of Rous sarcoma virus, *Virology,* 46, 485, 1971.
30. Sarkar, N. H., Moore, D. H., and Nowinski, R. C., The symmetry of the nucleocapsid of the oncornaviruses in RNA viruses, in *The Host Genome in Oncogenesis,* Emmelot, P. and Bentvelzen, P., Eds., North-Holland, Amsterdam, 1970.
31. Cheung, K. S., Smith, R. E., Stone, M. P., and Joklik, W. K., Comparison of immature (rapid harvest) and mature Rous sarcoma virus particles, *Virology,* 50, 851, 1972.
32. Sarkar, N. H. and Moore, D. H., The internal structure of mouse mammary tumor virus as revealed after tween-ether treatment, *J. Microsc.,* 7, 539, 1968.
33. Manning, J. S., Schaffer, F. L., and Soergel, M. E., Correlation between murine sarcoma virus buoyant density, infectivity and viral RNA electrophoretic mobility, *Virology,* 49, 804, 1972.
34. Shibley, G. P., Durr, F. E., Schidlovsky, G., Wright, B. S., and Schmitter, R., Leukemogenic activity of ether extracted Rauscher leukemia virus, *Science,* 156, 1610, 1967.
35. Duesberg, P. H., Physical properties of Rous sarcoma virus RNA, *Proc. Natl. Acad. Sci. U.S.A.,* 60, 1511, 1968.
36. Baltimore, D., Tumor viruses . . . 1974, *Cold Spring Harbor Symp. Quant. Biol.,* 40, 1187, 1975.

61

37. Strand, M., Billello, J. A., Shapiro, S. Z., and August, J. T., Genetic expression of mammalian RNA tumor viruses, in *Tumor Virus Infections and Immunity,* University Park Press, Baltimore, 1973.
38. Roy-Burman, P., Pal, B. K., Gardner, M. B., and McAllister, R. M., Structural polypeptides of primate derived type-C RNA tumor viruses, *Biochem. Biophys. Res. Commun.,* 56, 543, 1974.
39. Bolognesi, D. P., Huper, G., Green, R. W., and Graf, T., Biochemical properties of oncornavirus polypeptides, *Biochim. Biophys. Acta,* 355, 220, 1974.
40. August, J. T., Bolognesi, D. P., Fleissner, E., Gilden, R. V., and Nowinski, R. C., A proposed nomenclature for the virion proteins of oncogenic RNA viruses, *Virology,* 60, 585, 1974.
41. Baltimore, D., Viruses, polymerases and cancer, *Science,* 192, 632, 1976.
42. Baltimore, D. and Smoler, D., Primer requirement and template specificity of the DNA polymerase of RNA tumor viruses, *Proc. Natl. Acad. Sci. U.S.A.,* 68, 1507, 1971.
43. Spiegelman, S., Burny, A., Das, M. R., Keydar, J., Schlom, J., Travnicek, M., and Watson, K., Characterization of the products of RNA directed DNA polymerases in oncogenic RNA viruses, *Nature,* 227, 563, 1970.
44. Abrell, J. W. and Gallo, R. C., Purification, characterization and comparison of the DNA polymerases from two primate RNA tumor viruses, *J. Virol.,* 12, 431, 1973.
45. Temin, H. M., Ribonucleic acid directed deoxyribonuclei acid synthesis in virus and cells, *Acc. Chem. Res.,* 7, 169, 1974.
46. Hurwitz, J. and Leis, J. P., RNA dependent DNA polymerase activity of RNA tumor viruses, *J. Virol.,* 9, 116, 1972.
47. Molling, K., Bolognesi, D. P., Bauer, H., Busen, N., Plasman, H. W., and Hausen, P., Association of the viral reverse transcriptase with an enzyme degrading the RNA moiety of RNA-DNA hybrids, *Nature London New Biol.,* 234, 240, 1971.
48. Parks, W., Scolnick, E., Ross, J., Todaro, G., and Aaronson, S., Immunologic relationships of reverse transcriptase from ribonucleic acid tumor viruses, *J. Virol.,* 9, 110, 1972.
49. Miyamoto, K. and Gilden, R. D., Electronmicroscopic studies of tumor viruses. I. Entry of murine leukemia viruses into mouse embryo fibroblasts, *J. Virol.,* 7, 395, 1971.
50. Kakefuda, T., Lovinger, G. G., Gilden, R. D., and Hatanaka, M., Electron-microscopic studies of circular DNA in mouse embryo fibroblasts infected by Rauscher leukemia virus, *J. Virol.,* 21, 792, 1977.
51. Fan, H. and Baltimore, D., RNA metabolism of murine leukemia virus: Detection of virus-specific RNA sequences in infected and uninfected cells and identification of virus-specific RNA, *J. Mol. Biol.,* 80, 93, 1973.
52. Baltimore, D., Viral genetic systems, *Trans. N.Y. Acad. Sci.,* 33, 327, 1971.
53. Hardy, W. D., Old, L. J., Hess, P. W., Essex, M., and Cotter, S., Horizontal transmission of feline leukemia, *Nature,* 244, 266, 1973.
54. Huebner, R. J. and Todaro, G. J., Oncogenes of RNA tumor viruses as determinants of cancer, *Proc. Natl. Acad. Sci. U.S.A.,* 64, 1087, 1969.
55. Fischinger, P. J., Schafer, W., and Seiffert, E., Detection of murine leukemia virus antigens in virus particles derived from 3T3 cells transformed by murine sarcoma virus, *Virology,* 47, 229, 1972.
56. Aulakh, J. S. and Gallo, R. C., Rauscher leukemia-virus-related sequences in human DNA: Presence in some tissues of some patients with hematopoietic neoplasias and absence in DNA of other tissues, *Proc. Natl. Acad. Sci. U.S.A.,* 74, 353, 1977.
57. Todaro, G. J. and Gallo, R. C., Immunologic relationship of DNA polymerase of human acute leukemia cells and primate and mouse leukemia virus reverse transcription, *Nature,* 244, 206, 1973.
58. Desai, L. S., Short, D. L., Friedman, O. M., and Foley, G. E., Human leukemic cells: RNA-directed polymerase, *Eur. J. Biochem.,* 47, 453, 1974.
59. Strand, M. and August, J. T., Type-C RNA virus gene expression in human tissue, *J. Virol.,* 14, 1584, 1974.
60. Snyder, H. W., Jr., Pincus, G., and Fleissner, E., Specificities of human immunoglobulins reacted with antigens in preparations of several mammalian type-C viruses, *Virology,* 75, 60, 1976.
61. Gilden, R. V., Parks, N. P., Todaro, G. J., and Huebner, R., Group-specific antigen in human cell lines containing type C viruses, *Nature,* 233, 102, 1971.
62. Sherr, C. J. and Todaro, G. J., Primate type C virus p30 antigen in cells of human acute leukemia, *Science,* 187, 855, 1975.
63. Mak, T. W., Mansaster, J., Howatson, A. F., McColloch, E. A., and Till, J. E., Particles with characteristics of Leukoviruses in cultures of marrow cells from leukemic patients in remission and relapse, *Proc. Natl. Acad. Sci. U.S.A.,* 71, 4336, 1974.
64. Theilen, G. H., Gould, D., Fowler, M., and Dungworth, D. J., Type C virus in tissues of a woolly monkey (*Lagothrix* sp.) with fibrosarcoma, *J. Natl. Cancer Inst.,* 47, 881, 1971.
65. Kawakami, T., Hof, S., Buckely, P., Dungworth, D. J., Snyder, S., and Gilden, R. V., C-type virus associated with gibbon lymphosarcoma, *Nature London New Biol.,* 235, 170, 1972.
66. Goldberg, R. J., Scolnik, E. M., Parks, W. P., Yakovleva, I. A., and Lapin, B. A., Isolation of a primate type C virus from lymphomatous baboon, *Int. J. Cancer,* 14, 722, 1974.
67. Wolfe, L. G., Deinhardt, F., Theilen, G. H., Rabin, H., Kawakami, T., and Busted, L. K., Induction of tumors in marmoset monkeys by simian sarcoma virus, type 1, (*Lagothrix*): A preliminary report, *J. Natl. Cancer Inst.,* 47, 1115, 1971.

68. Wolfe, L. G., Smith, R. K., and Deinhardt, F., Simian sarcoma virus type 1 (*Lagothrix*): Focus assay and demonstration of non-transforming associated virus, *J. Natl. Cancer Inst.*, 48, 1905, 1972.

69. DiPaoli, A. and Garner, S., Acute lymphocytic leukemia in a white cheeked gibbon (*Hylobates concolor*), *Cancer Res.*, 28, 2559, 1968.

70. Gilden, R. V., Frank, K., Hansen, M., Bladen, S., Toni, R., and Crozlan, S., Similarity between gibbon ape and woolly monkey type C virus internal antigens by quantitative microcomplement fixation, *Intervirology*, 2, 360, 1974.

71. Benveniste, R. and Todaro, G. J., Homology between type C viruses of various species as determined by molecular hybridization, *Proc. Natl. Acad. Sci. U.S.A.*, 70, 3316, 1973.

72. Todaro, G., Scherr, C., Benveniste, R., Lieber, M., and Melnick, J., Type C viruses of baboons: isolation from normal cell cultures, *Cell*, 2, 55, 1974.

73. Scherr, C. J. and Todaro, G. J., Radioimmunoassay of the major group specific protein of endogenous baboon type C viruses: Relation to the RD114/CCC group and detection of antigen in normal baboon tissues, *Virology*, 61, 168, 1974.

74. Benveniste, R., Heinemann, R., Wilson, R., Callahan, R., and Todaro, G. J., Detection of baboon type C viral sequences in various tissues by molecular hybridization, *J. Virol.*, 14, 56, 1974.

75. Chopra, H. C. and Feller, W. F., Viruslike particles in human breast cancer, *Tex. Rep. Biol. Med.*, 27, 945, 1969.

76. Seman, G. and Dmochowski, L., Electronmicroscope observation of viruslike particles in comedocarcinoma of the human breast, *Cancer*, 32, 822, 1973.

77. Sun, C., Byre, G. E., and Pinkerton, H., *Experientia*, 29, 100, 1973.

78. Niwa, O., DeCleve, A., and Kaplan, H. S., Potentiating effect of iododeoxyuridine on MuLV replication in mouse embryo fibroblasts, *Virology*, 67, 158, 1975.

79. Hsiung, G. D., Activation of Guinea pig C type virus particles in a culture of spleen cells by 5-bromo-2-deoxyuridine, *J. Natl. Cancer Inst.*, 49, 567, 1972.

80. Silagi, S., Beju, D., Wrathall, J., and DeHarven, E., Tumorigenicity, immunogenicity and virus production in mouse melanoma cells treated with 5-bromo-2-deoxyuridine, *Proc. Natl. Acad. Sci. U.S.A.*, 69, 344, 1972.

81. Svoboda, J. and Dourmashkan, K. R., Rescue of Rous sarcoma from virogenic mammalian cells associated with chicken cell and treated with Sendai virus, *J. Gen. Virol.*, 4, 523, 1969.

82. Levy, J., Xenotropic viruses: murine leukemia virus associated with NIH Swiss, NZB and other strains, *Science*, 182, 1151, 1973.

83. Gallagher, R. E., Slalhuddin, S. Z., Hall, W. T., McCreadie, K. P., and Gallo, R. C., Growth and differentiation in culture of leukemic leukocytes from patients with acute myelogenous leukemia and reidentification of type C virus, *Proc. Natl. Acad. Sci. U.S.A.*, 72, 4137, 1975.

84. Mak, T. W., Mamaster, J., Howatson, A. F., McCulloch, E. A., and Till, J. E., Particles with characteristics of leukoviruses in cultures of marrow cells from patients in remission and relapse, *Proc. Natl. Acad. Sci. U.S.A.*, 71, 4336, 1974.

85. Dmochowski, L., Yumoto, T., and Grace, B. E., Electronmicroscopic studies of human leukemia and lymphoma, *Cancer*, 20, 760, 1967.

86. Morton, D. L., Hall, W. T., and Malmgren, R. A., Human liposarcomas: tissue cultures containing foci of transformed cells with viral particles, *Science*, 165, 813, 1969.

87. Priori, E. S., Dmochowski, L., Meyers, B., and Wilber, J. R., Constant production of type C virus particles in a continuous tissue culture derived from pleural effusion cells of a lymphoma patient, *Nature London New Biol.*, 232, 61, 1971.

88. Gallo, R. C., Savin, P. S., Allen, P. T., Newton, W. A., Priori, E. S., Bower, J. M., and Dmochowski, L., Reverse transcriptase and type C particles of human origin, *Nature London New Biol.*, 232, 140, 1971.

89. Gilden, R. V., Parks, W. B., Huebner, R. J., and Todaro, G. J., Murine leukemia virus group specific antigen in a type C virus containing human cell line ESP-1, *Nature*, 233, 102, 1971.

90. Scolnick, E. M., Parks, W. P., Todaro, G. J., and Aaronson, S. A., Immunological characterization of primate C type virus reverse transcriptases, *Nature London New Biol.*, 235, 35, 1972.

91. McAllister, R. M., Nicholson, M., Gardner, M. B., Rongey, R. W., Rasheed, S., Sarma, P. S., Huebner, R. J., Hatanaka, M., Crozlan, S., Gilden, R. V., Kabigting, A., and Vernon, L., Type C virus released from cultured human rhabdomyosarcoma cells, *Nature London New Biol.*, 235, 3, 1972.

92. McAllister, R. M., Nelson-Rees, W. A., Johnson, W. A., Rongey, E. W., and Gardner, M. B., Disseminated rhabdomyosarcomas formed in kittens by cultured rhabdomyosarcoma cells, *J. Natl. Cancer Inst.*, 47, 603, 1971.

93. Sarma, P., Tiang, J., Lee, Y., and Gilden, R. V., Virus similar to RD114 in cat cells, *Nature London New Biol.*, 244, 56, 1973.

94. Baluda, M. and Roy-Burman, R., Partial characterization of RD114 virus by DNA-RNA hybridization studies, *Nature London New Biol.*, 244, 59, 1973.

95. Gallagher, R. E. and Gallo, R. C., Type C RNA tumor viruses isolated from cultured human acute myelogenous leukemia cells, *Science*, 187, 350, 1975.

96. Teich, N. M., Weiss, R. A., Salahuddin, S. Z., Gallagher, R. E., Gillispie, D. A., and Gallo, R. C., Infective transmission and characterization of C type virus released by cultured human myeloid leukemia cells, *Nature*, 256, 551, 1976.

97. Gallagher, R. E., Salahuddin, S. Z., Hall, W. T., McCreadie, K. B., and Gallo, R. C., Growth and differentiation in culture of leukemic leukocytes from a patient with acute myelogenous leukemia and reidentification of type C virus, *Proc. Natl. Acad. Sci. U.S.A.*, 72, 4137, 1975.

98. Mondel, H., Gallagher, R. E., and Gallo, R. C., RNA directed DNA polymerase from human leukemic blood cells and from primate type C virus producing cells: high and low molecular weight forms with variant biochemical and immunological properties, *Proc. Natl. Acad. Sci. U.S.A.*, 72, 1194, 1975.

99. Reitz, M. S., Miller, N. R., Wong-Stahl, F., Gallagher, R. E., Gallo, R. C., and Gillespie, D. H., Primate type C nucleic acids sequences (woolly monkey and baboon type) in tissues of patients with acute myelogenous leukemia and in viruses isolated from cultured cells from the same patient, *Proc. Natl. Acad. Sci. U.S.A.*, 73, 2113, 1976.

100. Nooter, J., Aarsen, A. M., Bentvelzen, P., Degroot, F. G., and Van Pelt, F. G., Isolation of infection C-type oncornavirus from human leukemic bone marrow cells, *Nature*, 256, 595, 1975.

101. Klement, V., Rowe, W. P., Hartley, J. W., and Pugh, W. E., Mixed culture cytopathogenicity: A new test for growth of murine leukemia viruses in tissue culture, *Proc. Natl. Acad. Sci. U.S.A.*, 63, 753, 1969.

102. McGrath, C. M., Furmanski, P., Russo, J., McCormack, J. J., and Rich, M. A., A candidate human breast cancer virus, in *Critical Factors in Cancer Immunology*, Academic Press, New York, 1975, 734B.

103. Panem, S., Prowchownik, E., Reale, F. R., and Kirsten, W., Isolation of type C virions from a normal human fibroblast strain, *Science*, 189, 297, 1975.

104. Mak, T. W., Kurtz, S., Mamaster, J., and Housman, D., Viral related information and oncornavirus like particles isolated from cultures of human cells from leukemic patients in relapse and remission, *Proc. Natl. Acad. Sci. U.S.A.*, 72, 623, 1975.

105. Gabelman, N., Waxman, S., and Douglas, S., Oncornavirus-like particles in cultures of human tumor cells cocultivated with rat cells, *Clin. Res.*, 22, 484, 1974.

106. Gabelman, N., Ong, S., and Waxman, S., Cocultivation of human tumor and XC cells as a method for induction of C-type particles, *Clinical Res.*, 23, 273A, 1975.

107. Gabelman, N., Waxman, S., Smith, W., and Douglas, S. D., Appearance of C type virus particles after cocultivation of human lung tumor and rat (XC) cells, *Int. J. Cancer*, 16, 355, 1975.

108. Wolfe, L. G. and Deinhardt, F., Oncornaviruses associated with spontaneous and experimentally induced neoplasia in non human primates. A review, in *Medical Primatology*, Vol. 3, Goldsmith, E. I. and Moor-Jankowski, J., Eds., Karger, Basel, 1972, 176.

109. Gabelman, N., Smith, W., Geller, S., Prystowsky, M., Ong, S., and Waxman, S., Induction of a reticulum cell sarcoma by a primate virus (v-L104) induced by cocultivation of rat and human tumor cells, *Proc. Am. Soc. Hematol.*, 1976.

110. Benveniste, R. and Todaro, G., Evolution of C-type viral genes: inheritance of exogenously acquired viral genes, *Nature*, 252, 456, 1974.

111. Axel, R., Schlom, J., and Spiegelman, S., Presences in human breast cancer of RNA homologous to mouse mammary tumor virus RNA, *Nature*, 235, 32, 1972.

112. Hehlman, R., Kufe, D., and Spiegelman, S., RNA in human leukemia cells related to the RNA of a mouse leukemia virus, *Proc. Natl. Acad. Sci. U.S.A.*, 69, 435, 1972.

113. Wong-Stahl, F., Gillespie, D., and Gallo, R. C., Proviral sequences of baboon endogenous C type RNA virus in DNA of human leukemic tissues, *Nature*, 262, 190, 1976.

114. Aaronson, S. A. and Stephenson, J. R., Widespread natural occurrence of high titers of neutralizing antibodies to a specific class of endogenous type C virus, *Proc. Natl. Acad. Sci. U.S.A.*, 71, 1957, 1974.

115. Essex, M., Horizontally and vertically transmitted oncornaviruses of cats, *Adv. Cancer Res.*, 21, 175, 1975.

116. Kawakami, T. G., Buckely, T. M., McDowell, T., and DiPaoli, A., Antibodies to simian C-type virus antigen in sera of gibbons (*Hylobates*, sp.), *Nature London New Biol.*, 246, 105, 1973.

117. Hersh, E. M., Hanna, M. C., Jr., Gutterman, J. V., Mavligit, J., Yurkonic, M., Jr., and Gschwind, C. R., Human immune response to active immunization with Rauscher leukemia virus. II. Humoral immunity, *J. Natl. Cancer Inst.*, 53, 327, 1974.

118. Strand, M. and August, J. T., Type-C virus expression in human tissue, *J. Virol.*, 14, 1584, 1974.

119. Scherr, C. J., Todaro, G. J., Type-C viral antigens in man. I. Antigens related to endogenous primate virus in human tumors, *Proc. Natl. Acad. Sci. U.S.A.*, 71, 4703, 1974.

120. Charman, H., White, M. H., Rukhsana, R., and Gilden, R. V., Species and interspecies radioimmunoassays for rat type C virus p30: interviral comparisons and assay of human tumor extracts, *J. Virol.*, 17, 51, 1976.

121. Prowchownik, E. and Kirsten, W. H., Inhibition of reverse transcriptases of primate C-type viruses by 7S immunoglobulin from patients with leukemia, *Nature*, 260, 64, 1976.

122. Snyder, H. W., Jr., Pincus, T., and Fleissner, S., Specificities of human immunoglobulins reactive with antigens in preparations of several mammalian type-C viruses, *Virology*, 75, 60, 1976.

123. Stephenson, J. R. and Aaronson, S. A., Search for antigens and antibodies cross-reactive with type C viruses of the Woolly Monkey and Gibbon Ape in animal models and in humans, *Proc. Natl. Acad. Sci. U.S.A.*, 73, 1725, 1976.

124. Gabelman, N., Robinson, A., Ong, S., and Waxman, S., Antibodies to an oncornavirus (v-L104) isolated from human tumor cells cocultivated with rat cells, *Proc. Am. Assoc. Cancer Res.*, 18, 135, 1977.

125.   **Rowe, W. P.,** Genetic factors in the natural history of murine leukemia virus infection, G.H.A. Clowes Memorial Lecture, *Cancer Res.,* 33, 3061, 1973.

126.   **Hirschhorn, K., Price, P. M., Gabelman, N., and Waxman, S.,** The evolutionary significance of the persistance of latent oncogenic virus information in vertebrates, *Lancet,* 1, 58, 1973.

127.   **Whitmeyer, C. E. and Huebner, R. J.,** The inhibition of chemical carcinogenesis by viral vaccines, *Science,* 177, 60, 1972.

128.   **Salerno, R. A., Whitmire, C. E., Garcia, I. M., and Huebner, R. J.,** Chemical carcinogenesis in mice inhibited by interferon, *Nature,* 239, 31, 1972.

129.   **Price, P. J., Bellow, T. M., King, F. V., Freeman, A. E., Gilden, R. V., and Huebner, R. J.,** Prevention of viral-chemical co-carcinogenesis *in vitro* by type specific antiviral antibody, *Proc. Natl. Acad. Sci. U.S.A.,* 73, 152, 1976.

Chapter 6
FRIEND LEUKEMIA AS A MODEL FOR STUDYING LEUKEMIA CELLS AND LEUKEMIA CELL MATURATION

Harvey Preisler

TABLE OF CONTENTS

I. INTRODUCTION

In clinical medicine there appears to be a relationship between the degree of differentiation of malignant cells and the duration of patient survival. There is at least one report of a patient with neuroblastoma whose long-term survival appeared to result from the spontaneous differentiation of the patient's tumor.[1] Two other examples illustrate the converse situation. While chronic myelocytic leukemia and polycythemia vera are neoplastic diseases, they become truly malignant diseases only when their bone marrow stem cells lose the capacity to undergo "normal" differentiation and blastic transformation supervenes.

These three examples of differentiation of neoplastic cells are not unique. Auer rods are occasionally seen in morphologically normal granulocytes in patients with acute myeloblastic leukemia and have been interpreted as providing evidence that the leukemic cell can spontaneously mature beyond the blastic stage. Studies by Cline and Metcalf[2] of an acute myelomonocytic leukemia in mice have demonstrated that under the proper conditions these leukemic cells can differentiate into morphologically normal granulocytes and monocytes. Furthermore, studies with this myelomonocytic leukemia have also demonstrated that the replication of the leukemic stem cell is not endogenously fixed, but is affected by environmental influences, since the number of leukemic stem cells in a tumor mass is influenced by the site at which the tumor is growing.[3]

Ichikawa[4] has established a suspension culture cell line from an SL mouse with a spontaneous acute myeloblastic leukemia. The leukemic cells grow as undifferentiated blasts and their leukemogenicity can be demonstrated by inoculation back into the SL mice. When these blast cells are cultured in the presence of conditioned medium for 48 hr, the cells develop the ability to phagocytize india ink particles, and stop replicating.[5] The leukemogenicity of the suspension culture is also significantly decreased. Furthermore, in the author's laboratory, we have recently been able to induce these myeloid leukemic cells to differentiate in suspension culture into mature granulocytes and macrophages. Human leukemic myeloblasts growing in suspension culture have shown morphologic evidence of a limited degree of differentiation.[6]

Studies in the allied field of tumor viruses lend support to the basic thesis that malignant cells retain the capacity to differentiate. Cells transformed by temperature-sensitive mutants of Rous sarcoma virus[7] and murine sarcoma virus[8] become phenotypically normal when cultured in vitro at the nonpermissive temperature and are less malignant in vivo. Furthermore, these revertent cells manifested decreased tumorigenicity in vivo despite the persistence of the viral gs antigen.[9] These studies demonstrate not only that the malignant change is reversible, but also that reversal can occur despite the persistence of the oncogenic viral genome.

The current approach to the treatment of acute leukemia involves the use of cytotoxic drugs to kill the leukemic stem cell. Unfortunately, these drugs are also toxic to normal tissues; hence, the treatment itself results in significant morbidity and mortality. An alternate approach to the treatment of leukemia would be highly desirable. Treatment by inducing the differentiation of leukemic cells would have several advantages over cytotoxic chemotherapy. Even if only a portion of the leukemic cells could be induced to differentiate fully, the resultant granulocytes would make the patient more resistant to infection (the major cause of morbidity and mortality in this disease). Another potential advantage of this therapy is illustrated by the reduction or loss of malignancy of the erythroleukemic cells which occurs despite the continued production of leukemia virus (*vide infra*). Hence, the problem posed by the possible relationship between the vertical transmission of the leukemia virus (oncogene) and the etiology of the disease would not be a factor in this form of therapy. Furthermore, the significance of this approach is not limited to leukemia, since neoplasms of other organs, such as the breast, have been shown to possess the potential to differentiate.

This chapter will describe a murine leukemia system in which chemically induced differentiation has been achieved. Studies of the cell biology and molecular biology of leukemic cell differentiation will be discussed, and preliminary attempts at treating the leukemia in vivo with agents which induce in vitro differentiation will be described.

II. FRIEND LEUKEMIA IN VIVO

A. Biological Characteristics of the Disease

In Friends's original description,[10] the intraperitoneal inoculation of adult Swiss mice with either a filtrate of or cells from the spleens of mice with Friend leukemia resulted in a fatal hematologic disorder. The disease was characterized by progressive splenomegaly, anemia, and an increase in the number of nucleated cells in the peripheral blood. The peripheral blood contained "large mononuclear cells with a rounded, lobed, or horseshoe-shaped nucleus." Nucleated erythrocytes also appeared in the peripheral blood during advanced stages of the disease. The spleen, bone marrow, and liver were infiltrated with mononuclear cells which were similar to those found in the blood. Death of the animals was often due to splenic rupture.

Metcalf, et al.[11] also characterized Friend leukemia. Their findings agreed with those of Friend. These investigators emphasized the progressive anemia which accompanied the disease. They also found that there was initially a progressive increase in peripheral white blood cell count which they felt was primarily due to an increase in lymphocytes and "Friend cells." The "Friend cells" constituted 10 to 20% of the circulating white blood cells and were described as being similar in size to large lymphocytes with a scanty to moderate amount of deep blue cytoplasm which was devoid of granules. They also described an increase in the peripheral blood of cells with "doughnut nuclei" which they believed to be unrelated myeloid precursors.

Metcalf et al.[11] reported that the first histologic sign of the disease was the appearance of reticulum cells in the subcapsular region of the spleen. The reticulum cell foci in the spleen rapidly enlarged and coalesced, and there were foci of erythroblasts amid the infiltrating reticulum cells. A similar infiltrate of reticulum cells occurred in the liver. The bone marrow was characterized as consisting of primarily immature myeloid and erythroid cells with some infiltration of reticulum cells.

Buffet and Furth[12] as well as Friend and Haddad[13] reported that fragments of leukemic liver or spleen implanted subcutaneously produced tumors at the site of implantation. The tumors consisted of large mononuclear cells with basophilic cytoplasm and spherical, indented, or slightly lobed nuclei. The subcutaneous tumors were transplantable. The cells were similar and felt to be identical to the "Friend" or "reticulum" cells which characterized Friend leukemia. The tumors were devoid of erythroid activity. Tumors growing subcutaneously in Swiss mice were occasionally accompanied by full-blown Friend leukemia. DBA/2 mice carrying subcutaneous tumors almost invariably developed Friend leukemia. These investigators classified the subcutaneous tumors as reticulum cell sarcomas.

B. Friend Virus

The disease caused by the initial isolates of Friend virus was characterized by a progressive anemia.[10,11] Mirand[14] demonstrated, however, that some strains of Friend virus produced a disease which was characterized by polycythemia and hypervolemia. He also found that the polycythemic strains of Friend virus could initiate erythropoiesis in mice rendered polycythemic by hypertransfusion, while the anemia-inducing strains of Friend virus could not induce erythropoiesis under these conditions. The existence of

both anemia- and polycythemia-inducing strains of virus should be noted, since all the long-term suspension culture cell lines apparently have been derived (as can best be determined by reports in the literature) from animals made leukemic by anemia-inducing strains of Friend virus.

The Friend virus has been found to be more complex than was originally believed. Inoculation of the polycythemia variant of Friend virus into Ha/ICR or DBA/2 mice resulted in the appearance of discrete focal lesions on the surface of the spleens of the mice 9 days later.[15] These lesions were called spleen foci, and the virus could be titered in terms of spleen focus forming units. Inoculation of Friend virus into rats or C57Bl mice, both resistant to the Friend disease which occurs in DBA/2 or Swiss mice, caused lymphatic leukemia.[16] Recovery of virus from the rats or from the C57Bl mice followed by inoculation back into DBA/2 or Swiss mice also resulted in lymphatic leukemia. Hence, a viral component essential for the production of Friend disease was removed by passage through C57 black mice or rats. The spleen focus forming virus (SFFV) could be removed from the lymphatic leukemia virus (LLV) by dilution past the endpoint for the SFFV.[16]

Friend virus strains which produced marked polycythemia in Swiss mice demonstrated high titers of SFFV.[17] On the other hand, Friend virus strains which produced mild to severe anemia had lower titers of SFFV. Hence, the question as to the nature of the Friend virus was and still is in itself a very complex problem. In any event, it appears that the SFFV is a defective virus which is responsible for Friend disease and the LLV functions as its helper virus.[18] Furthermore, it appears that the genes which confer resistance or sensitivity to Friend virus (FV-1 and FV-2) act by the former gene regulating LLV function and the latter affecting SFFV function.[19]

C. The Nature of Friend Disease

While Friend leukemia is currently considered to be an "erythroleukemia" (the term should really be acute erythremia, since this disease is believed to be an acute proliferation of erythroid elements), the initial reports on Friend disease did not characterize the leukemia as erythroid in nature. Rather, the erythroid component was felt to represent a minor manifestation of the disease. Gradually, the disease became known as an erythroleukemia. The change most probably resulted from two observations. A small proportion of Friend leukemia cells growing in suspension culture spontaneously underwent erythroid maturation, as evidenced by morphologic criteria and the presence of benzidine-positive material in cell extracts (evidence of the synthesis of heme).[20] Secondly, the inoculation of tissue culture cells into lethally irradiated Swiss mice resulted in "erythroid" spleen colonies.[21]

It is unfortunate that the paper reporting the latter phenomenon did not relate the proportion of spleen colonies which contained erythroid elements, nor did it relate the proportion of cells in the colonies which were erythroid. There was simply a statement that the majority of cells were primitive Friend cells and the remainder of cells were "proerythroblasts and erythroblasts in various stages of maturation." However, the authors went on to state that the ratio of differentiated to undifferentiated cells was somewhat higher in the spleen colony population than it was in the tissue culture population. Since the proportion of spontaneously differentiating erythroid cells in tissue culture is usually <1%, it is clear that recognizable erythroid cells in the spleen colonies must have been quite uncommon.

While there was evidence that erythroid differentiation occurred when Friend cells were growing either in tissue culture or in the spleens of irradiated mice, the "reticulum cell sarcomas" which grew as a result of the subcutaneous inoculation of fragments of spleen taken from leukemic mice were devoid of erythroid activity.[22] Of interest was the observation that when cells from the subcutaneous tumors were inoculated into lethally irradiated mice, the spleen colonies which formed contained erythroid elements. Similarly, placing the cells of the subcutaneous tumors into tissue culture resulted in cultures containing some maturing erythroblasts. Hence, it appeared that the environment in which the Friend cells grew determined to some extent whether or not there would be accompanying differentiation. These early studies had two deficiencies. In the first place, the nature of the "Friend" cells or the reticulum cells themselves was unclear, and second, the absence of karyotypic studies left open the possibility that more than one cell population could have been present. One subpopulation could preferentially grow subcutaneously and be devoid of erythroid activity. A second population could be present whose pro-

liferation was favored by the splenic or tissue culture environment and whose progeny could differentiate along erythroid lines. The proportion of cells present from each population could vary greatly depending upon the environment.

Recent studies in our laboratory have reopened the question of the nature of Friend disease.[23] We inoculated DBA/2 mice subcutaneously with 1×10^6 tissue culture cells. A tumor appeared at the site of inoculation which grossly and by Giemsa staining appeared identical to that which had been previously described as being a reticulum cell sarcoma. Recent advances in hematologic pathology, however, have led to the recognition that without special stains it is virtually impossible to distinguish between a reticulum cell sarcoma and a myeloblastoma. The subcutaneously growing Friend leukemic cells gave a positive reaction for chloroacetate esterase (CAE) and peroxidase, two enzymes found only in cells of the granulocytic series and specifically not present either in reticulum sarcoma cells or in erythroid precursors.[24] The majority of the cells was CAE positive, and a minority was peroxidase positive. Furthermore, similar studies of mice which were inoculated intravenously with Friend cells and in which Friend disease was produced (massive hepatosplenomegaly; anemia; infiltration of the spleen, marrow, and liver by "Friend cells") demonstrated that the majority of Friend cells growing in the spleen were also CAE positive.

To our surprise, virtually all of the cells growing in suspension culture were also CAE positive.[25] The induction of erythroid differentiation (see below) in the culture did not reproducibly decrease the proportion of cells which were CAE positive. Furthermore, we found many cells which stained strongly positive for both heme and CAE. Hence, the same cells which were CAE positive could also be induced to differentiate along the erythroid pathway. This observation has been confirmed by karyotypic studies in which we demonstrated that the undifferentiated CAE-positive suspension culture cells, the benzidine-positive heme-containing tissue culture cells which had been induced to differentiate along the erythroid pathway, and the subcutaneously growing CAE-positive tissue culture cells had the same karyotypic abnormalities and hence were members of the same cell line.[25] Therefore, the Friend cells which grow in tissue culture have features of both the granulocytic and erythrocytic cell lines.

Reconsideration should also be given to the nature of the target cell of the Friend virus. Most investigators concluded that the target cell must be a cell which is already committed to erythroid differentiation and that it is the same for all Friend viruses be they the anemic or polycythemic strains. Recent studies by Okunewick and Phillips [26] and Wendling et al.[27] have demonstrated that spleens from mice with Friend leukemia contained increased numbers of colony-forming units (CFU-s). Wendling et al. directly compared the disease caused by the anemic and polycythemic variants of Friend virus and found several differences. While both diseases were characterized by leukocytosis and thrombocytopenia, the hematocrit fell in animals infected with the anemic variant (FVA), while it rose in those infected with the polycythemic variant (FVP). The effects of these two virus complexes on the splenic CFU-s also differed, with the FVP variant causing a much greater increase in the number of CFU-s present in the peripheral blood and spleen. The splenic CFU-s of mice made leukemic by either virus variant were able to form granulocytic, erythroid, and mega-karyocytic colonies.

Hence, it appears likely that the multipotential CFU-s is one of the targets for the Friend virus complex. The FVP variant may differ from the FVA variant in either directly stimulating the CFU-s to produce erythroid progeny or by infecting a committed erythroid stem cell as well as the CFU-s. This possibility is certainly compatible with the recent observations of Liao and Axelrad [28] and Horoszewicz et al.,[29] who found that the spleen cells removed from mice shortly after infection with the FVP variant formed erythroid colonies in vitro in the absence of erythropoietin. These studies suggest that viral-induced Friend disease may not be an "erythroleukemia" as has been believed for many years. The original descriptions of Friend disease[10,11] reported the appearance of cells with doughnut-shaped nuclei (photographs of these cells demonstrate that they are indistinguishable from murine metamyelocytes), and, in fact, in Metcalf's paper 2 pathologists (out of 14) classified Friend cells as myeloid. Recent studies by Golde et al.[30] have further emphasized that Friend leukemia is a true erythroleukemia consisting of malignantly transformed erythrocytic and granulocytic cells. This group studied the granulocyte potential of the cells of the spleens of DBA/2 mice with Friend leukemia which had been induced by inoculation with Friend virus (FVA). They found that the in vitro colony-forming efficiency of the leukemic spleen cells was tenfold greater than that of normal spleen cells and that leukemic cells produced normal granulocytic and macrophage colonies in agar and normal granulocytic cells in suspension culture. Differentiation of the leukemic cells in both systems was dependent upon the presence of colony-stimulating factor. One additional interesting aspect of these studies was the fact that the spleens were obtained from leukemic mice with advanced disease (24 to 48 hr prior to death), and at this time more than 97% of the cells were undifferentiated blasts.

Taken together, these data suggest that the malignant cells of Friend disease (FVA origin) as well as Friend leukemia cells growing in vitro are probably not committed erythroid elements, but rather are more primitive, with both a granulocytic and erythrocytic potential. The ability of the tissue culture lines studied to date to undergo granulocytic differentiation appears to be more restricted than their ability to undergo erythroid differentiation.

FRIEND LEUKEMIA CELLS (FLC) IN TISSUE CULTURE

A. Characteristics

Several investigators have established long-term suspension culture cell lines from mice infected with friend virus.[20,31,32] The cells grow as undifferentiated basophilic blast cells, with a small percentage of the cells spontaneously undergoing erythroid differentiation (Figure 1). Differentiation is manifested by a decrease in nuclear-cytoplasmic ratio, a decrease in the size of the cell, and the development of benzidine positivity (Figure 2). Benzidine positivity indicates the presence of heme in these cells. Cultures which contain benzidine-positive cells synthesize hemoglobin which is indistinguishable from the hemoglobin present in normal DBA/2 mice, the mouse strain from which the cells were derived.[33] The proportion of cells which spontaneously undergo erythroid differentiation varies from cell line to cell line (usually <1%). The addition of dimethyl-sulfoxide (DMSO),[35] any one of a variety of other cryoprotective compounds,[35,36] or butyric acid[37] induces the differentiation of a high proportion of the cells of inducible Friend cell lines

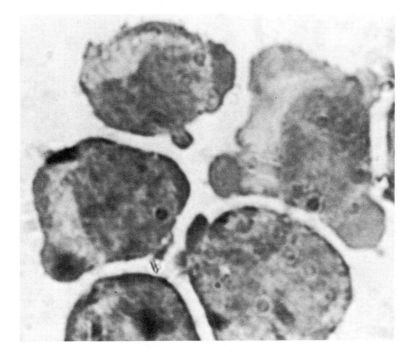

FIGURE 1. Friend leukemia cells grown in tissue culture. Note immaturity of cells with fine chromatin patterns and high nuclear:cytoplasmic ratio.

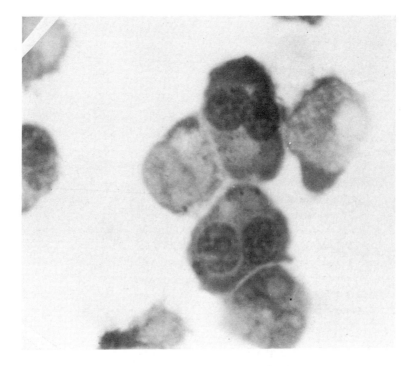

FIGURE 2. Friend leukemia cells undergoing erythroid differentiation. Two binucleate cells in center were strongly benzidine positive. Note clumped nuclear chromatin and small nuclear:cytoplasmic ratio.

(see below for discussion of different cell lines) (Figure 3).

The differentiation of these cells is characterized by morphological, biochemical, and functional alterations. During chemically induced differentiation, the morphologic changes are identical to those which occur during spontaneous differentiation, with many cells becoming morphologically indistinguishable from orthochromatophilic erythroblasts. Electron micrographic studies have demonstrated several alterations which occur during the differentiation of these cells.[38] Nuclear chromatin becomes condensed, and the total number of cytoplasmic ribosomes decreases and many become arranged in small clusters. Complex vacuolar structures appear in the cytoplasm, and the number of viruses budding from the cell membrane appears increased.

B. Biochemical Aspects of Differentiation

The original studies of the effects of DMSO on the erythroid differentiation of FLC employed line 707.[34] In this cell line, there was a detectable increase in the proportion of benzidine-positive cells (B+) after 72 hr of culture in the presence of DMSO. Biochemical studies demonstrated an increase in heme synthesis 24 hr earlier (after 48 hr of culture), and hemoglobin synthesis was first detected at 72 hr. After 72 hr of culture, DMSO-treated cells were synthesizing 20 times as much heme and 12 times as much hemoglobin as control cells, and at 96 hr heme synthesis was 60 times greater and hemoglobin synthesis was 40 times greater than control values. Using a different line of FLC, Ebert et al.[39] found an increase in Δ-aminolevulinic acid synthetase (Δ-ALA synthetase) after 28 hr of culture in the presence of DMSO. Of particular interest was their observation that allylisopropylacetamide, which was as effective an inducer of Δ-ALA synthetase activity as was 1% DMSO, did not stimulate hemoglobin synthesis.

DMSO-stimulated FLC synthesized hemoglobin which was indistinguishable by polyacrylamide gel electrophoresis from that present in DBA/2 mice.[34] The globin chain synthesized by these cells was indistinguishable by column chromatography and tryptic peptide digestion studies from the globin chains present in DBA/2 mice.[32,40] Studying Friend leukemia cell lines 707 and 745A, Boyer et al.[40] found that the ratio of α and β chains was 1:1. One the other hand, Gaedicke et al.,[71] using

two different FLC cell lines (FSD-1/clone F4 and FSD-1) reported that α and β globin chain synthesis was balanced in the former but unbalanced in the latter cell line (α:β = 1:4). Kabat et al.[41] have repeated these studies using lines 745A and FSD-1 and confirmed the findings of Boyer et al.[40] in that the α:β ratio in these leukemic cells was 1:1. The former investigators also determined the ratio of β-major:β-minor globin chains. In adult DBA/2 mouse erythrocytes the ratio was 4:1, while in DMSO-treated 745A cells it was 1.3 and in FSD-1 cells it was 9. These authors failed to detect any free hemin in the differentiating cells. Since the amounts of hemoglobin and globin were very similar, they concluded that heme and globin were synthesized coordinately. Hemoglobin synthesis in these lines was not "normal" because of the differences between the ratios of β-major and β-minor globin chains in these cell lines and in the normal mouse.

During studies of clone 745A globin synthesis was first detected 48 hr after the initiation of culture in the presence of DMSO.[42] In this cell line, this was the same time at which there were detectable changes in the polyribosome patterns of the cells[43] and there was a detectable increase in the amount of globin mRNA in the cells.[42,44] In cell lines 707 and 745A, approximately one ninth of the total protein synthesized during 4 days of culture in the presence of DMSO was globin. Using an immunoprecipitation technique, Boyer et al.[40] estimated that the average FLC in a culture grown in the presence of DMSO for 100 hr contained 8.5 pg hemoglobin, approximately one half of that present in a normal adult erythrocyte. Similar data has been reported by Ostertag et al.,[32] who found that globin comprised 25% of the labeled soluble cytoplasmic protein being synthesized by FSD-1 cells after 4 days of culture in the presence of DMSO. Kabat et al.,[41] have found that 6% of the total soluble protein of FLC (FSD-1 or 745A) present after 120 hr of culture in the presence of DMSO was globin.

Several other biochemical changes occurred during DMSO-induced differentiation. There was a measurable increase in cytidine deaminase activity (a similar increase occurs during normal erythroid differentiation), and there appeared to be a decrease in the activity of enzymes that are involved in the early steps in the *de novo* synthesis of purines.[45] As in the normal erythroid differentiation, there was an increase in carbonic

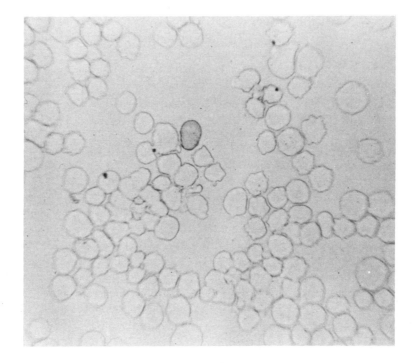

A

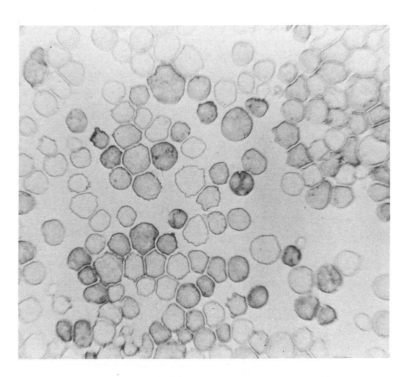

B

FIGURE 3.   (a) Low-power view of control culture of Friend leukemia cells. The single dark cell in the center is benzidine positive. (b) Low-power view of Friend leukemia cells cultured for 5 days in the presence of tetramethyl urea. Most of the cells are benzidine positive.

anhydrase activity; however, neither pyruvate kinase nor 2,3-diphosphoglycerate mutase activity was detectable in differentiating FLC.[41] In addition to the accumulation of globin mRNA during differentiation, Agris[46] has found an alteration in tRNAs with the appearance of three and possibly six new or modified tRNAs in these cells.

The above discussion of the biochemical events which accompany the differentiation of FLC was derived from studies which employed DMSO as the agent which induced differentiation. For reasons discussed below, some of the events which occur during DMSO-induced differentiation may be more characteristic of the effects of DMSO per se than of FLC differentiation.

C. General Biological Effects of DMSO-induced Differentiation

The rates of macromolecule synthesis (DNA, RNA, and protein) of cells cultured in the presence of DMSO is less than that of control cultures.[47] In control cultures, there was a rapid increase in macromolecule synthesis after the culture was seeded, and the maximal rate of DNA, RNA, and protein synthesis occurred 24 hr after seeding. These rates of synthesis declined with continued incubation. In cultures containing DMSO, there was little increase in macromolecule synthesis 24 hr after seeding (as compared to the zero time rate of the 3- or 4-day-old cells used to seed the cultures). The rate of DNA synthesis was increased at 48 hr (and was higher than that of control cultures at this time) and declined thereafter. The rate of synthesis of RNA and protein, however, remained low and never exceeded that of control cells.

Several factors were probably responsible for these observations. The lag in the increase in DNA synthesis was primarily a reflection of the 24-hr lag in the onset of cell replication which occurred when cells were seeded in culture in the presence of 2% DMSO.[34] This lag was reflected by a delay in the initiation of DNA synthesis by individual cells in these cultures.[48] During DMSO-induced differentiation, there was a progressive decrease in cell size which may also have played a role in the lower rates of macromoleculer synthesis.[49] Finally, the rates of macromolecule synthesis were measured by determining the incorporation of tritium-labeled thymidine, uridine, and leucine into DNA, RNA, and protein. The rates of uptake and incorporation may not have accurately reflected the rate of macromolecular synthesis, since pool sizes of the corresponding normal metabolites may have been altered by differentiation per se or by DMSO and hence may not have been the same as those of control cells.

In the initial communication on DMSO-induced differentiation, Friend et al.[34] reported that DMSO-induced differentiation was accompanied by a decrease in the malignancy of the cells. The study is difficult to evaluate. While the differences in the mean survival of mice receiving 5×10^5 control cells subcutaneously as compared to the same number of DMSO-treated cells (cultured for 4 days) appeared to be substantial (38 days vs. 56 days), each group consisted of only five mice. Furthermore, there did not appear to be a substantial difference in the mean survival of mice which received 5×10^4 cells subcutaneously. Even if there was truly a decrease in malignancy, these studies did not differentiate between the several possible explanations for the observations. An increase in survival of mice which received DMSO-treated cells could have been the result of (1) differentiation of the DMSO-treated cells with consequent decreased malignancy, (2) a toxic effect of DMSO on the cells, or (3) an increase in or change in the immunogenicity of DMSO-treated cells.

Studies of cells cultured in the presence of DMSO have demonstrated that within 24 hr there was a decrease in the clonogenicity of the cells in soft agar in vitro.[48] After 96 hr of culture, the clonogenicity of the DMSO-treated cells was only 1% of that of control cells. Hence, the clonogenicity experiments were compatible with the studies which reported decreased malignancy upon culture in the presence of DMSO. This observation suggested that altered immunogenicity was not the cause of the decreased malignancy. The explanation for the decreased clonogenicity is not clear. It could have been a result of cumulative DMSO toxicity or due to DMSO-induced erythroid differentiation, since erythroid precursors will not form colonies in vitro in the absence of erythropoietin.

Several observations suggest that the decline in clonogenicity was not the result of DMSO toxicity.[48] For example, between the end of the first and second days of culture there was a 2½-fold decline in clonogenicity. This decline occurred at a time when the cell number was increasing exponentially, when more than 99% of the cells excluded trypan blue, and when 92% of the cells were engaged in DNA synthesis.

On the other hand, the continuation of DNA synthesis and cell replication is not de facto evidence of an absence of DMSO-toxicity. It is known that supralethally damaged cells can in some instances engage in DNA synthesis and go through several cell divisions prior to dying.

We have found that the ATP pool size of cells seeded in the presence of DMSO decreased rapidly and that within 24 hr it had fallen to 50% of that of control levels.[50] Continued culture in the presence of DMSO resulted in a continued fall in ATP pool size. Other more potent inducers of FLC differentiation (tetramethylurea) caused a much lesser decline in the pool sizes. Furthermore, when FLC were incubated simultaneously with DMSO and bromodeoxyuridine (BUdR), the BUdR inhibited DMSO-induced erythroid differentiation but did not inhibit DMSO-induced decrease in ATP pool size. Hence, the effects of DMSO on ATP pool size appeared to be a result of toxicity per se and not due to differentiation. One additional observation also suggested that DMSO toxicity was biologically significant. Compounds which had less of an effect on ATP pool size (tetramethylurea for example) caused less of a lag in initial cell growth than that which was observed in cultures containing DMSO.[36]

From the above observations it is apparent that many of the already complete studies, particularly those of biological phenomena (the studies demonstrating decreased malignancy or clonogenicity, for example), that accompany DMSO-induced differentiation should be repeated using inducers of differentiation other than DMSO to permit a distinction to be made for alterations which are truly associated differentiation and those which are due to inducer toxicity.

DMSO-induced differentiation was accompanied by an additional phenomenon characteristic of normal erythroid maturation. The addition of erythropoietin (Ep) to control suspension cultures of FLC had no effect on the rates of DNA, RNA, protein, or heme synthesis.[51] On the other hand, culture of cells in the presence of DMSO for 48 hr rendered the suspension cultures responsive to Ep (as manifested by an increase in heme, protein, and RNA synthesis.[52] In fact, responsiveness to Ep could be detected 24 hr earlier if the cells were placed into plasma clots

in the presence of Ep and the proportion of erythroid colonies determined.[53] Similarly, the process of differentiation was also characterized by the appearance of normal erythrocyte membrane antigens.[54]

D. Effect of DMSO-induced Differentiation on Virus Release

All FLC tissue culture lines reported to date release Friend leukemia virus. Ikawa[54] reported that FLC cultures containing DMSO produced 200 times as many viruses as did control cultures. Dube et al.,[55] reported that in their cell line the increase in the release of viruses paralleled the increase in synthesis of globin mRNA. The induction and release of virus in DMSO-containing cultures was temporary and began to decline after 2 to 3 days of growth in the presence of DMSO, and after 5 to 6 days of culture the DMSO-treated cells released less virus than did control cells. They also reported that DMSO failed to increase virus release in a cell line which was resistant to DMSO induction of differentiation. Differentiation did not depend upon virus release, since the addition of interferon to differentiating FLC cultures markedly reduced virus release but had no effect on globin synthesis.[56] Unexpectedly it appeared that DMSO induced the release of an endogenous N-tropic virus and not the virus which is released by control cells.[55]

E. Chemical Inducers of Differentiation

DMSO and dimethylformamide[57] are basic aproteic polar solvents with cryoprotective properties. Many cryoprotective agents can induce the differentiation of FLC (Table 1). Inspection of this list leads to the conclusion that a variety of physical structures are possible for a compound to induce differentiation. The compounds could be linear, branched linear, or cyclic. The presence of methyl groups was not essential. All had a low molecular weight. Studies with families of inducers (tetramethylurea [TMU], dimethylurea [DMU], and urea [U], dimethylformamide, methyl-formamide, formamide, etc.) have led to several conclusions.[36] When considering different families of compounds, an increase in basicity was associated with an increase both in inducing ability and in cryoprotective ability TMU>DMU>U, for example). Members of different families of compounds which are both cryoprotective and inducing agents differ in their optimal inducing

TABLE 1

Inducers of FLC Differentiation Compounds with Known or Theoretical Cryoprotective Ability

Inducer	B+ Cells (%)[a]
Control	0.3
Diethylene glycol	7
Pyridazine	10
Dimethylurea	13
Acetamide	16
Dimethylformamide	30
Dimethylsulfoxide	55
Pyridine N-oxide	55
N-methylacetamide	55
Dimethylacetamide	70
Tetramethylurea	70

[a]Percent of benzidine-positive cell after 5 days of culture in the presence of the inducing agent.

concentration (optimal concentration of dimethylacetamide is 0.02 M, while that of DMSO is 0.22 M).

Several other groups of investigators have looked at the ability of various compounds to induce FLC differentiation. Sugano et al.,[58] using the appearance of erythrocyte membrane antigens as an indicator of differentiation, found that N-demethylrifampicin and bleomycin as well as cytosine arabinoside and glycerol induced FLC differentiation. They related that the most effective concentrations were those which moderately damaged the cells. Evaluation of these studies is difficult. It has not been demonstrated that the appearance of erythrocytic antigens during FLC differentiation is a result of *de novo* synthesis or may merely be the result of the unmasking of proteins already present on the cell surface. If the latter were correct, perhaps the moderate damage to the cells caused by these agents caused unmasking of the erythrocyte antigens, and hence the "differentiation" induced by these agents would clearly be a different category from that produced by the cryoprotective inducers.

Both Tanaka et al.[59] and Bernstein et al.[49] have also investigated agents which induce FLC differentiation. The former group recognized several inducing agents on the basis of their high polarity but failed to recognize the role played by differences in basicity in determining the inducing

ability of related polar compounds. For example, Tanaka et al. could not explain why two equally polar compounds, i.e., methylpyrrolidone and pyrrolidone, differed in inducing ability. Recognition that the former is more basic than the latter makes the former compound's greater potency understandable.[36] Bernstein et al.[49] have studied a similar group of compounds and found that the ability of these compounds to induce differentiation also correlated to some extent with their octanol/water coefficient. This latter group of investigators also recognized that glycolic acid, a compound with little if any inducing ability, potentiated the inducing effects of DMSO. This observation is similar to that of our previous studies in which we found that compounds such as glycerol and urea, with little inducing ability of their own, potentiated the effects of DMSO.[35]

Leder and Leder[37] recognized the inducing ability of butyric acid. This compound was effective at low concentration (0.002 M), and the kinetics of induction appeared similar to that of DMSO. Butyric acid and DMSO were antagonistic with regard to induction of differentiation. Apparently with respect to inducing fatty acids, a three-carbon straight aliphatic chain attached to a carboxyl group provided optimal inducing ability. This compound does not appear to fit into the pattern relating cryoprotective ability and Lewis basicity with the ability to induce differentiation.

F. Initiation and Fixation of Differentiation

The initial report relating DMSO induction of differentiation contained two seemingly contradictory observations.[34] On the one hand, it was reported that exposure of FLC to DMSO for as little as 1 hr resulted in the induction of differentiation in some of the cells. On the other hand, when new cultures were seeded with cells which had been cultured in the presence of DMSO for 4 days, the resultant culture consisted of only undifferentiated cells. This latter observation suggested that DMSO-induced differentiation may be reversible.

We approached this problem by incubating FLC in the presence of DMSO for varying periods of time, washing the cells with DMSO-free media and resuspending the cells in fresh media and then determining the proportion of differentiated cells after additional culture in DMSO-free media.[60] If cells were exposed to DMSO for less than 24 hr, we could not detect any subsequent DMSO-induced differentiation. This observation has also been reported from two other laboratories.[61,62] Exposure of cells to DMSO for increasing periods of time greater than 24 hr followed by subsequent culture in DMSO-free media led to an increasingly great number of differentiated cells in the culture.[60] These studies demonstrated that once DMSO-induced differentiation was begun, the vast majority of cells continued to differentiate even after removal of DMSO from the medium. Hence, exposure to DMSO for at least 24 hr was necessary to initiate the differentiation of FLC. In addition, once differentiation was initiated, the process continued even after the cells were transferred to DMSO-free media (i.e. the process became fixed). This left unanswered the question of why new cultures seeded with cells which had been cultured for 4 days with DMSO ended up containing only undifferentiated cells.

To approach this problem, the following studies were carried out. Cells were cultured for 4 days in the presence of DMSO and then resuspended from the culture in fresh DMSO-free media for 6 days. Cells were removed from the culture each day for counting and the determination of the proportion and absolute number of benzidine-positive cells (B+). During this period of secondary culture, the total number of cells in the culture increased and the proportion of B+ cells declined from 68% to 20 to 30%. The initial decline (first 3 days) in the proportion of B+ cells was only a relative decline, for in fact the absolute number of B+ cells was unchanged. Hence, the decline in percentage of B+ cells represented simply the rapid division of undifferentiated cells in the culture. In addition, during the first 3 days of secondary culture, the differentiated cells became more strongly B+, and the total amount of heme in the culture doubled. This indicated that the individual cells continued to synthesize and accumulate heme during secondary culture. After the third day, the differentiated cells became increasingly vacuolated and appeared to die. Hence, cultures containing undifferentiated cells were produced when cultures were seeded with differentiated cells as a result of two phenomena: (1) the more rapid proliferation of undifferentiated cells, and (2) the apparent death of the differentiated cells.

The studies described above (especially the observation that cells had to be exposed to DMSO for more than 24 hr for differentiation to occur and the fact that increasing durations of exposure resulted in an increase in the proportion of differentiated cells) suggested that cells might have to be exposed to DMSO during a "sensitive" phase in the cell cycle if differentiation were to occur. Studies by McClintock and Papaconstantinou are in accord with this possibility.[63] Clone 745A cells were synchronized by seeding in isoleucine-deficient media. After 40 hr, the cells were released by diluting the suspensions with normal media and adding isoleucine. The degree of synchronization obtained was excellent and persisted through at least three cell cycles. When the cells were released by seeding into media containing DMSO, hemoglobin was not detected until the cells had gone through two cell cycles. To demonstrate that the number of cycles was the significant variable, FLC were grown in medium containing 7.5 and 2.5% fetal calf serum (instead of 15%). The generation time of cells grown under these conditions was 36 hr and 48 hr, respectively, as compared to 24 hr for media containing 15% FCS. Under these conditions, the onset of hemoglobin synthesis was detected at 72 hr and 96 hr, respectively. These studies were interpreted as having demonstrated that two rounds of DNA synthesis and/or two mitoses in the presence of DMSO were essential for differentiation of FLC to be induced.

This work is very intriguing; however, it is dependent in part upon the studies conducted with cells cultured in media containing less than optimal concentrations of fetal calf serum. Work carried out in our laboratory raises questions with regard to the interpretation of this aspect of the studies.[35] We cultured line 745A cells in media containing 15% fetal calf serum which had previously been dialyzed. Cell replication was somewhat impaired, since after 5 days of growth the cultures made with dialyzed fetal calf serum contained half as many cells as did conventional cultures ($1.03 \pm 0.089 \times 10^6$ cells vs. $2.1 \pm 0.295 \times 10^6$ cells/ml, respectively). However, since the cultures were initially seeded at a cell concentration of 1×10^5/ml, the cells grown in the presence of dialyzed fetal calf serum went through slightly more than three cycles in the presence of DMSO. Despite having gone through more than three cell cycles, the amount of heme synthesized per cell was one third less for cells in the culture containing dialyzed fetal calf serum than in cells grown in conventional media.

A possible explanation for the apparent conflict

between the two studies is that the extra cell cycle through which conventionally grown cells went as compared to cells grown in the presence of dialyzed fetal calf serum could have accounted for the greater amount of heme present in the cultures containing nondialyzed FCS. However, the studies reported by McClintock and Papconstantinou[63] using dibutyryl cyclic AMP (BtcAMP) suggested that this explanation is not correct. When these investigators added BtcAMP to cultures containing DMSO which had been previously grown for 48 hr, there was an inhibition of cell replication so that after 96 hr of growth these cultures contained half as many cells as identical cultures to which BtcAMP were not added. Yet the amount of hemoglobin present in both cultures was identical. Therefore, an alternate explanation should be considered. Perhaps fetal calf serum contains a factor which is necessary for the optimal growth and differentiation of FLC grown in Eagle's basal medium. If this were so, the use of dialyzed fetal calf serum or the growth of cells in low concentrations of fetal calf serum could result in impairment of both proliferation and differentiation, with the former not necessarily being causally related to the latter.

Levy et al.[62] have also studied the possible relationship between cell cycle and DMSO-induced differentiation. These investigators attempted to utilize double thymidine blockade to synchronize FLC. These studies present a fundamental problem in interpretation. No data are provided which would permit evaluation of the degree of synchrony which was obtained, and in contrast to McClintock and Papconstantinou's studies,[63] the degree of synchrony appears to be poor, since there was virtually no second wave of DNA synthesis, and this even prevented determination of the generation time of the cells.[62] Furthermore, given the evident difficulty in achieving synchrony and the apparent prevention of cell replication, studies designed to determine the site in the cell cycle at which cells were arrested would have permitted more reliable interpretation of the data, since all the cells may not have been arrested at the G_1/S interface. These difficulties notwithstanding, the investigators carried out several studies of interest. From 3 to 5% of cells exposed to double thymidine blockade in the presence of DMSO and then released by seeding into fresh media in the absence of DMSO became B+. From 85 to 94% of cells seeded into fresh media

containing DMSO became B+. Since they calculated the duration of S to be 4 hr, the next series of studies involved the release of thymidine-blockaded cells into fresh media containing DMSO for 4 hr and then transfer to fresh DMSO-free media. This resulted in 13 to 65% B+ cells.

The technical problems notwithstanding, the conclusions reached by both McClintock and Papaconstantinou[63] and Levy et al.,[62] contradict those reached by other investigators. Conkie et al.[61] using clone 707, found that cells which were taken from a stationary culture and seeded at low density in the presence of DMSO did not divide. Nevertheless, the majority of cells became hemoglobinized. Of even greater importance are the studies by Leder et al.[64] who, using cell line T3C12 and butyric acid as the inducer of differentiation, demonstrated that stationary phase cells could be induced to differentiate. Furthermore, butyric acid could induce the differentiation of these cells even when cell replication and DNA synthesis were inhibited by either hydroxyurea or cytosine arabinoside. Thus, it appears that the reports of the requisite nature of DNA synthesis and cell division may be related more to the effects of DMSO than to the process of differentiation per se. On the other hand, the contradictory results of the studies of Conkie et al.[61] as compared to those of the studies of McClintock and Papaconstantinou[63] may be the result of differences in the two cell lines studied. Conkie et al. studied clone 707, a cell line in which translational control may play a role in the regulation of differentiation (see below). McClintock and Papconstantinou studied line 745A, in which transcriptional control appears to be dominant.

Finally, Levy et al.[62] attempted to measure the rate of uptake of ^{3}H-DMSO into cell water. They report that the intracellular concentration of DMSO did not equilibrate with that of the tissue culture medium for 24 to 30 hr. Since they felt that this intracellular concentration was critical (2% v/v) for differentiation to occur, they concluded that this observation may have accounted for the fact that cells incubated with DMSO for shorter periods of time are not induced to differentiate. The reported data are difficult to evaluate. In the first place, the results of only a single experiment are given. The investigators suggest that there is a significant difference between an intracellular concentration of DMSO of 1.7% (intracellular concentration achieved sometime between 14 and 22 hr of incubation), and 2%. Without confidence limits around the individual points, a difference of 0.3% is impossible to evaluate. Furthermore, since line 745A will differentiate to a significant degree in the presence of 1% DMSO, and since from the given data this concentration is reached within the cells at some time between 2 and 14 hr of incubation, it is difficult to understand why 24- to 30-hr exposure to DMSO before the "critical S-phase" of the cell cycle is necessary. Despite these difficulties the study is of interest. In view of the irreversibility of DMSO-induced differentiation, it would be of interest to determine if the intracellular concentration in DMSO falls when the cells are placed in DMSO-free media. This experiment would also answer another question raised by these studies. If DMSO takes 24 to 30 hr to attain an intracellular concentration equivalent to that in the media, and assuming that upon transfer to DMSO-free media there would be a gradual fall in intracellular DMSO concentration, then why are so few cells induced to during thymidine blockade? In other words, if it is true that DMSO must be present at a critical intracellular concentration during S phase, and if DMSO does not disappear immediately upon seeding in fresh media, then the synchronization of cells in the presence of DMSO followed by release in DMSO-free media followed by a S period of only 4 hr should induce a substantial number of cells to differentiate. Yet it does not.

G. Essential Metabolic Events During Differentiation

Ross et al.[65] have looked at the effects of metabolic inhibitors on DMSO-induced differentiation. Actinomycin D, cyclohexamide, or puromycin were added to FLC cultures either prior to or after the addition of DMSO, and the effects of these inhibitors on the accumulation of globin mRNA were determined. When added prior to the addition of DMSO, these inhibitors prevented the initiation of globin mRNA synthesis. When added to cells synthesizing globin mRNA, the synthesis of the mRNA immediately ceased. The basic problem with these studies as well as those described below is the fact that these inhibitors have multiple metabolic effects and are quite toxic. Hence, it is difficult to know whether the inhibition of globin mRNA synthesis was due specifically to actinomycin D effects on RNA

synthesis. Similar questions can be raised about whether the effects of cycloheximide and puromycin on protein synthesis were responsible for the inhibition of globin mRNA synthesis or whether some other toxic effects were operative.

We observed that if FLC were incubated in the presence of DMSO for 24 hr (primary culture) and then cultured in DMSO-free media for 2 days (secondary culture), there was a doubling of both the rate of ^{59}Fe incorporation into heme and in the total amount of heme/cell in the culture.[66] Hence, for at least some cells during the initial 24 hr, there was initiation and fixation of differentiation. This provided us with the opportunity to determine the effects of various metabolic inhibitors on the processes of initiation and fixation. Cells were seeded in primary culture in the presence of either hydroxyurea (5×10^{-4} M/ml) or cycloheximide (2.5×10^{-5} M/ml). At 1 hr later, when hydroxyurea had significantly inhibited DNA synthesis or when cycloheximide had significantly inhibited protein synthesis (Table 2), DMSO was added to half of the cultures. At 24 hr later the cultures were harvested and the cells washed and counted and resuspended in secondary culture at a cell concentration of 2 to 3×10^6 cells/ml in triplicate plates. At 2 days later, 1×10^6 cpm of ^{59}Fe bound to mouse transferrin was added to each plate, and 4 hr later the cultures were harvested, the heme extracted, and iron incorporation into heme determined. Each experiment was carried out at least four times.

After 2 days of secondary culture, cells which had been cultured in the presence of DMSO during primary culture were synthesizing heme at twice the rate as identically treated cultures of cells which had never been exposed to DMSO (Table 3). Inhibition of DNA synthesis by hydroxyurea during exposure to DMSO had no effect on DMSO stimulation of heme synthesis. On the other hand, cycloheximide inhibition of protein synthesis prevented DMSO stimulation of heme synthesis. A variation of these studies was also conducted in which cells were cultured in the presence of DMSO for 24 hr and then resuspended in fresh medium in the presence or absence of 5-bromo-2'-deoxyuridine (3 μg/ml). Secondary culture in the presence of BUdR decreased DMSO stimulation of heme synthesis (Table 3).

These studies led to several unexpected observations. Secondary cultures of cells exposed to only hydroxyurea or cycloheximide during primary

TABLE 2

Effect of Metabolic Inhibition on DMSO-induced Differentiation

Group	Isotope	% Inhibition	Group	Isotope	% Inhibition
(1 Hr)			(24 Hr)		
Control	^{3}H-TdR	—	Control	^{3}H-TdR	—
HU		99	HU		99
Cycloheximide		96	Cycloheximide		99
Control	^{3}H-UdR	—	Control	^{3}H-UdR	—
HU		10	HU		87
Cycloheximide		61	Cycloheximide		92
Control	^{3}H-leu	—	Control	^{3}H-leu	—
HU		40	HU		89
Cycloheximide		98	Cycloheximide		99

Note: The cells were seeded at 5×10^5 cells/ml in the presence of the appropriate inhibitor. After 1 hr, 3 μCi of the appropriate isotope was added and the culture was made 2% DMSO (v/v). At 40 min later, the incorporation of isotope was measured. At 24 hr after the addition of DMSO, the rates of macromolecule synthesis were measured in these cultures. Each experimental point represents the mean % inhibition of triplicate plates.

TABLE 3

Effect of Metabolic Inhibitors on DMSO-induced Differentiation

Group	Number of experiments	Mean stimulation ± standard error (%)
DMSO	10	111 ± 37
Hydroxyurea (HU) + DMSO	5	108 ± 66
Cordycepin + DMSO	3	62 ± 11
Cycloheximide + DMSO	4	−15 ± 11.8
DMSO − → BUdR	4	18 ± 13

Note: In each experiment, cells exposed in primary culture to a metabolic inhibitor served as the control for cells exposed to DMSO in the presence of the inhibitor. For example, cells were exposed during primary culture to either hydroxyurea or hydroxyurea + DMSO. After 24 hr the cells were washed and seeded into fresh DMSO-free media. Two days later the rate of heme synthesis was measured. To calculate the percent stimulation the following was carried out:

$$\frac{\text{CPM − heme in DMSO + HU cells − CPM heme in HU cells}}{\text{CPM Heme in HU-exposed cells}} \times 100$$

culture contained more heme (more than two and a half times) than control cultures (cells cultured in the absence of a metabolic inhibitor) in five out of five experiments for cells exposed to hydroxyurea and in three of four experiments for cells exposed to cycloheximide. It is not clear whether the metabolic inhibitors truly stimulated heme synthesis per se or whether there was selective survival of cells which were differentiating spontaneously. These studies are, however, reminiscent of those of Sugano et al.[58] which have already been discussed.

The problem of these inhibitor studies is

exemplified by the following observations. Cells grown in primary culture in the presence or absence of DMSO for 24 hr resulted in a doubling of the cell number. The number of cells also doubled during secondary culture whether or not the cells had been exposed to DMSO during primary culture. During primary culture in the presence of either hydroxyurea or cycloheximide (whether or not DMSO was present), the number of cells fell by 50%. Similarly, during the secondary culture of cells previously exposed to hydroxyurea, the number of cells fell by 30% in five of seven experiments. There was an identical fall of

30% in cell number during the secondary culture of cells previously exposed to cycloheximide in three of four experiments. Hence, both inhibitors were quite toxic to cells.

The following study was conducted to test the proposition that cycloheximide might selectively kill a subpopulation of cells which is responsive to DMSO. Cells were placed in primary culture in the presence of cycloheximide and DMSO for 24 hr. They were washed and placed in secondary culture at 1×10^5 cells/ml in the presence or absence of DMSO (2% v/v). At 4 and 6 days of culture, the cells were counted and the proportion of B+ cells determined. Cells which were placed in secondary culture in the absence of DMSO grew normally. On the other hand, cells placed in secondary culture in the presence of DMSO did not increase in number, so that at 4 and 6 days the total cell count was 0.8 and 0.75×10^5 cells/ml respectively (control cultures contained more than 10^6 cells/ml). Despite a lack of growth, 12% of the cells were B+ on Day 4 and 22% on Day 6. The proportion of B+ cells in control cultures (incubated in primary culture in the absence of cycloheximide) was 64 and 78% on Days 4 and 6. Thus, cells simultaneously exposed to cycloheximide and DMSO were "damaged," so that exposure to DMSO during secondary culture impaired cell proliferation and prevented optimal differentiation. When cells which had grown for 4 days in fresh DMSO-free medium during secondary culture were reseeded into fresh medium in the presence or absence of DMSO, both cell growth and differentiation were indistinguishable from control cells. Hence, 3 days of growth in DMSO-free media was sufficient either to reverse the DMSO-cycloheximide-induced damage or to permit replacement of the damaged cells.

These studies are compatible with the following interpretation. When FLC are induced to differentiate by exposure to DMSO for 24 hr, the synthesis of DNA during this period of time is not essential. On the other hand, protein synthesis during this period is essential for the initiation and "fixation" of differentiation. As described below, BUdR inhibits DMSO-induced differentiation by preventing the accumulation of globin mRNA. Therefore, the BUdR experiments described above suggest that the differentiation of FLC after exposure to DMSO for 24 hr was dependent upon the accumulation of globin mRNA during culture in the absence of DMSO. These observations are compatible with those reported by Ross et al.,[65] which have already been described. It is not known whether DMSO or one of its metabolites is present in the cells during secondary culture in DMSO-free media or, if present, whether it is necessary for differentiation to continue.

We attempted similar studies with inhibitors of RNA synthesis, but actinomycin D, a-amanitin, and camptothecin caused irreversible cell damage and led to 100% cell death when they were added at concentrations which significantly inhibited RNA synthesis. Cordycepin, at 25 μg/ml, decreased RNA synthesis by 30% and did not prevent DMSO-stimulation of heme synthesis (Table 3). Of further interest was the observation that in two of three experiments, secondary cultures of cells exposed only to cordycepin during primary culture synthesized more heme than secondary cultures of control cells.

H. Different FLC Lines

The FLC lines used by Ikawa, Ross, and Leder (the T3C lines) were derived from a spleen focus in DDD mice bearing Friend leukemia. The lines used by Friend, ourselves, Paul,[61] Levy,[62] and Tanaka[59] (745A and 707) originated from subcutaneous Friend cell tumors grown in DBA/2 mice.[20] The FSD family of cell lines used by Ostertag and Dube[32] originated from the spleens of leukemic mice (DBA/2). Hence, a variety of methods was used to establish these cell lines. In reviewing the work done in this field, the question naturally arises as to the biological differences between the cell lines studied by the various laboratories.

Paul and Hickey[67] reported studies employing two Friend cell lines (707 and Fw) which differed in their ability to differentiate in vitro. Clone 707 cells were induced to differentiate by inclusion of DMSO in the culture media, while line Fw cells did not respond to DMSO. The latter cells were still capable of some degree of erythroid differentiation, since 7 to 8% of these cells became B+ when cultured in intraperitoneal perfusion chambers in Porton strain Swiss mice.

We have compared several FLC lines with regard to ability to differentiate and responsiveness to various inducing agents. 745D (a subclone of line 745A) was not induced to differentiate by DMSO.[36] However, culture in the presence of other cryoprotective agents (pyridine *N*-oxide, dimethylformamide, dimethylacetamide, or tetramethylurea) resulted in a doubling of the heme content of the cultures.[36] Even more impressive was the observation that culture in the presence of butyric acid resulted in the differentiation of 41% of these cells.[36] In fact, clone 745D cells responded better to butyric acid than did 745A cells (15% B+). Therefore, refractoriness of a particular FLC line to one inducing agent does not mean that the cell line is incapable of undergoing erythroid differentiation. These findings are compatible with those of Orkin et al.[68] who studied two FLC clones which, while differing significantly with regard to their responsiveness to DMSO, contained the same number of globin genes per cell.

These observations clearly suggest that it may not be valid to extrapolate the properties of one Friend leukemic cell line to another; thus, conflicts in the observations of different groups of investigators may relate to differences in the cell lines under study.

I. Theoretical Aspects of the Regulation of Differentiation of Various FLC Clones In Vitro

An observation which is consistent in the reports of all investigators is that the greater duration of exposure to DMSO (up to 4 days) the greater the proportion of FLC which differentiate. Furthermore, even in clonal cell lines, DMSO does not induce all of the cells to differentiate. If the remaining undifferentiated cells in the culture are used to seed fresh cultures, the resulting cell population has the same responsiveness to DMSO as did the original culture.[34] The nonequivalent responsiveness of cells which are presumably genetically identical is further emphasized by the work of Orkin et al.[68] These investigators studied the responsiveness of the secondary subclones of FLC line 745A to DMSO. More than 90% of the subclones of this line FLC contained a majority of B+ cells (upon exposure to DMSO), while the remaining clones contained 25 to 50% B+ cells. Hence, as was observed in the mass culture, even between and within subclones there was differing responsiveness to DMSO.

It remains possible that cells exposed to DMSO must traverse a sensitive phase in the cell cycle for differentiation to occur. As was already discussed, the reported studies of this possibility are inconclusive. An observation made in our laboratory[39] raises additional questions about whether the determinant for the differentiation of an individual cell is related to simple exposure to DMSO during a particular phase in the cell cycle.[39] We found that at least 92% of the cells synthesized DNA between the end of the first and end of the second day of culture in the presence of DMSO, and yet the proportion of differentiated cells 3 days later was less than 50%. Between the end of Days 1 and 4, the cell count increased from 1.2×10^5 to 1.1×10^6. Therefore, virtually all of the cells went through at least one and probably three cell cycles in the presence of DMSO. It appears that if there is cell cycle sensitivity to DMSO, there must be an additional determinant of whether or not the cell will differentiate. The concept of quantal[69] divisions could explain why cells of a single clone going through a complete cell cycle differ in their response to DMSO. In this concept there are two classes of mitosis: proliferative and quantal. The daughter cells of the former are identical with the parent cells, while after quantal mitosis the daughter cells differ from the parent cell and are now able to respond to factors which induce differentiation.

Whether or not DNA synthesis or mitosis is necessary for the differentiation of FLC, it is apparent that for each cell line there is a probability of responsiveness to DMSO and that this probability is indeed determined by stable genetic or epigenetic factors.[68] This may be another way of stating that the probability of a mitosis being of the quantal variety may vary from cell line to cell line and may determine the proportion of cells which can be induced by chemical agents to differentiate in vitro.

This concept probably applies not only to cells cultured in the presence of DMSO but to their progeny as well. We exposed FLC to DMSO for 24 to 48 hr and then seeded them in plasma clots (which were free of DMSO). The erythroid colonies formed by these cells consisted of erythroid cells of differing degrees of differentiation.[53] In addition, the observation that the same clone of cells can be differentially sensitive to several inducers of differentiation further complicates the situation, since this differential sensitivity requires the presence of additional genic or genetically determined factors and possibly different mechanisms of action for different inducing compounds.

Another aspect of the regulation of differentiation relates to whether the same factors which control spontaneous differentiation also control DMSO-induced differentiation. Our earlier studies[57] of the effects of BUdR suggested that this may not be the case. While BUdR significantly inhibited both DMSO- and DMF-induced differentiation, it appeared to have no effect upon spontaneous differentiation.[57] Furthermore, the addition of BUdR to control cell cultures appeared to have a small but significant stimulatory effect upon the amount of globin mRNA present in cells grown in the absence of DMSO (? further evidence of differentiation induced by yet another metabolic inhibitor). Further evidence for a fundamental difference between spontaneous and DMSO-induced differentiation is found in the cell hybridization studies reported by Orkin et al.[68] In hybrids formed between a cell line which responded well to DMSO (745A) and a cell line minimally responsive to DMSO (the T3C variant discussed above), the amount of globin mRNA present in control cultures was intermediate between that of both parent types. On the other hand, the responsiveness of the hybrids to DMSO was significantly limited. Hence, this apparent dissociation between the mechanisms which regulate spontaneous differentiation and those which regulate DMSO-induced differentiation suggests that not only are there a variety of factors (regulatory phenomena) which determine differences in responsiveness between various clones but also that within a cell there may be different mechanisms which control spontaneous and induced differentiation.

J. Possible Mechanisms of Action of Inducers of Differentiation

1. Level of Control of Globin Synthesis

The differentiation of FLC is characterized by a variety of morphologic, biochemical, and functional changes. The earliest detectable changes include the development of responsiveness to erythropoietin and decreased clonogenicity in agar, both detectable after 24 hr of growth in the presence of DMSO. Shortly thereafter there is an increase in Δ-aminolevulinic acid synthetase activity. For most cell lines, differentiation seems to correlate with the synthesis of and/or the accumulation of globin in mRNA. Heme synthesis is not rate limiting with regard to hemoglobin synthesis, and globin mRNA accumulation apparently precedes globin synthesis. For FLC lines 745A,[70] FSD 1/44,[31] and M2, globin mRNA content increases by at least 25 to 100 times during differentiation. Gilmour et al.[72] have studied FLC line M2 with regard to the possible site of regulation of globin mRNA accumulation. They found that in a cell-free system, chromatin extracted from DMSO-treated cells was transcribed by *Escherichia coli* RNA polymerase to produce globin mRNA, while chromatin extracted from control M2 cells did not produce globin mRNA. Hence, in this cell line and perhaps in most other FLC lines, globin mRNA accumulation during differentiation seems to be (at least in part) the result of DMSO-induced transcription of DNA sequences which code for globin mRNA. However, these studies did not rule out additional DMSO effects upon the processing and degradation of globin mRNA.

Harrison et al.[73] have studied FLC line 707. In contradistinction to their observations using line M2, these authors found evidence for significant regulation at the level of translation. Cytoplasmic globin mRNA content increased only tenfold during differentiation, and radioautographic studies demonstrated a significant amount of cytoplasmic globin mRNA even in uninduced cells (similar studies with the M2 clone failed to reveal any cytoplasmic globin in mRNA in uninduced cells.) Furthermore, chromatin extracted from control cells directed globin mRNA synthesis in a cell-free system. Thus, in this cell line, the control of differentiation was not limited to the regulation of the transcription of genes which code for globin mRNA. The possibility of posttranscriptional regulation in FLC was further reinforced by the studies of Cimadevilla et al.,[74] who have found a protein in FLC (FDS-1/clone 4) grown in the absence of DMSO which inhibits protein synthesis by lysates of rabbit reticulocytes and by a fractionated system programed with reticulocyte mRNA.

Therefore, although the following discussion emphasizes transcriptional events, this does not mean that translational phenomena may not be significant. It merely indicates that more is known about potential transcriptional events. Furthermore, it does not include a discussion of the phenomena which render an individual cell responsive to the inducer be it quantal mitoses or some other phenomenon, since there is virtually nothing known about these theoretical processes.

2. Possible Direct Effects on Transcription of Globin mRNA

5'-Bromodeoxyuridine (BUdR) inhibits differentiation in a larger number of systems. BUdR also inhibits DMSO- and DMF-induced differentiation at concentrations which did not significantly inhibit cell growth. As in the other differentiating systems, BUdR must be incorporated into DNA for inhibition to occur. Holtzer[69] suggested that BUdR affects a regulatory portion of the genome. Our observations are in accord with Holtzer's predictions, since we[70] found that BUdR inhibited with FLC differentiation by inhibiting globin mRNA accumulation while having no demonstrable effect on globin mRNA size or base sequences. Furthermore, the inhibition in globin mRNA accumulation (70%) appeared to be proportional to the inhibition in the number of differentiating cells in the culture (also 70% inhibition).

Studies by Lin and Riggs[75] demonstrated that BUdR-substituted lac-operon DNA bound lac repressor more tightly than did normal lac-operon DNA. These observations suggested a model which could explain the effects of both DMSO and BUdR of FLC differentiation. FLC growing in vitro may not differentiate because of the presence of a repressor of those portions of the genome which direct erythroid differentiation. DMSO could induce differentiation either by decreasing the affinity of repressor for operon (through DMSO interaction with either repressor or operon) or by decreasing the amount of repressor present. BUdR, by increasing the affinity of repressor for operon, could inhibit DMSO-induced differentiation by directly opposing the effects of DMSO or by making lower intracellular levels of repressor more efficient inhibitors. Lapeyre and Bekhor[76] have studied the effects of BUdR and DMSO on chromatin extracted from Krebs II ascites tumor cells, and their findings are compatible with this hypothesis. They found that DMSO induced chromatin to transform into a more relaxed state, possibly by modifying the interaction between histones and DNA. When BUdR had been previously incorporated into the DNA of the chromatin, the collapsing effect of DMSO on chromatin was significantly decreased. The studies of Travers[77] are also compatible with the above hypothesis, since DMSO was found to increase the rate of RNA synthesis in a cell-free system.

Recent studies have further defined the potential physical effects of DMSO (and other cryoprotective inducers). We have found, as described previously, that there is a correlation between Lewis basicity and the inducing potency of cryoprotective agents. These compounds are also small and considerably hydrophilic. Taken together, these properties can be employed to explain the interaction of the inducing agents with two classes of molecules which are suspected to function as regulators of genic expression. This class of inducing agents has the potential to interfere with the binding of histones to DNA by disrupting the structure of water in the region of nucleoprotein and hence altering hydrophobic bonding. The basicity of these compounds could also permit the direct interaction of these compounds with acidic nucleoproteins or even directly disrupt the internal hydrogen bonding within the DNA helix and thus permit the DNA to unwind.

This concept regarding the regulation of FLC differentiation has several limitations. It is dependent upon the transcription itself and not any posttranscriptional events being the predominant regulator of the globin mRNA content of the cell. Even if it is valid for globin mRNA, it may not be valid for other mRNAs whose functioning is necessary for differentiation to occur.

3. Possible Membrane Effects of Cryoprotective Inducing Agents

The fact that many inducing agents are effective cryoprotectors of erythrocytes led us to study the effects of these compounds on the transition temperature (Tc) which characterizes the change of an artificial phospholipid from the solid crystal to liquid crystal state.[78] An increase in the Tc is associated with decreased lipid fluidity and increased stability, while the converse is true for a decrease in Tc. While the cryoprotective agents studied had differing effects on the standard Tc (TMU, DMU, DMF, PNO, DMSO tested), all of the agents caused the appearance of a new and previously unrecognized Tc which was present at a much higher temperature than the conventional Tc. We interpreted these findings as being indicative of a decrease in membrane fluidity. The importance of the basicity of the compounds was emphasized by our finding that the more acidic the phospholipid membrane the larger the effects of the inducers on the Tc.[79]

Since topical anesthetics had been found to increase membrane fluidity (lower the Tc),[80] we studied the interaction of the inducing agents and the topical anesthetics. The topical anesthetics prevented the inducing agents from causing the appearance of the upper Tc. Calcium, an ion known to interfere with the effects of the topical anesthetics on cell membranes,[81] prevented the anesthetics from interfering with the effects of the inducing agents on the artificial membranes. Furthermore, the addition of either Ca^{+2} or Mg^{+2} to the test system potentiated the effects of the inducing agents in the phospholipid membranes.

We then studied the effects of topical anesthetics and divalent cations on the differentiation of FLC (clone 745A) in vitro.[78] An increase in the concentration of either magnesium or calcium ions in the tissue culture media potentiated the inducing ability of either DMSO or TMU (when present in one half optimal concentration). The addition of either dibucaine or procaine to cultures containing either DMSO or TMU at one half optimal concentration decreased both the proportion of benzidine-positive cells in the culture and also decreased the intensity of benzidine positivity in the differentiated cells in the culture. As predicted by the phospholipid membrane studies, an increase in the concentration of calcium in the tissue culture medium prevented the inhibitory effects of the topical anesthetics.

The inhibition of FLC differentiation by the topical anesthetics may be fundamentally different from that produced by BUdR. In cultures in which DMSO-induced differentiation was inhibited by BUdR, there was no apparent effect on the degree of benzidine positivity of those cells which differentiated. Rather, the proportion of differentiated cells was affected. This was different from the effects of the anesthetics which appeared to decrease the degree of benzidine positivity of the differentiated cells. While BUdR apparently inhibited differentiation by interfering with the accumulation of globin mRNA, perhaps the topical anesthetics inhibited differentiation through their membrane effects. For example, they could interfere with heme synthesis in mitochondria, or they could inhibit the translation of globin in RNA by membrane-bound polyribosomes. Hence, it remains to be determined whether topical anesthetics inhibit all aspects of FLC differentiation or whether they merely affect the benzidine positivity of cells.

IV. COMMENTS

The membrane effects of these inducing agents are not necessarily incompatible with the postu-

lated effects of these agents on transcription. In fact, the interaction of the agents with the phospholopid membranes may be a manifestation of the same physical interactions that occur within the nucleus, since they both can be related to acid-base interactions and/or effects on the structure of water.

There are several additional possibilities which warrant consideration. Even if differentiation is associated with or dependent upon the transcription of globin mRNA, there is no evidence that this is a primary effect of the inducing agents. For example, the interaction of the inducing agent with the cell membrane may be the primary event, with the subsequent release of a secondary intracellular messenger (like cAMP) which effects the transcriptional events. In fact, one report claims that the addition of cAMP to FLC cultures induces differentiation.[71] There are, however, two reports which contradict this observation.[58,63] Despite their penetrant carrier properties, the agents do not apparently induce differentiation by enabling regulating macromolecules to enter the cell, since Kluge et al.,[82] have induced differentiation with DMSO in serumless media. Alternatively, the inducing agents could have more than one effect on the cells. They could, for example, directly affect transcription while simultaneously interacting with the external and intracellular cell membranes to alter such cellular functions as the transport of materials and the functioning of membrane-bound polyribosomes and membrane-bound enzymes.

Finally, the question remains as to why some cell lines respond to some inducing agents and not to others. For example, line 745A responded well to all the cryoprotective agents tested, and its responsiveness to these agents was closely paralleled by our phospholipid membrane studies. By contrast, line 745D is virtually unresponsive to DMSO and barely responsive to other cryoprotective agents. Hence, the phospholipid membrane studies do not correlate with the responsiveness of this cell line. Furthermore, butyric acid, a compound apparently without similarities in physical properties with the cryoprotective inducers, is an extremely potent inducer of 745D differentiation. Butyric acid does induce the differentiation of line 745A. Several different hypotheses could account for these observations. For example, the mechanisms of action of the cryoprotective inducers and butyric acid may be identical, but the 745D cells may exclude or rapidly metabolize the cryoprotective inducers. Alternatively, the cryoprotectors and butyric acid may have different mechanisms of inducing differentiation, and the 745D cells may differ from 745A cells in that the events triggered by the cryoprotectors in inducing differentiation in 745A cells either do not occur or simply do not produce differentiation in these cells. Several observations favor the existence of more than one mechanism whereby differentiation is induced. The actions of butyric acid and DMSO are antagonistic with respect to FLC clone T3C.[37] Even within the cryoprotective family of inducers, there may be some differences in their mechanisms of action, since some combinations of inducers appear to be additive, while others are "synergistic."[35] Finally, at least one cell line which is completely refractory to DMSO in vitro can be induced to differentiate in vivo by as yet unknown factors.[36]

V. IN VIVO CHEMOTHERAPY

The recognition that low concentrations of N-methyl acetamide and tetramethylurea were potent inducers of differentiation permitted the initiation of in vivo chemotherapy studies.[83,84] DBA/2 mice were inoculated either subcutaneously or intravenously with FLC which were responsive to these agents in vitro. After 7 days, inoculation with either inducing agent was begun and continued until death. While these agents only occasionally prolonged the survival of the mice, in every instance the massive splenomegaly which accompanied Friend disease was absent. Studies in which mice were serially sacrificed during therapy demonstrated that after as little as one inoculation of N-methylacetamide the proliferation of FLC in the spleen was halted. However, at no time did we find evidence that FLC differentiation was induced in vivo.

Neither inducing agent had any effect upon the proliferation of FLC growing subcutaneously. The inoculation of normal mice with N-methylacetamide caused a decrease in spleen size. Hence, to date, we have not been able to induce the differentiation of FLC in vivo but have been able to inhibit the proliferation of these cells in vivo. Perhaps changes in the schedule of drug administration in the inducing agents employed will permit induction of differentiation in vivo.

VI. SUMMARY

The study of the mechanisms which regulate the differentiation of neoplastic cells is obviously of great significance with respect both to the potential therapy of the diseases and to increased understanding of the nature of neoplasms. While the Friend leukemia system has been the most carefully studied system to date, many fundamental questions remain. The identity of the target cell of the Friend virus is not known, nor is it clear whether the disease is an acute erythremia or a true erythroleukemia. Studies employing a variety of FLC lines and inducing agents have demonstrated that there are several levels at which differentiation is controlled. For example, the mechanism(s) which determine the level of spontaneous differentiation in vitro does not appear to be identical to that which determines whether or not cells can be induced to differentiate in vitro by chemical agents. Similarly, the proportion of cells which can be induced to differentiate can vary from cell line to cell line and from inducing agent to inducing agent. A line which is very responsive to one agent can be totally refractory to another agent, and the reverse can be true for a different FLC line.

Recognition of differences between inducing agents has raised the possibility that some in vitro alterations associated with DMSO induction of differentiation may be related to toxic effects of DMSO and not a manifestation of leukemic cell differentiation. Hence, many of the initial experiments relating to the DMSO-induced differentiation of the FLC must be repeated. Taken together, the ability to induce FLC to differentiate in vitro and the ability of the tissue culture cells to cause leukemia in vivo should provide the first test of the possibility of treating leukemia through the induction of differentiation of neoplastic cells in vivo.

REFERENCES

1. Cushing, H. and Wolback, S. B., The transformation of a malignant paravertebral sympathicoblastoma into a benign ganglioneuroma, *Am. J. Pathol.,* 3, 203, 1927.
2. Cline, M. J. and Metcalf, D., Cellular differentiation in a murine myelomonocytic leukemia, *Blood,* 42, 771, 1972.
3. Metcalf, D. and Moore, M. A. S., Factors modifying stem cell proliferation of myelomonocytic leukemic cells in vitro and in vivo, *J. Natl. Cancer Inst.,* 44, 801, 1970.
4. Ichikawa, Y., Differentiation of a cell line of myeloid leukemia, *J. Cell. Physiol.,* 74, 223, 1969.
5. Ichikawa, Y., Further studies on the differentiation of a cell line of myeloid leukemia, *J. Cell. Physiol.,* 76, 175, 1970.
6. Clarkson, B., Continuous culture of seven new cell lines (SK-LI to 7). From patients with acute leukemia, *Cancer,* 21, 926, 1967.
7. Pluznik, D. H. and Sachs, L., The cloning of normal "mast" cells in tissue culture, *J. Cell. Physiol.,* 66, 319, 1965.
8. Bradley, T. R. and Metcalf, D., The growth of mouse bone marrow cells in vitro, *Aust. J. Exp. Med. Sci.,* 44, 287, 1966.
9. Metcalf, D., Moore, M. A. S., and Warner, N. L., Colony formation in vitro by myelomonocyte leukemic cells, *J. Natl. Cancer Inst.,* 43, 983, 1969.
10. Friend, C., Cell-free transmission in adult Swiss mice of a disease having the character of a leukemia, *J. Exp. Med.,* 105, 307, 1957.
11. Metcalf, D., Furth, J., and Buffet, R. A., Pathogenesis of mouse leukemia caused by Friend virus, *Cancer Res.,* 19, 52, 1959.
12. Buffet, R. F. and Furth, J., A transplantable reticulum-cell sarcoma variant of Friend's viral leukemia, *Cancer Res.,* 19, 1063, 1959.
13. Friend, C. and Haddad, J. R., Tumor formation with transplants of spleen or liver from mice with virus-induced leukemia, *J. Natl. Cancer Inst.,* 25, 1279, 1960.
14. Mirand, E. A., Erythropoietic response of animals infected with various strains of Friend virus, *Natl. Cancer Inst. Monogr.,* 22, 483, 1966.
15. Axelrad, A. A. and Steeves, R. A., Assay for Friend leukemia virus: rapid quantitative method based on enumeration of macroscopic spleen foci in mice, *Virology,* 24, 513, 1964.
16. Steeves, R. A., Eckner, R. J., Bennett, M., Mirand, E. A., and Trudel, P. R., Isolation and characterization of a lymphatic leukemia virus in the Friend virus complex, *J. Natl. Cancer Inst.,* 46, 1209, 1971.
17. Mirand, E. A., Steeves, R. A., and Avila, L., Spleen focus formation by polycythemic strains of Friend leukemia virus, *Proc. Soc. Exp. Biol. Med.,* 127, 900, 1968.
18. Steeves, R. A., Spleen focus-forming virus in Friend and Rauscher leukemia virus preparations, *J. Natl. Cancer Inst.,* 54, 289, 1975.
19. Lilly, F. and Pincus, T., Genetic control of murine viral leukemogenesis, *Adv. Cancer Res.,* 17, 231, 1973.
20. Friend, C., Patuleia, M. C., and De Harven, E., Erythrocytic maturation in vitro of Murine (Friend) virus-induced leukemia cells, *Natl. Cancer Inst. Monogr.,* 22, 505, 1966.
21. Rossi, G. B. and Friend, C., Erythrocytic maturation of (Friend) virus-induced leukemic cells in spleen clones, *Proc. Natl. Acad. Sci. U.S.A.,* 58, 1373, 1967.
22. Rossi, G. B. and Friend, C., Further studies on the biological properties of Friend virus-induced leukemic cells differentiating along the erythrocytic pathway, *J. Cell. Physiol.,* 76, 159, 1970.
23. Preisler, H. D., Bjornsson, S., Mori, M., and Barcos, M., Granulocyte differentiation by Friend leukemia cells, *Cell Differ.,* 4, 273, 1975.
24. Yam, L. T., Li, C. Y., and Crosby, W. H., Cytochemical identification of monocytes and granulocytes, *Am. J. Clin. Pathol.,* 55, 283, 1971.
25. Preisler, H. D., Shiraishi, Y., Mori, M., and Sandberg, A. A., Individual clones of Friend leukemia cells: differences in karyotypes and responsiveness to inducers of differentiation, *Cell Differ.,* submitted for publication.
26. Okunewick, J. P. and Phillips, E. L., Change in marrow and spleen CFU compartments following leukemia virus infection: comparison of Friend and Rauscher virus, *Blood,* 42, 885, 1973.
27. Wendling, F., Tambourin, P., Gallien-Lartigue, O., and Charon, M., Comparative differentiation and numeration of CFUs from mice infected either by the anemia- or polycythemia-inducing strains of Friend viruses, *Int. J. Cancer,* 13, 454, 1974.
28. Liao, S. K. and Axelrad, A. A., Erythropoietin-independent erythroid colony formation in vitro by hemopoietic cells of mice infected with Friend virus, *Int. J. Cancer,* 15, 467, 1975.
29. Horoszewicz, J., Leong, S. S. and Carter, W. A., Friend leukemia: rapid development of erythropoietin-independent hematopoietic precursors, *J. Natl. Cancer Inst.,* 54, 265, 1975.
30. Golde, D. W., Faille, A., Sullivan, A., and Friend, C., Granulocytic stem cells in Friend leukemia, *Cancer Res.,* 36, 115, 1976.
31. Furusawa, M., Ikawa, Y., and Sugano, H., Phenotypic changes in Friend tumor cells, *Gann. Monogr. Cancer Res.,* 12, 231, 1972.

32. Ostertag, W., Melderis, H., Steinheider, G., Kluge, N., and Dube, S., Synthesis of mouse haemoglobin and globin mRNA in leukaemic cell cultures, *Nature (London) New Biol.*, 239, 231, 1972.

33. Scher, W., Holland, J. G., and Friend, C., Hemoglobin synthesis in murine virus-induced leukemic cells in vitro. I. Partial purification and identification of hemoglobins, *Blood,* 37, 428, 1971.

34. Friend, C., Scher, W., Holland, J. G., and Sato, T., Hemoglobin synthesis in murine virus-induced leukemic cells in vitro: stimulation of erythroid differentiation by dimethyl sulfoxide, *Proc. Natl. Acad. Sci U.S.A.,* 68, 378, 1971.

35. Preisler, H. D. and Lyman, G., Differentiation of erythroleukemic cells in vitro: properties of chemical inducers, *Cell Diff.,* 4, 179, 1975.

36. Preisler, H. D., Christoff, G., and Taylor, E., Cryoprotective agents as inducers of erythroleukemic cell differentiation in vitro, *Blood,* 47, 363, 1976.

37. Leder, A. and Leder, P., Butyric acid, a potent inducer of erythroid differentiation in cultured erythroleukemic cells, *Cell,* 5, 319, 1975.

38. Sato, T., Friend, C., and de Harven, E., Ultrastructural changes in Friend erythroleukemia cells treated with dimethyl sulfoxide, *Cancer Res.,* 31, 1402, 1971.

39. Ebert, P. S. and Ikawa, Y., Induction of Δ-aminolevulinic acid synthetase during erythroid differentiation of cultured leukemia cells, *Proc. Soc. Exp. Biol. Med.,* 146, 601, 1974.

40. Boyer, S. H., Wuu, K. D., Noyes, A. N., Young, R., Scher, W., Friend, C., Preisler, H. D., and Bank, A., Hemoglobin biosynthesis in murine virus-induced leukemic cells in vitro: structure and amounts of globin chains produced, *Blood,* 40, 823, 1972.

41. Kabat, D., Sherton, C. C., Evans, L. H., Bigley, R., and Koler, R. D., Synthesis of erythrocyte-specific proteins in cultured Friend leukemia cells, *Cell,* 5, 331, 1975.

42. Friend, C., Scher, W., and Preisler, H. D., Hemoglobin biosynthesis in murine virus-induced leukemia cells in vitro, *Ann. N.Y. Acad. Sci.,* 241, 582, 1974.

43. Preisler, H. D., Scher, W., and Friend, C., Polyribosome profiles and polyribosome-associated RNA of Friend leukemia cells following DMSO-induced differentiation, *Differentiation,* 1, 27, 1973.

44. Ross, J., Ikawa, Y., and Leder, P., Globin messenger-RNA induction during erythroid differentiation of cultured leukemia cells, *Proc. Natl. Acad. Sci. U.S.A.,* 69, 3620, 1972.

45. Reem, G. H. and Friend, C., Purine metabolism in murine virus-induced erythroleukemic cells during differentiation in vitro, *Proc. Natl. Acad. Sci. U.S.A.,* 72, 1630, 1975.

46. Agris, P. F., Alterations of transfer RNA during erythroid differentiation of murine virus-induced leukemia cells, *Arch. Biochem. Biophys.,* 170, 114, 1975.

47. Friend, C., Scher, W., Preisler, H. D., and Holland, J. G., Studies on erythroid differentiation of Friend virus-induced murine leukemic cells, *Bibl. Haematol. (Pavia),* 39, 916, 1973.

48. Preisler, H. P., Lutton, J., Giladi, M., Goldstein, K., and Zanjani, E. D., Loss of clonogenicity in agar by differentiating erythroleukemic cells, *Life Sci.,* 16, 1241, 1975.

49. Bernstein, A., Boyd, A. A., Crichley, V., and Lamb, V., Induction and inhibition of Friend leukemic cell differentiation: the role of membrane-active compounds, in press.

50. Preisler, H. D. and Rustum, Y. M., Differing effects of inducers of differentiation on the ribonucleotide pool sizes of Friend leukemia cells, *Life Sci.,* 17, 1287, 1975.

51. Friend, C., Scher, W., and Rossi, G., The biosynthesis of heme in Friend virus-induced leukemia cells in vitro, in *The Biology of Large RNA Tumor Viruses,* Mahy, B. W. K., and Barry, R., Eds., Academic Press, London, 1970.

52. Preisler, H. D. and Giladi, M., Erythropoietin responsiveness of differentiating Friend leukemia cells, *Nature,* 251, 645, 1974.

53. Goldstein, K., Preisler, H. D., Lutton, J., and Zanjani, E. D., Erythroid colony formation in vitro by dimethylsulfoxide-treated erythroleukemic cells, *Blood,* 44, 831, 1974.

54. Ikawa, Y., Furusawa, M., and Sugano, H., Erythrocyte membrane-specific antigens in Friend-virus induced leukemia cells, *Bibl. Haematol.* (Pavia), 39, 955, 1973.

55. Dube, S. K., Pragnell, I. B., Kluge, N., Gaedicke, G., Steinheider, G., and Ostertag, W., Induction of endogenous and of spleen focus-forming viruses during dimethylsulfoxide-induced differentiation of mouse erythroleukemia cells transformed by spleen focus-forming virus, *Proc. Natl. Acad. Sci. U.S.A.,* 72, 1863, 1975.

56. Swetly, P. and Ostertag, W., Friend virus release and induction of haemoglobin synthesis in erythroleukaemic cells respond differently to interferon, *Nature,* 251, 642, 1974.

57. Scher, W., Preisler, H. D., and Friend, C., Hemoglobin synthesis in murine virus-induced leukemic cells in vitro. III. Effects of 5-bromo-2'-deoxyuridine, dimethylformamide, and dimethylsulfoxide, *J. Cell. Physiol.,* 81, 63, 1973.

58. Sugano, H., Furusawa, M., Kawaguchi, T., and Ikawa, Y., Enhancement of erythrocytic maturation of Friend virus-induced leukemia cells in vitro, *Bibl. Haematol.* (Pavia), 39, 943, 1973.

59. Tanaka, M., Levy, J., Terada, M., Breslow, R., Rifkind, R. A., and Marks, P. A., Induction of erythroid differentiation in murine virus-infected erythroleukemia cells by highly polar compounds, *Proc. Natl. Acad. Sci. U.S.A.,* 72, 1003, 1975.

60. Preisler, H. D. and Giladi, M., Differentiation of erythroleukemic cells in vitro: irreversible induction by dimethyl sulfoxide, *J. Cell. Physiol.,* 85, 537, 1975.

61. Conkie, D., Affara, N., Harrison, P. R., Paul, J., and Jones, K., *In situ* localization of globin messenger RNA formation. II. After treatment of Friend virus-transformed mouse cells with dimethyl sulfoxide, *J. Cell Biol.,* 63, 414, 1974.

62. Levy, J., Terada, M., Rifkind, R. A., and Marks, P. A., Induction of erythroid differentiation by dimethylsulfoxide in cells infected with Friend virus: relationship to cell cycle, *Proc. Natl. Acad. Sci. U.S.A.,* 72, 28, 1975.

63. McClintock, P. R. and Papaconstantinou, J., Regulation of hemoglobin synthesis in a murine erythroblastic leukemic cell: the requirement for replication to induce hemoglobin synthesis, *Proc. Natl. Acad. Sci. U.S.A.,* 71, 4551, 1974.

64. Leder, A., Orkin, S., and Leder, P., Differentiation of erythroleukemic cells in the presence of inhibitors of DNA synthesis, *Science,* 190, 893, 1975.

65. Ross, J., Gielen, J., Packman, S., Ikawa, Y., and Leder, P., Globin gene expression in cultured erythroleukemic cells, *J. Mol. Biol.,* 87, 697, 1974.

66. Preisler, H. D. and Giladi, M., The effect of metabolic inhibitors on DMSO-induced differentiation of Friend leukemic cells in vitro, in Proc. American Society of Hematologists, 17th Annual Meeting, December 7 to 10, 1975, Abstr. No. 370.

67. Paul, J. and Hickey, I., Haemoglobin synthesis in inducible, uninducible and hybrid Friend cell clones, *Exp. Cell Res.,* 87, 20, 1974.

68. Orkin, S. H., Harosi, F. I., and Leder, P., Differentiation in erythroleukemic cells and their somatic hybrids, *Proc. Natl. Acad. Sci. U.S.A.,* 72, 98, 1975.

69. Holtzer, H., Proliferative and quantal cell cycles in the differentiation of muscle, cartilage and red blood cells, in *Current Topics in Developmental Biology,* Vol. 7, Moscona, A. A. and Monroy, A., Eds., Academic Press, New York and London, 1972, 229.

70. Preisler, H. D., Housman, D., Scher, W., and Friend, C., Effects of 5-bromo-2′-deoxyuridine on production of globin messenger RNA in dimethyl-sulfoxide stimulated Friend leukemia cells, *Proc. Natl. Acad. Sci. U.S.A.,* 70, 2956, 1973.

71. Gaedicke, G., Abidin, Z., Dube, N., Kluge, N., Neth, N., Steinheider, G., Weinmann, B. J., and Ostertag, W., Control of globin synthesis during DMSO-induced differentiation of mouse erythroleukemic cells in culture, in *Modern Trends in Human Leukemia,* Neth, R., Gallo, R., Stohlman, F., and Spiegelmann, S., Eds., Grune & Stratton, New York, 1973.

72. Gilmour, R. S., Harrison, P. R., Windass, J. D., Affara, N. A., and Paul, J., Globin messenger RNA synthesis and processing during haemoglobin induction in Friend cells. I. Evidence for transcriptional control in clone M2, *Cell Diff.,* 3, 9, 1974.

73. Harrison, P. R., Gilmour, R. S., Affara, N. A., Conkie, D., and Paul, J., Globin messenger RNA synthesis and processing during haemoglobin induction in Friend cells. II. Evidence for post-transcriptional control in clone 707, *Cell Diff.,* 3, 23, 1974.

74. Cimadevilla, J. M., Kramer, G., Pinphanichakarn, P., Konecki, D., and Hardesty, B., Inhibition of peptide chain initiation by a nonhemin-regulated translational repressor from Friend leukemia cells, *Arch. Biochem. Biophys.,* 171, 145, 1975.

75. Lin, S. Y. and Riggs, A. D., *Lac* operator analogues: bromodeoxyuridine substitution in the *lac* operator affects the rate of dissociation of the *lac* repressor, *Proc. Natl. Acad. Sci. U.S.A.,* 69, 2574, 1972.

76. Lapeyre, J. and Bekhor, I., Effects of 5-bromo-2′-deoxyuridine and dimethyl sulfoxide on properties and structure of chromatin, *J. Mol. Biol.,* 89, 137, 1974.

77. Travers, A., On the nature of DNA promoter conformations: the effects of glycerol and dimethylsulphoxide, *Eur. J. Biochem.,* 47, 435, 1975.

78. Lyman, G., Preisler, H. D., and Papahadjopoulos, D., Studies of the membrane action of DMSO and other chemical inducers of Friend leukemia cell differentiation, *Nature,* submitted for publication.

79. Lyman, G. H., Papahadjopoulos, D., and Preisler, H. D., Phospholipid membrane stabilization by DMSO and other inducers of Friend leukemic cell differentiation, *Biochim. Biophys. Acta,* submitted for publication.

80. Papahadjopoulos, D., Jacobson, K., Poste, G., and Sheperd, G., Effects of local anaesthetics on membrane properties. I. Changes in the fluidity of phospholipid bilayers, *Biochim. Biophys. Acta,* 394, 504, 1975.

81. Jacobson, K. and Papahadjopoulos, D., Phase transitions and phase separations in phospholipid membranes induced by changes in temperature, pH and concentrations of divalent cations, *Biochemistry,* 14, 152, 1975.

82. Kluge, N., Gaedicke, G., Steinheider, G., Dube, S., and Ostertag, W., Globin synthesis in Friend-erythroleukemia mouse cells in protein- and lipid-free medium, *Exp. Cell Res.,* 88, 257, 1974.

83. Preisler, H. D., Bjornsson, S., Mori, M., and Lyman, G., In vivo therapy of Friend leukemia with agents which induce differentiation in vitro, Abstr. American Society of Hematologists, Dallas, December 1975.

84. Preisler, H. D., Bjornsson, S., Mori, M., and Lyman, G. H., Inducers of erythroleukemic cell differentiation in vitro. Effects of in vivo administration, *Br. J. Cancer,* in press.

Chapter 7

CELLULAR KINETICS IN THE LEUKEMIAS*

Michael L. Greenberg

TABLE OF CONTENTS

I. INTRODUCTION

Considerable information is available concerning the proliferation and turnover of leukemic cells in various types of leukemia. In some cases, information regarding the behavior of morphologically mature bone marrow or peripheral blood cells is also available. This chapter will review data derived from in vitro or in vivo studies of human leukemic cells but will not summarize studies of the various animal leukemias that are often used as models for hu-

man disease, since the applicability of animal studies to man is necessarily uncertain. The review of published material is meant to be comprehensive in terms of concepts, but will not include all individual articles on each subject.

II. ACUTE LEUKEMIAS

A. Studies of Leukocyte Colony-forming Units, Colony-stimulating Factor, and Other Factors

The formation of a colony in vitro is gener-

* This work was supported in part by NCI Grant CA 10515.

ally taken as evidence that a stem cell existed, i.e., a CFU, and that the number of colonies seen reflects the number of stem cells present in the specimen being cultured. Various authors have often used different culture techniques, however, so that their results are often not strictly comparable. Since the morphologic identity of colonies is often uncertain or not mentioned, not all reported leukocyte CFUs are necessarily typical granulocyte-macrophage colonies. Also, whether the leukocyte CFUs are derived from leukemic or normal cell lines is usually unknown.

Bone marrow from patients with acute myelocytic leukemia (AML), acute myelomonocytic leukemia (AMML), chronic myelocytic leukemia (CML) in blast crisis, or acute lymphocytic leukemia (ALL) usually had decreased concentrations of leukocyte CFUs in comparison to bone marrow from normals.[1-12] Some patients formed many clusters which were too small to meet the criteria for colonies.[2,5,6,10,12] Leukemic leukocyte CFUs had an abnormally light bouyant density,[5,6] and leukemic leukocyte CFUs had a smaller fraction in DNA synthesis than did normal CFU.[5] Cytogenetic analysis suggested that CFU-C and cluster-forming cells are leukemic.[13] Leukocyte CFU-producing granulocyte-macrophage colonies do have significant differences as compared to leukocyte CFUs derived from normal bone marrow cells. Also, the optimal conditions for cultures of these abnormal leukocyte CFUs may differ from those for leukocyte CFUs from normal individuals so that quantitation of in vitro studies may not accurately reflect the physiologic capacity of those cells. Patients with no persisting cells in culture had a good prognosis to respond to therapy in one series[12] and a poor prognosis in another;[6] both studies found a good prognosis in patients with persisting single cells or small clusters. During remission, leukocyte CFUs generally returned to normal in numbers,[1,2,5,7-9] bouyant density,[5] and fraction of cells in DNA synthesis.[5] Poor colony formation during remission often presaged relapses.[3,4] By comparison, bone marrow cells from patients with AML[14,15] or CML in blast crisis[15] cultured with phytohemagglutinin produced colonies of primitive leukemic cells at diagnosis or during relapse; these colonies were not found during remission. Thus, measurement of the numbers

and in vitro growth characteristics of such cells could often define the clinical state and prognosis for the individual patient.

CFU-C have also been measured from peripheral blood cells. The number of leukocyte CFUs was increased in many patients with AML[16,17] and ALL[6,8] in some studies, but in other studies decreased numbers of leukocyte CFUs were found in patients with AML[5,6] and ALL.[17] Again, leukocyte CFUs had an abnormally light bouyant density, and only a small fraction was in DNA synthesis.[5,11] Patients in relapse had no correlation between the concentrations of leukocyte CFUs in the bone marrow and in the peripheral blood.[8,11] The peripheral blood may be unrelated to the bone marrow because some cells in the peripheral blood may be derived from extramedullary sites, because only a subpopulation of bone marrow leukocyte CFUs is released to the peripheral blood, because the peripheral blood milieu differs from that in the bone marrow in terms of ability to sustain leukocyte CFUs, or because a steady state may not have existed at the time of the studies.

The growth of fresh AML cells in a suspension culture depended upon two populations of cells which were separable by velocity gradient sedimentation.[18,19] Phytohemagglutinin stimulated proliferation of one population, and leukocyte-conditioned medium (including supernates from the first population) stimulated the other population. Karyotypic analysis suggested that the proliferating cells were leukemic. These studies, as well as others mentioned below, suggest that leukemic growth is regulated, though abnormal.

Many patients with AML and ALL had high levels of a factor, colony-stimulating factor, in serum or urine which stimulated colony formation in vitro by cells derived from normal bone marrow or peripheral blood.[6,20] Peripheral blood cells from most patients with acute monoblastic leukemia[21] and some patients with AML,[22] AMML,[21,23] and CML in blast crisis[21] were a source of colony-stimulating factor. Adherent cells within the leukemic population were primarily responsible for colony-stimulating factor production,[23] suggesting that the responsible cells may be residual normal cells or partially differentiated normal cells. Patients with AML liberated only one of the three molecular weight species of colony-stimulating factor which normals liberate, however, even though all three species were found in their cell membranes.[24] Some patients with AML, AMML, and CML in blast crisis produced a colony-stimulating factor which stimulated mouse but not human cells,[25] at least under standard conditions of culture. Cells from most patients with AML[2,21] and ALL[7,17] did not produce colony-stimulating factor unless remission was obtained.[2] The absence of colony-stimulating factor in the peripheral blood cells was associated with a poor prognosis.[22]

Both high[26,27] and low or absent[17,18] levels of serum or peripheral blood cellular inhibitors of granulocyte-macrophage colony formation by normal bone marrow cells have been found. In one study,[29] segmented neutrophils from normal individuals inhibited colony formation, but acute leukemic peripheral blood segmented neutrophils failed to inhibit leukocyte CFUs. None of these authors have stated whether the inhibitor might be chalone, but the granulocytic chalone was able to induce regression of leukemia in five of seven patients with AML or CML in blast crisis, including one complete remission.[30] Some of the disparate findings in relation to stimulating and inhibiting substances may be the result of using different techniques, but these factors may be unrelated to the primary disease processes.

B. Studies of Proliferation of the Leukemic Blasts

As has been reviewed,[31] leukemic cells had a low stathmokinetic index (rate of accumulation of cells in mitosis after exposure to an agent which blocked cells in mitosis), a low mitotic index (fraction of cells in mitosis), and a low labeling index (fraction of cells which labeled with ^{3}H-thymidine, i.e., cells in DNA synthesis). Also, there was a slow return of the level of leukemic cells in the peripheral blood after leukapheresis. The observation that large blasts were more likely to be in DNA synthesis than small ones[32] was followed by observations that large bone marrow blasts produced smaller ones[33] and that at least some small lymphoblasts[34,35] enlarged and divided again.[34] Thus, those lymphoblasts may have been acting as stem cells with an infinite capacity for self-replication and maintenance of the total popula-

tion. Also, these observations demonstrated that blasts cannot be considered as a single, homogeneous population. Leukemic myeloblasts may[36] or may not[37] have such self-maintaining kinetics, but nearly all have the potential for DNA synthesis.[38] If one considered only large leukemic myeloblasts, the labeling index for leukemics was within the range reported for normal myeloblasts,[31] suggesting that at least that population of leukemic blasts may replicate in a manner similar to normal myeloblasts. Another suggestion of blasts with various replicative behaviors was the observation that markedly monocytoid myeloblasts had a much lower labeling index than did less monocytoid or nonmonocytoid myeloblasts.[37,42]

The time required for a complete cell generation cycle has been estimated to be 15 to 370 hr,[31,36,39-44,46] but many different techniques were used in data collection and calculation. Those techniques which require that all cells be in continuous cell cycle during the period of observation have given generation times only up to 58 hr.[31] One group[45] reexamined original data from a study which had proposed generation times of 49 and 83 hr.[41] By eliminating resting postmitotic cells from the calculations, they recalculated generation times of 25 hr. The proper interpretation of the generation cycle and its subdivisions requires that only replicating cells be considered. If, however, cells return to the cycle after prolonged rest periods, the cell cycle may have more importance in designing optimal therapy for remission induction than for cure.

Estimates of DNA synthesis time have also varied widely: 4.7 to 29 hr.[31,39-41,43,44] Premitotic rest times have been 1 to 5½ hr.[31,39-41] The mitotic times have been calculated to be 0.47 to 2.4 hr,[39-41] but actual measurements with microcinematography gave measurements of 77±7 min.[46] The postmitotic rest time has been variable and has not been measured directly. Although few hematologically normal individuals have been studied, these values for subdivisions of the leukemic cell generation cycle were not very dissimilar to values for normal hematopoietic cells in vivo.[31]

Labeling index and mitotic index were greater in the bone marrow than in the peripheral blood in patients with all types of acute leukemia,[36,39,41,42,46] except for some patients with

ALL who had a higher labeling index in the peripheral blood than in the bone marrow.[37,43,47] Although bone marrow blasts generally feed into the peripheral blood, the dominant migration may have been in the opposite direction in some of the ALL patients.[37,47] The labeling index declined as untreated AML progressed[48] and was higher at relapse than at time of diagnosis in both ALL and AML,[49-51] although mitotic index was unchanged.[50] The labeling index may reflect the total number of cells in the population, since less crowding is associated with a greater fraction of cells in the generation cycle in many replicating systems and greater crowding decreases the fraction actively reproducing. An increase in the labeling index of myeloblasts when patients with AML went into remission[52] may have represented a return to the usual physiologic state or may have been a result of drug effects. Small diurnal variations were seen in the bone marrow of some patients, with the maximal labeling index usually at noon to 6:00 p.m. and the maximal mitotic index at 6:00 p.m. to midnight.[50] It is unclear whether these changes were of sufficient magnitude to result in a therapeutic advantage with cell-cycle-specific agents to be given at the maxima.

Labeling index and mitotic index may have some prognostic value. An initial labeling index greater than 9% gave a significantly greater chance for a complete remission than an labeling index below 9% in one study,[48] but labeling index had no influence in another.[53] An increasing labeling index with chemotherapy was also associated with more complete remissions,[54] while a declining mitotic index was associated with progressive disease.[55]

In addition to labeling index being related to size of the blasts, as noted previously, markedly monocytoid myeloblasts had a much lower labeling index than less monocytoid or nonmonocytoid blasts.[37,42]

The growth fraction, i.e., all cells involved in cellular replication, of bone marrow blasts has been calculated to be 13 to 65% of the total blasts.[39] The calculation used required that the labeling index be derived only from cells which were proliferating. Since nonproliferating cells were often included, as discussed in relation to generation time calculations above, the estimates for growth fraction must be considered maximal in those patients, but calculations[31] in

other patients gave similar results. If noncycling cells are able to reenter the cell cycle at a later date, the potential growth fraction might truly be as large as 100%.

The rates of replacement of proliferating bone marrow blasts were calculated to be 0.65 to 3.0% per hour,[31,44] while the rate of replacement of nonproliferating blasts was estimated at 0.2 to 1.9% per hour.[39] Continuous infusion or repetitive injections of ³H-thymidine over 5 to 10 days[36,42,56] labeled some subpopulations completely, but up to 36% of all leukemic blasts were unlabeled, indicating that the complete population had still not been replaced and had not replicated for that period of time. Some quiescent cells may serve as potential stem cells for eventual relapse of the disease, but others may be end-stage cells destined to die.

C. Leukemic Blasts in the Peripheral Blood

Blasts entered the peripheral blood within the first few hours after injection of ³H-thymidine.[39,41,42,57] It is uncertain whether cells entered the peripheral blood while in DNA synthesis, but some cells in the peripheral blood were synthesizing DNA. Since some peripheral blood blasts may be derived from extramedullary sites whose contribution is not measurable, one cannot determine from published studies whether release of blasts from the bone marrow is random or perhaps follows (at least in part) a maturation sequence as in normal hematopoiesis. ³H-thymidine-labeled cells entered the peripheral blood in waves in some patients, with peaks seen at about 1 to 2 days and 3 to 4 days.[57] This periodicity suggests the existence of either some control mechanism for bone marrow release or sequential release from different sites, but one patient had no leukemic cells released to the peripheral blood from an ovarian leukemic mass. The usual slow return of leukemic cells in the peripheral blood over several days after leukapheresis[58] demonstrated that there usually was no extravascular compartment readily mobilizable into the peripheral blood. The fact, mentioned above, that labeling index was usually higher in the bone marrow than in the peripheral blood is consistent with either input from sites with kinetics different from the bone marrow, with different survival characteristics in the peripheral blood of cells in different parts of the cell cycle, or with preferential retention in the bone marrow of cells in DNA synthesis. The rarity of mitoses in the peripheral blood[39] and the smaller size of blasts in the peripheral blood[39,42] may be similarly explained.

Studies of labeled peripheral blood blasts suggested that they left the peripheral blood in a random fashion with a half-life of approximately 1 to 6 days.[36,37,41,42,59,60] Some labeled cells were seen in the peripheral blood at least 16 days later.[59] It is unknown whether those cells remained continuously in the peripheral blood or recirculated back to the peripheral blood after entering a noncirculating intra- or extravascular site. A rapid equilibrium did exist, however, between circulating intravascular blasts and a noncirculating pool.[59] At least part of the noncirculating pool is presumed to be the intravascular marginal pool. Calculations of turnover of blasts in the peripheral blood of 9.15 to 86.4 × 10⁷/kg/day[59] assumed that recirculation was not occurring. It is interesting that these values are less than those for peripheral blood neutrophils in normal man. Leukemic blasts are obviously not comparable to normal mature neutrophils, but the comparison draws attention to the fact that effective cell production is not as great as might be expected. The accumulation of cells in both the peripheral blood and the bone marrow reflects a balance between production, life span, migration, and destruction or other modes of cell loss.

Some peripheral blood blasts were able to return to the bone marrow in patients with ALL[60] and may[61] or may not[62] have done so in patients with AML. These findings suggest the possibility of repopulating the bone marrow with leukemia from extramedullary sites of growth, as has appeared to have occurred in some patients.

D. Granulocytic, Erythrocytic, and Megakaryocytic Cell Systems

Granulocytic stem cell activity as measured in various culture systems was discussed above. Morphologically more mature cells have also been studied, but it is unknown whether these are derived from leukemic or normal stem cells. Myelocytes and promyelocytes from three patients with AML or promyelocytic leukemia had significantly lower labeling indexes than were found during remission or in normal patients.[63] A heterogeneous population in relation to cellular replication may exist, as noted above for leukemic blasts, but it is also possible that the leukemic milieu prevents normal replication by nonleukemic cells.

The time required for all myelocytes and their progeny labeled with ³²P-diisopropylfluorophosphate to leave the bone marrow and traverse the peripheral blood in untreated patients with AML or AMML was 17 to 34+ days as opposed to 17 to 22 days in normals.[64,65] After complete remission the prolongation remained,[64] suggesting that bone marrow granulocytic precursors and their progeny have greater difficulty in fully maturing to the point of egress from the bone marrow. An alternative explanation that the total population is expanded seems less likely.

Various patients with AML or AMML had measured values of the total blood neutrophil pool, the total blood neutrophil turnover per day, and the half-life of survival of neutrophils in the blood below, within, or above the range for normal individuals.[65] The intravascular disappearance of labeled cells was frequently complex, perhaps due to multiple populations with differing abilities to enter tissues. Patients with ALL and AML tested for neutrophil mobilization from bone marrow to peripheral blood by etiocholanolone had decreased mobilization in about two thirds of patients in relapse prior to therapy and in about one half prior to monthly maintenance therapy in remission.[66] Peripheral blood neutrophils migrated poorly into tissues (abraded skin).[119] These results, taken as a whole, suggest that the morphologically mature and maturing neutrophils have considerable kinetic derangements in production and migration and do not always revert to normal even in complete remission. These cells, like erythrocytic cells (vide infra), may be leukemic. Alternatively, they may have functional defects induced in the leukemic milieu or, later, by antileukemic therapy.

Erythroid marrow precursors in AML may be leukemic since the same chromosomal abnormalities were found in these cells as in nonerythroid leukemic cells from the same patients.[67] Erythropoietin-responsive cells were present in the bone marrow in ALL[68] and in the erythroid phase of erythroleukemia,[69] but they were nearly absent in the bone marrow in

AML[68] and in the terminal leukemic phase of erythroleukemia.[69] In some patients with AML,[41,70,71] AMML,[70] promyelocytic leukemia,[71] and erythroleukemia,[70-72] the labeling index of the polychromatophilic normoblasts and of megaloblastoid cells was diminished as compared to the labeling index of polychromatophilic normoblasts from hematologically normal patients. The labeling index returned to normal in remission.[70,71] Mitotic index was also low in bone marrow erythrocytic precursors in AML, promyelocytic leukemia, and erythroleukemia and returned to normal levels in remission in one study.[71] Mitotic index was higher than normal in another study,[73] however. The DNA synthesis time was prolonged in polychromatophilic normoblasts in a patient with AML.[74] Most of these studies are consistent with ineffective erythropoiesis[72,74] during the leukemic state.

In patients with AML, the labeling index of megakaryocytes was usually lower than in those from normal individuals, and the labeling index reached normal levels in remission.[75] Polyploidization in relapse was less than in normals in some patients, but hyperploidy was noted in others.[75] The total bone marrow megakaryocytic mass and effective platelet production were normal or increased in most patients before treatment, but the intravascular platelet life span was short, resulting in thrombocytopenia even in those patients who did not have a demonstrable decrease in the total megakaryocytic mass.[76]

E. Therapy and Cytokinetics

Removal of AML cells from the peripheral blood by extracorporeal irradiation of the blood[77] or leukapheresis[78] usually produced an increase of the labeling index and the mitotic index in the bone marrow[77,78] and peripheral blood,[78] suggesting that leukemic bone marrow cells responded appropriately to depletion of peripheral blood blasts by increasing cell production. Some cells labeled in vivo prior to leukapheresis were still circulating 42 days later,[78] however, demonstrating the possibility for a long life span of such cells.

Most studies in relation to therapy, however, involve drugs. Several reviews have been written in the last few years.[79-82] The effects of individual drugs and the effect of drug combinations or sequences will be discussed. Some therapeutic attempts to utilize these effects to take advantage of synchronization within the generation cycle and/or recruitment of quiescent cells into the cell cycle will be reviewed.

Daunomycin both inhibited DNA synthesis and arrested blasts in the premitotic rest phase so that both labeling index and mitotic index decreased in patients with AML and AMML, but a randomized cytocidal effect was also evident.[79,81-84] In addition, daunomycin appeared to hinder cells blocked in the premitotic rest phase from leaving the bone marrow and entering the blood.[84] In those studies, as with others to be mentioned below, it is important to note that the various techniques used for these studies do not distinguish between perfectly intact cells, cells which are dying but have not yet been removed, and cells which have been damaged but may still have a limited replicative ability. If one could isolate those cells which were undamaged and were still capable of adversely affecting the patient, different conclusions might be drawn.

Cytosine arabinoside used in patients with AML, AMML, and ALL markedly decreased both labeling index and mitotic index within 1 to 4 hr with recovery in 6 to 72 hr, labeling index usually recovering before mitotic index.[79,81,82] In some patients there was synchronization of surviving cells so that at peak recovery of DNA synthesis the labeling index in the blasts was higher than that before therapy.[79] No direct effect on the cell cycle other than inhibition of DNA synthesis has been found.[81]

Methotrexate in AML and ALL also inhibited DNA synthesis, but the labeling index initially increased in some patients because only the *de novo* pathway of DNA synthesis was blocked.[79,81,82,85,86] ^{3}H-thymidine entered DNA via the salvage pathway, which continued to operate in cells which remained alive and in cells which were newly recruited into the cell cycle. In contrast, cytosine arabinoside blocked at a more distal site (DNA polymerase) so that thymidine was not incorporated into DNA. Cells were not inhibited from entering DNA synthesis. Mitotic index decreased abruptly because cells were unable to progress beyond DNA synthesis. Cells out of the DNA synthetic phase were not affected.[86]

Hydroxyurea in AML also blocked cells in

DNA synthesis without blocking entry into that phase so that the labeling index rose progressively,[87] similar to what was seen with methotrexate.

L-Asparaginase in ALL inhibited postmitotic blasts from entering DNA synthesis in some studies[79,82] and blocked and then destroyed cells in DNA synthesis in another study.[88] The drug also destroyed cells independent of their phase in the cell cycle.[79,87] Both labeling index and mitotic index fell in both bone marrow and peripheral blood after an initial rise in the first few hours.[88]

Corticosteroids in ALL, but not in AML, destroyed cells independent of the cell cycle but also blocked entry of cells into DNA synthesis.[79,81,82] There was no direct effect on DNA synthesis; therefore, the labeling index decreased only gradually. These results suggest that one should not give an agent specific for DNA synthesis shortly after corticosteroids, since fewer cells would be sensitive to such a drug at that time.

Cyclophosphamide in ALL has had multiple effects: inhibition of DNA synthesis, arrest in mitosis, and inhibition of cell entry into DNA synthesis.[79] The labeling index was markedly diminished in AML blasts 24 hr after giving the drug in responders, but the labeling index was unchanged or increased in nonresponders.[89]

Vincristine has been studied in ALL, AML, and AMML.[79-82,89] A rapid increase in mitotic index was seen with a peak at 5 to 24 hr after a bolus injection[79-82] or by the end of a 24- to 48-hr infusion[89] because the drug has a profound effect on the mitotic spindle. After a bolus injection, the labeling index often fell after the peak mitotic index,[79,81,82] probably because daughter cells of those held up or destroyed in mitosis did not proceed into the next generation cycle. After prolonged infusions, variable changes in labeling index were seen, probably reflecting balances in individual patients between cell destruction and recruitment of new cells into cycle. The stathmokinetic effect on erythrocytic precursors was even greater than that on the blast cells.[81,89] The drug also destroyed cells independent of the cell cycle,[90,91] and this action may be the primary cytocidal drug effect.

Many schemes have been devised to make use of cell-cycle changes induced by drugs to treat leukemic patients.[79,80,82,85,87,89,92-94] The details of individual treatment programs will not be discussed, but the principles being used by various investigators are few. Drugs with effects in different parts of the cell cycle can be given simultaneously for additive effect, but most investigators have left those attempts to the biochemical pharmacologists. Recruitment of quiescent cells into cycle where they could then be killed by cycle-active agents has been attempted frequently. The first drug may be cycle active or may be independent of the cell cycle. Recruitment is the result of a stimulus to new cell production as a result of the destruction of large numbers of blasts by the first drug. Synchronization to get an increased fraction of cells into a sensitive portion of the cell cycle may be a result of recruitment or may be the result of a temporary accumulation of cells at a certain point of the cycle followed by a release of the block (either by merely discontinuing the first drug or by giving a drug which bypasses the metabolic block of the first drug, e.g., folinic acid following methotrexate). Following recruitment and/or synchronization, a second drug (perhaps the same drug as used initially) is given at the time when maximal synchronization at the sensitive portion of the generation cycle is expected. Although some efforts have been remarkably successful,[89,94] more information on the kinetic effects on both leukemic and residual normal cells is clearly required.

III. CHRONIC MYELOCYTIC LEUKEMIA IN THE CHRONIC PHASE

A. Introduction

Although only 80 to 90% of the patients have the Philadelphia chromosome, this fact has not always been considered when kinetics were studied; therefore, the conclusions derived from the studies to be reviewed may not apply equally well to all patients. The presence of the Philadelphia chromosome in granulocytic, erythrocytic, and megakaryocytic cell lines does allow one to set the leukemic process at a pluripotent stem cell level. Most studies, however, have been concerned only with the granulocytic line.

B. Studies of Leukocyte CFUs, Colony-Stimulating-Factor and Other Factors

The in vitro assay systems for granulocytic cells have allowed studies of both colony-stimulating factor and leukocyte CFUs, as in the acute leukemias. Urine[20,95] and serum[95] from most patients had a high level of colony-stimulating factor[20,95] without any correlation with the white blood count or clinical stage. One patient with spontaneous cycles of the peripheral blood leukocyte levels, however, had cyclic fluctuations of colony-stimulating factor levels which were out of phase with those leukocyte levels.[127] Serum levels of colony-stimulating factor were also frequently high.[95] In these CML patients, colony-stimulating factor was produced by peripheral blood and bone marrow leukocytes, apparently by monocytes, although perhaps in amounts somewhat less per cell than normal.[23,96,97] In contrast, an inhibitor of colony formation by normal and CML leukocyte CFUs appeared to be present in mature granulocytes from both control and most CML patients to equal degrees,[98] but CML neutrophils were less efficient in suppressing granulopoiesis than were normal neutrophils in a diffusion chamber culture.[99] These stimulators and inhibitors appeared to be present at what would be physiologically appropriate times and levels if one assumed that the patient's granulocytes should be maintained at their observed elevated levels in the peripheral blood. Therefore, whatever mechanism(s) measures and regulates the production and the peripheral blood granulocyte level may be faulty. Another possibility is that abnormal leukocyte CFUs (*vide infra*) may be unable to respond to those factors and/or moderate the usual feedback controls in a normal fashion.

The number of leukocyte CFUs was moderately increased in the peripheral blood and was markedly increased in the bone marrow in comparison to normals,[5,16,97,98,100] the number usually being related to the white blood count.[16,97,98,100] The concentration of leukocyte CFUs returned to normal in remission.[5,100] Some investigators found a smaller fraction of leukemic than normal leukocyte CFUs in DNA synthesis,[5] but others found a decrease only in advanced disease.[101] Leukocyte CFUs from both bone marrow and peripheral blood had an abnormally light buoyant density.[101] Thus, the granulocyte-macrophage stem cells also appear to differ from normal quantitatively and qualitatively, but they do respond to appropriate humoral stimuli.

C. Studies of Cellular Proliferation

Cell cycle characteristics have been studied in granulocytic precursors from several sites. The reported labeling indexes of myeloblasts and promyelocytes ranged from 4.5 to 80%,[44,52,102,104,105] while 5.3 to 41% of myelocytes were in DNA synthesis.[44,102,103,107] The mean values, especially for myeloblasts, were generally lower than for myeloblasts from the bone marrow of normal individuals. The labeling index of peripheral blood[105,107-109] and spleen[103,105] myelocytes was usually the same as for bone marrow myelocytes in these patients, whereas peripheral blood blasts usually had a lower labeling index than did bone marrow blasts.[105,109] Furthermore, the labeling index of bone marrow myelocytes was similar to values from normal controls.[52] The labeling index was lower in neutrophilic precursors from spleen and liver than in those from the bone marrow.[110] The mitotic index for bone marrrow myeloblasts may have been less than for comparable cells from normal patients.[109] Some calculations of cell fluxes suggest partially ineffective granulopoiesis.[44] These data suggest that the milieu either affects the proliferation of cells or influences the presence of different clones with varying proliferative potentials in each site. On the other hand, the mere existence of these cells in extramedullary sites is abnormal, and the presence of immature granulocytes in the peripheral blood suggests that the release from the bone marrow is abnormal or that release from extramedullary sites differs from that of the bone marrow. Furthermore, cells which mature to myelocytes seem to be less abnormal than earlier precursors.

The labeling index of bone marrow myeloblasts was independent of the white blood count above $40,000/\mu l$ but was significantly lower than when the white count was less than $20,000/\mu l$,[52,108] the latter being similar to bone marrow myeloblasts from normal control patients.[52] The labeling index of splenic myelocytes increased with increasing white blood counts.[103] Thus, there appeared to be at least some feedback regulation of production.

DNA synthesis times of 8.9 to 26 hr have been calculated,[44] similar to or somewhat lower than values in normals: such values were the same in bone marrow and peripheral blood cells.[107] Generation times, on the other hand, were generally longer than in normals,[44] but the calculations depended upon all of the cells being continuously replicating, an unlikely event.

As maturation of granulocytic cells became progressively impaired during the disease and blasts and promyelocytes accumulated, erythrocytic precursors showed similar changes with accumulation of basophilic erythroblasts.[111] The milieu affected cellular growth as judged by the fact that the spleen had a higher proportion of erythroblasts with a lower mitotic index and more megaloblastic changes than did the bone marrow.[112] Chromosomal analysis of splenic cells showing a greater fraction with abnormalities than in bone marrow cells during or prior to the blast crisis may have reflected a greater incidence of onset of new clones in the spleen or merely a preferential growth of cells with karyotypic abnormalities migrating into the spleen.[113-115] These clonal differences may explain many of the findings listed above.

D. Peripheral Blood Cells — Life Span, Migration, Turnover

The total bone marrow granulocyte pool was obviously enlarged, as noted by microscopic examination, and the number of granulocytes entering and leaving the peripheral blood per day was also increased — up to at least nine times normal.[116-118] The bone marrow neutrophilic compartment (myelocytes and more mature cells) fed into and remained in the peripheral blood longer than in normals.[64] The total blood granulocyte pool was enlarged up to at least 88 times normal,[116] roughly in proportion to the white blood count. As in normal individuals, the intravascular neutrophils were found in two pools which were in dynamic equilibrium. One pool was circulating, while the other, slightly larger on average, was marginated along vascular walls (thought to be mainly in small capillaries). The ratio of circulating to marginating cells was within the normal range.[116-118] The marginal pool was mainly in the spleen.[120,121]

The granulocytes remained in the peripheral blood up to 15 times longer than normal[118] and migrated into a skin abrasion at a slower than normal rate.[119] Labeled blood granulocytes left the peripheral blood at a single exponential rate or with a biphasic or multiphasic disappearance

while in relapse. In remission, the disappearance followed the normal pattern of a single exponential decline in some patients but had a small slow component (residual leukemic cells?) in others.[64,117,118] The intravascular life span of mature neutrophils was measured by various techniques and was shorter than,[118] longer than,[116,121] or the same as[117] that of immature neutrophils. It was similar to[118] or, more commonly, longer than that of normal neutrophils in nonleukemic individuals. Cross-transfusion studies with labeled leukocytes suggested that the prolonged intravascular survival was due to an intrinsic defect in the leukemic cell, although the leukemic milieu probably also had some effect.[117,118] Some of the immature peripheral blood granulocytes apparently migrated into the bone marrow parenchyma, resided there for some time, matured (and perhaps replicated), and then returned to the peripheral blood.[121-124] A similar process may have occurred in the spleen. At least a portion of the measurement of a prolonged and often complex intravascular survival may be accounted for by this complex compartmentalization.

As judged by the frequently poor granulocyte response to an injection of endotoxin[125] or the slow return of granulocytes after leukapheresis,[58] the considerable number of mature bone marrow neutrophils seen morphologically is not readily mobilizable into the peripheral blood. The decreases in the sizes of the spleen and liver in some patients with repeated leukaphereses[126] suggested that a part of the slowly mobilizable pool resides in those organs. Although the extravascular pool was not readily mobilizable, it fed into the peripheral blood for many days longer than in control patients.[64]

The studies summarized in this section point to the abnormal intravascular life span and migration patterns present even in the morphologically mature neutrophils. No real comparison is possible for the immature cells since their counterparts in normal individuals do not circulate.

E. Cyclic Phenomena

Cyclic fluctuations in the leukocytosis were seen in some patients. The periodicity was between 1 and 4 months in various patients.[127-132] The nadirs were stable in some patients and rose progressively in others. Urinary and serum colony-stimulating factor levels showed an inverse relationship to the white blood count.[127,132] Immature cells increased in the peripheral blood in association with the rise in the white blood count.[127] Changes in white blood counts were due to changes in the total blood granulocyte pools rather than to changes in the fraction of marginating cells.[129] Leukocytes labeled in vitro with ^{32}P-diisopropylfluorophosphate disappeared most rapidly from the peripheral blood when the white count was at its nadir.[127,129] Both cyclic thrombocytopenia[128,130] and cyclic thrombocytosis,[129,131,132] as well as cyclic reticulocytosis,[132] have been seen associated with cyclic leukocytosis on occasion, the first associated with hydroxyurea therapy[128] or occurring spontaneously.[130] The labeling index of the peripheral blood granulocytic precursors varied with the white blood count.[132] A mathematical model including an increased granulocyte maturation time and increased precursor input was consistent with these findings.[133] Even if the model is incorrect, the cycling phenomena imply a type of feedback control of proliferation and/or release of cells to the peripheral blood.

F. Drug Effect

As in acute leukemics (Section II.E), cytosine arabinoside produced a profound decrease in both mitotic index and labeling index, with labeling index recovering first.[134]

IV. CHRONIC LYMPHOCYTIC LEUKEMIA

Cellular kinetics were comprehensively reviewed in 1968.[132] Although much more information is now available, chronic lymphocytic leukemia (CLL) remains the least well studied of the common leukemias. Furthermore, the investigations below were performed on a mixed population of cells without even separating them into B and T cells; thus, it is frequently impossible to know the degree to which the data reflect residual normal lymphocytes rather than the leukemic cell population.

Cellular production has been studied with ^{3}H-thymidine; 0.2% (mean) of peripheral blood cells were in DNA synthesis.[136-138] In comparison, normal individuals had 0.1% of peripheral blood and 0.5% of lymph node lymphocytes in DNA synthesis.[139] Since the total number of lymphocytes is much larger in CLL, these results suggest that the total number of cells produced per unit time is greater in CLL than in normals. Much larger fractions of large lymphocytes were in DNA synthesis (mean 4.4%) than of small lymphocytes.[138]

Several early studies of the rate of replacement of unlabeled peripheral blood lymphocytes by cells labeled with various radioactive substances demonstrated multiple populations of lymphocytes with apparent life spans ranging from 3 to more than 300 days.[135] The apparent turnover time of ^{32}P-labeled CLL cells was longer than for peripheral blood lymphocytes in normal individuals. One study suggested a rate of formation of only 0.1% per day.[140] Peripheral blood studies of labeling patterns after single injections of ^{3}H-thymidine in vivo suggested two patterns: (1) patients without organomegaly and lower peripheral blood lymphocyte counts had a small, proliferating population which resided only briefly in the peripheral blood and a large, long-lived population and (2) patients with organomegaly and higher peripheral blood lymphocyte counts had nearly a pure population of nonproliferating, long-lived cells.[138] Radiotherapy in one patient and splenectomy in another appeared to preferentially remove the long-lived population.[138] In a study of two patients who received continuous infusions of ^{3}H-thymidine over 7 days, about 95% of small peripheral blood lymphocytes were long-lived with turnover times greater than a year, but 50 to 62% of the large peripheral blood lymphocytes were turned over during the week of infusion.[141] In those patients, no peripheral blood lymphocytes of any size and no small bone marrow or lymph node lymphocytes were in DNA synthesis. In the same study, 3.5 to 7.5% of large bone marrow and lymph node lymphocytes were in DNA synthesis, and 34 to 48% were turned over in 1 week. About two thirds of lymph node blast cells were in DNA synthesis, and 77 to 98% were turned over in 1 week. Thus, only certain subpopulations replicate, and these populations may not circulate in advanced disease.

The thoracic duct and its lymphocytes have been studied at some length. In contrast to nonleukemic patients, a lower concentration of lymphocytes was present in the thoracic duct than in the peripheral blood in nearly all patients studied.[142,143] The flux from the thoracic duct could replace no more than 5% of the peripheral blood lymphocytes per day.[142] Several studies were done in patients after the intravenous infusion of their autologous lymphocytes which had been radiolabeled in vitro. Within 24 hr, 95% of thoracic duct CLL lymphocytes left the blood,[144] results similar to those seen in normals with peripheral blood lymphocytes which, like thoracic duct lymphocytes, are mostly T cells. In contrast, only 60 to 80% of autologous peripheral blood CLL lymphocytes left the peripheral blood by 24 hr in most patients studied.[144-146] Peripheral blood CLL lymphocytes appeared in the thoracic duct within 1 to 6 hr of reinfusion in five patients[147] but not until 96 hr in another.[143] Only 0.4 to 1.0% of peripheral blood lymphocytes appeared in the thoracic duct lymph within 2 days (4.6% in a normal individual).[147] These data suggest that peripheral blood CLL lymphocytes recirculate poorly through the lymph (as expected, since they are B cells in most patients) and that the thoracic duct lymphocytes are probably nonleukemic.

In other studies, reinfused peripheral blood CLL lymphocytes rapidly equilibrated with a pool of cells estimated to be 0.33 to 50 times as large as the intravascular circulating compartment.[135,145,146,148-153] The anatomic site of this pool of dilution probably included lymph nodes,[149] an intravascular marginating pool,[146,152] spleen,[146,153-155] liver,[155] and bone marrow.[146,153] The absolute size of the rapidly equilibrating pool of dilution correlated better with the degree of splenomegaly[146,153] and marrow infiltration[146] than with the blood lymphocyte count, although it proportionately decreased as blood lymphocytosis increased.[149] Clearance of labeled lymphocytes from the peripheral blood was decreased in relation to the total peripheral blood lymphocyte pool, but there appeared to be a normal total flux.[153] This finding is consistent with the idea that total production may have been adjusted to maintain the normal number of lymphocytes entering tissues.

Many patients treated by leukapheresis[150,151] or extracorporeal irradiation of the blood,[152] modalities which directly removed or destroyed only peripheral blood cells, also demonstrated the equilibrium of the peripheral blood with the spleen and lymph nodes since those organs frequently shrank after those procedures. There also appeared to be a slowly exchanging pool of lymphocytes of unknown size and site and also an immobile tissue pool.

Peripheral blood CLL lymphocytes did not generally disappear as a single exponential function after initial equilibration. Approximate half-lives have been 1.0 to 34 days after the initial equilibration,[146,154-157] and the values were unrelated to the size of the blood lymphocyte pool.[146] In comparison, studies of lymphocytes of lymphocytes in nonleukemic patients suggested a half-life of 1.7 to 20 days.[155,158,159] Thus, although studies within the first 24 hr, listed above, suggested a slow initial disappearance of peripheral blood CLL lymphocytes, these studies failed to demonstrate a similarly prolonged life span over the next several days to weeks. More precise comparisons of lymphocyte life spans and migration patterns in both normals and CLL patients are required. T and B lymphocytes and, perhaps, specific subpopulations must be measured separately if one is to understand the kinetic differences between leukemic and normal lymphocytes.

V. SUMMARY

Detailed studies of cellular proliferation and of migration patterns of leukemic cells and of some of the normal hematopoietic elements aid our understanding of certain elements of pathophysiology, but these studies necessarily reflect the state extant only after expansion of the leukemic population has reached diagnostic levels, i.e., 10^{11} to 10^{12} cells. At that time there is no evidence of acceleration of the generation cycle, although the total number of new cells produced may exceed normal in some patients. The size and identity of the leukemic stem cell pool remain unknown. Since an expanding population implies an imbalance between production and destruction, the latter would appear to be inadequate. At the same time, production of normal hematopoietic elements may be ineffective, perhaps because those elements may be merely morphologically mature derivatives of a leukemic clone. Evidence for some persistence of normal control mechanisms exists, but those controls are obviously defective.

The design of treatment based upon kinetic principles has begun in the past few years, but more complete details are required before ideal programs can be devised.

REFERENCES

1. Brown, C. H. and Carbone, P. P.,*In vitro* growth of normal and leukemic human bone marrow, *J. Natl. Cancer Inst.*, 46, 989, 1971.
2. Greenberg, P. L., Nichols, W. C., and Schrier, S. L., Granulopoiesis in acute myeloid leukemia and preleukemia, *N. Engl. J. Med.*, 284, 1225, 1971.
3. Bull, J. M., Duttera, M. J., Stashick, E. D., Northrup, J., Henderson, E., and Carone, P. P., Serial *in vitro* marrow culture in acute myelocytic leukemia, *Blood*, 42, 679, 1973.
4. Duttera, M. J., Bull. J. M., Northrup, J. D., Henderson, E. S., Stashick, E. D., and Carbone, P. P., Serial *in vitro* marrow culture in acute lymphocytic leukemia, *Blood*, 42, 687, 1973.
5. Moore, M. A. S., Williams, N., and Metcalf, D., *In vitro* formation by normal and leukemic human hematopoietic cells: characterization of the colony-forming cells, *J. Natl. Cancer Inst.*, 50, 603, 1973.
6. Moore, M. A. S., Spitzer, G., Williams, N., Metcalf, D., and Buckley, J., Agar culture studies in 127 cases of untreated acute leukemia: the prognostic value of reclassification of leukemia according to *in vitro* growth characteristics, *Blood*, 44, 1, 1974.
7. Ragab, A. H., Gilkerson, E. S., and Myers, M. L., Granulopoiesis in childhood leukemia, *Cancer*, 33, 791, 1974.
8. Ragab, A. H., Gilkerson, E., Myers, M., and Choi, S. C., The culture of colony forming units from the peripheral blood and bone marrow of children with acute lymphocytic leukemia, *Cancer*, 34, 663, 1974.
9. Curtis, J. E., Cowan, D. H., Bergsagel, D. E., Hasselback, R., and McCulloch, E. A., Acute leukemia in adults: assessment of remission induction with combination chemotherapy by clinical and cell-culture criteria, *Can. Med. Assoc. J.*, 113, 289, 1975.
10. Sultan, C., Marguet, M., and Joffroy, Y., Etude des leucémies myéloides chroniques par culture de moelle "in vitro," *Nouv. Rev. Fr. Hematol.*, 15, 161, 1975.
11. Tebbi, K., Rubin, S., Cowan, D. H., and McCulloch, E. A., A comparison of granulopoiesis in culture from blood and marrow cells of nonleukemic individuals and patients with acute leukemia, *Blood*, 48, 235, 1976.
12. Spitzer, G., Dicke, K. A., Gehan, E. A., Smith, T., and McCredie, K. B., The use of the Robinson *in vitro* agar culture assay in adult acute leukemia, *Blood Cells*, 2, 139, 1976.
13. Moore, M. A. S. and Metcalf, D., Cytogenetic analysis of human acute and chronic myeloid leukemic cells cloned in agar culture, *Int. J. Cancer*, 11, 143, 1973.
14. Dicke, K. A., Spitzer, G., Cork, G., and Ahearn, M. J., *In vitro* colony growth of acute myelogenous leukemia, *Blood Cells*, 2, 125, 1976.
15. Spitzer, G., Schwarz, M. A., Dicke, K. A., Trujillo, J. M., and McCredie, K. B., Significance of PHA induced clonogenic cells in chronic myeloid leukemia and early acute myeloid leukemia, *Blood Cells*, 2, 149, 1976.
16. Paran, M., Sachs, L., Barak, Y., and Resnitzky, P., *In vitro* induction of granulocytic differentiation in hematopoietic cells from leukemic and non-leukemic patients, *Proc. Natl. Acad. Sci. U.S.A.*, 67, 1542, 1970.
17. Robinson, W. A., Kurnick, J. E., and Pike, B. L., Colony growth of human leukemic peripheral blood cells *in vitro*, *Blood*, 38, 500, 1971.
18. Aye, M. T., Till, J. E., and McCulloch, E. A., Interacting populations affecting proliferation of leukemic cells in culture, *Blood*, 45, 485, 1975.
19. Aye, M. T., Niho, Y., Till, J. E., and McCulloch, E. A., Studies of leukemic cell populations in culture, *Blood*, 44, 205, 1974.
20. Robinson, W. A. and Pike, B. L., Leukopoietic activity in human urine: the granulocytic leukemias, *N. Engl. J. Med.*, 282, 1291, 1970.
21. Goldman, J. M., Th'ng, K. H., Catovsky, D., and Galton, D. A. G., Production of colony-stimulating factor by leukemic leukocytes, *Blood*, 47, 381, 1976.
22. Granström, M. and Gahrton, G., Colony-forming and colony-stimulating cells in relation to prognosis in leukemia, *Acta Med. Scand.*, 196, 221, 1974.
23. Golde, D. W., Rothman, B., and Cline, M. J., Production of colony-stimulating factor by malignant leukocytes, *Blood*, 43, 749, 1974.
24. Price, G. B., Senn, J. S., McCulloch, E. A., and Till, J. E., The isolation and properties of granulocyte stimulating activities from medium conditioned by human peripheral leukocytes, *Biochem. J.*, 148, 209, 1975.

25. Lind, D. E., Bradley, M. L., Gunz, F. W., and Vincent, P. C., The non-equivalence of mouse and human marrow culture in the assay of granulopoietic stimulatory factors, *J. Cell. Physiol.*, 83, 35, 1974.
26. Chiyoda, S., Mizoguchi, H., Kosaka, K., Takaku, F., and Miura, Y., Influence of leukaemic cells on the colony formation of human bone marrow cells *in vitro Br. J. Cancer*, 31, 355, 1975.
27. Mintz, U. and Sachs, L., Differences in inducing activity for human bone marrow colonies in normal serum and serum from patients with leukemia, *Blood*, 42, 331, 1973.
28. Metcalf, D., Chan, S. H., Gunz, F. W., Vincent, P., and Ravich, R. B. M., Colony-stimulating factor and inhibitor levels in acute granulocytic leukemia, *Blood*, 38, 143, 1971.
29. Broxmeyer, H. E., Baker, F. L., and Galbraith, P. R., *In vitro* regulation of granulopoiesis in human leukemia: application of an assay for colony-inhibiting cells, *Blood*, 47, 389, 1976.
30. Rytömaa, T., Vilpo, J. A., Levanto, A., and Jones, W. A., Effect of granulocyte chalone on acute and chronic granulocytic leukaemia in man. Report of seven cases, *Scand. J. Haematol.*, Suppl. 27, 5, 1976.
31. Greenberg, M. L., Chanana, A. D., Cronkite, E. P., Giacomelli, G., Rai, K. R., Schiffer, L. M., Stryckmans, P. A., and Vincent, P. C., The generation time of human leukemic myeloblasts, *Lab. Invest.*, 26, 245, 1972.
32. Killmann, S. A., Cronkite, E. P., Bond, V. P., and Fliedner, T. M., Proliferation of human leukemic cells studied with tritiated thymidine *in vivo*, in *Proc. 8th Congr. Eur. Soc. Haematology*, S. Karger, Basel, 1962.
33. Gavosto, F., Pileri, A., Bachi, C., and Pegoraro, L., Proliferation and maturation defect in acute leukaemia cells, *Nature* (London), 203, 92, 1964.
34. Gabutti, U., Pileri, A., Tarocco, R. P., Gavosto, F., and Cooper, E. H., Proliferative potential of out-of-cycle leukaemic cells, *Nature* (London), 224, 375, 1969.
35. Saunders, E. F. and Mauer, A. M., Reentry of nondividing leukemia cells into a proliferative phase in acute childhood leukemia, *J. Clin. Invest.*, 48, 1299, 1969.
36. Clarkson, B., Fried, J., Strife, A., Sakai, Y., Ota, K., and Ohkita, T., Studies of cellular proliferation in human leukemia. III. Behavior of leukemic cells in three adults with acute leukemia given continuous infusions of ³H-thymidine for 8 or 10 days, *Cancer*, 25, 1237, 1970.
37. Gavosto, F., Pileri, A., Ponzone, A., Masera, P., Tarocco, R. P., and Gabutti, V., Different blast kinetics in acute myeloblastic and lymphoblastic leukaemia, *Acta Haematol.*, 41, 215, 1969.
38. Stryckmans, P., Delalieux, G., Manaster, J., and Socquet, M., The potentiality of out-of-cycle acute leukemia cells to synthesize DNA, *Blood*, 36, 697, 1970.
39. Killmann, S. A., Acute leukemia. The kinetics of leukemic blast cells in man, *Ser. Haematol.*, 1(3), 38, 1968.
40. Ogawa, M., Studies of cellular proliferation in acute leukemia using ³H-thymidine, *J. Nagoya Med. Assoc.*, 90, 91, 1967.
41. Clarkson, B., Ohkita, T., Ota, L., and Fried, J., Studies of cellular proliferation in human leukemia. I. Estimation of growth rates of leukemic and normal hematopoietic cells in two adults with acute leukemia given single injections of tritiated thymidine, *J. Clin. Invest.*, 46, 506, 1967.
42. Clarkson, B. D., Sakai, Y., Kimura, T., Ohkita, T., and Fried, J., Studies of cellular proliferation in human leukemia. II. Variability in rates of growth and cellular differentiation in acute myelomonoblastic leukemia and effects of treatment, in *The Proliferation and Spread of Neoplastic Cells*, Williams & Wilkins, Baltimore, 1968, 295.
43. Gavosto, F., Pilera, A., Gabutti, V., Tarocco, R. P., Masera, P., and Ponzone, A., Unusual blast proliferation and kinetics in acute lymphoblastic leukaemia, *Eur. J. Cancer*, 5, 343, 1969.
44. Gavosto, F., Granulopoiesis and cell kinetics in chronic myeloid leukaemia, *Cell Tissue Kinet.*, 7, 151, 1974.
45. Rubinow, S. I., Lebowitz, J. L., and Sapse, A. M., Parametrization of *in vivo* leukemic cell populations, *Biophys. J.*, 11, 175, 1971.
46. Rondanelli, E. G., Magliulo, E., Pilla, E., Falchi, F., and Barigazzi, G. M., Chronology of the mitotic cycle of acute leukaemia cells, *Acta Haematol.*, 42, 76, 1969.
47. Gavosto, F. and Masera, P., Different cell proliferation models in myeloblastic and lymphoblastic leukemia, *Blood Cells*, 1, 217, 1975.
48. Hart, J. S., Livingston, R. B., Murphy, W. K., Barlogie, B., Gehan, E. A., and Bodey, G. P., Neoplasia, kinetics and chemotherapy, *Semin. Oncol.*, 3, 259, 1976.
49. Foadi, M. D., Cooper, E. H., and Hardisty, R. M., Proliferative activity of leukaemic cells at various stages of acute leukaemia of childhood, *Br. J. Haematol.*, 15, 269, 1968.
50. Saunders, E. F., Lampkin, B. C., and Mauer, A. M., Variation of proliferative activity in leukemic cell populations of patients with acute leukemia, *J. Clin. Invest.*, 46, 1356, 1967.
51. Pileri, A., Gabutti, V., Masera, P., and Gavosto, F., Proliferative activity of the cells of acute leukaemia in relapse and in steady state, *Acta Haematol.*, 38, 193, 1967.
52. Stryckmans, P., Debusscher, L., Peltzer, T., and Socquet, M., Variations of the proliferative activity of leukemic myeloblasts related to the stage of the disease, *Blood Cells*, 1, 239, 1975.
53. Crowther, D., Beard, M. E. J., Bateman, C. J. T., and Sewell, R. L., Factors influencing prognosis in adults with acute myelogenous leukaemia, *Br. J. Cancer*, 32, 456, 1975.
54. Cheung, W. H., Rai, K. R., and Sawitzky, A., Characteristics of cell proliferation in acute leukemia, *Cancer Res.*, 32, 939, 1972.
55. Sjögren, U., Prognostic value of mitotic studies in myeloid leukaemias, *Acta Med. Scand.*, 199, 289, 1976.

56. Greenberg, M. L., Chanana, A. D., Cronkite, E. P., Schiffer, L. M., and Stryckmans, P. A., Tritiated thymidine as a cytocidal agent in human leukemia, *Blood*, 28, 851, 1966.
57. Godwin, H. A., Zimmerman, T. S., and Perry, S., Peripheral leukocyte kinetic studies of acute leukemia in relapse and remission and chronic myelocytic leukemia in blast crisis, *Blood*, 31, 686, 1968.
58. Bierman, H. R., Marshall, G. J., Kelley, K. H., and Byron, R. L., Leukapheresis in man. III. Hematologic observations in patients with leukemia and myeloid metaplasia, *Blood*, 21, 164, 1963.
59. Hoelzer, D., Harriss, E. B., Fliedner, T. M., and Heimpel, H., The turnover of blast cells in peripheral blood after *in vitro* ^{3}H-cytidine labelling and retransfusion in human acute leukemia, *Eur. J. Clin. Invest.*, 2, 259, 1972.
60. Tarocco, R. P., Pileri, A., Ponzone, A., and Gavosto, F., Bone marrow return and division of circulating acute lymphoblastic leukemia cells, *Acta Haematol.*, 47, 277, 1972.
61. Killmann, S. A., Karle, H., Ernst, P., and Andersen, V., Return of human leukaemic myeloblasts from blood to bone marrow, *Acta Med. Scand.*, 189, 137, 1971.
62. Hoelzer, D., Fliedner, T. M., and Harriss, E. B., Investigations of the fate and RNA turnover of autotransfused ^{3}H-cytidine labeled leukaemic blast cells, in Abstr. 13th Int. Congr. of Hematology, August 1970, p. 226.
63. Wickramasinghe, S. N. and Moffatt, B., Disturbed myelocyte proliferation in acute leukaemia, *Scand. J. Haematol.*, 9, 477, 1972.
64. Galbraith, P. R. and Advincula, E. G., Observations on the myelocyte to tissue transit time (MTT) in acute leukaemia and other proliferative disorders, *Br. J. Haematol.*, 22, 453, 1973.
65. Galbraith, P. R., Chikkappa, G., and Abu-Zahra, H. T., Patterns of granulocyte kinetics in acute myelogenous and myelomonocytic leukemia, *Blood*, 36, 371, 1970.
66. Godwin, H. A., Zimmerman, T. S., Kimball, H. R., Wolff, S. M., and Perry, S., Correlation of granulocyte mobilization with etiocholanolone and the subsequent development of myelosuppression in patients with acute leukemia receiving therapy, *Blood*, 31, 580, 1968.
67. Blackstock, A. M. and Garson, O. M., Direct evidence for involvement of erythroid cells in acute myeloblastic leukaemia, *Lancet*, 2, 1178, 1974.
68. Chiyoda, S., Mizoguchi, H., Suzuki, S., Takaku, F., and Miura, Y., Effect of erythropoietin on human bone marrow cells *in vitro*. III. Studies of acute leukemia, *Proc. Soc. Exp. Biol. Med.*, 146, 684, 1974.
69. Yamada, H. and Hotta, T., Regulation of erythropoiesis in erythroleukemia: a study on the *in vitro* response of marrow cells to erythropoietin, in *Erythropoiesis*, Nakao, K., Fisher, J. W., and Tukaku, F., Eds., University of Tokyo Press, Tokyo, 1975, 187.
70. Queisser, W., Graubner, A., Hoelzer, D., Queisser, U., and Heimpel, H., Some characteristics of the proliferative activity of erythroblasts in untreated and treated acute leukaemia, *Acta Haematol.*, 49, 271, 1973.
71. Huber, C., Huber, H., Schmalzl, F., and Braunsteiner, H., Decreased proliferative activity of erythroblasts in granulocytic stem cell leukaemia, *Nature* (London), 229, 113, 1971.
72. Mitrou, P. S., Fisher, M., and Hubner, K., Some aspects of erythropoietic cell proliferation in erythroleukaemia, *Acta Haematol.*, 53, 65, 1975.
73. Sjögren, U., Erythroblastic islands and ineffective erythropoiesis in acute myeloid leukaemia, *Acta Haematol.*, 54, 11, 1975.
74. Dörmer, P., Hegemann, F., and Brinkmann, W., Proliferation and production of hemopoietic cells in two stages of disease: preleukemia and overt disease, *Klin. Wochenschr.*, 54, 461, 1976.
75. Queisser, W., Queisser, U., Ansmann, M., Brunner, G., Hoelzer, D., and Heimpel, H., Megakaryocyte polyploidization in acute leukaemia and preleukaemia, *Br. J. Haematol.*, 28, 261, 1974.
76. Cowan, D. H., Thrombokinetics in acute nonlymphocytic leukemia, *J. Lab. Clin. Med.*, 82, 911, 1973.
77. Chan, B. W. B. and Hayhoe, F. G. J., Changes in proliferative activity of marrow leukemic cells during and after extracorporeal irradiation of the blood, *Blood*, 37, 657, 1971.
78. Hoelzer, D., Kurrle, E., Dietrich, M., Meyer-Hamme, K.-D., and Fliedner, T. M., The effect of continuous cell removal on blast cell kinetics in acute leukaemia, *Scand. J. Haematol.*, 12, 311, 1974.
79. Lampkin, B. C., McWilliams, N. B., and Mauer, A. M., Cell kinetics and chemotherapy in acute leukemia, *Semin. Hematol.*, 9, 211, 1972.
80. Klein, H. O. and Lennartz, K. J., Chemotherapy after synchronization of tumor cells, *Semin. Hematol.*, 11, 203, 1974.
81. Killmann, S. A., Effect of cytostatic drugs on the kinetics of leukemic blast cells in man, *Schweiz. Med. Wochenschr.*, 104, 278, 1974.
82. Mauer, A. M., Cell kinetics and practical consequences for therapy of acute leukemia, *N. Engl. J. Med.*, 293, 389, 1975.
83. Ernst, P., Perturbation of generation cycle of human leukaemic blast cells *in vivo* by daunomycin, *Scand. J. Haematol.*, 11, 13, 1973.
84. Stryckmans, P. A., Manaster, J., Lachapelle, F., and Socquet, M., Mode of action of chemotherapy *in vivo* on human acute leukemia. I. Daunomycin, *J. Clin. Invest.*, 52, 126, 1973.
85. Greenberg, M. L. and Waxman, S., Sequential use of methotrexate, folinic acid, and cytosine arabinoside in the treatment of acute leukemia, *Eur. J. Cancer*, 12, 617, 1976.
86. Ernst, P. and Killmann, S.-A., Perturbation of generation cycle of human leukaemic myeloblasts *in vivo* by methotrexate, *Blood*, 38, 689, 1971.

87. **Sauer, H., Pelka, R., and Wilmanns, W.,** Zur Pharmakokinetik von unter Ausnutzung von synchronisations und Recruitment - Effekten, *Klin. Wochenschr.,* 54, 203, 1976.

88. **Pagliardi, G. L., Gabutti, V., and Gavosto, F.,** Mechanism of action of l-asparaginase on the cell cycle and growth in acute lymphoblastic leukemia, *Acta Haematol.,* 50, 257, 1973.

89. **Burke, P. J. and Owens, A. H., Jr.,** Attempted recruitment of leukemic myeloblasts to proliferative activity by sequential drug treatment, *Cancer,* 28, 830, 1971.

90. **Greenberg, M. L., Ferreira, P. P. C., and Holland, J. F.,** Perturbations of indices of cellular replication and survival induced by 24—48 hour vincristine infusions in human patients, *Cancer Res.,* submitted for publication.

91. **Stryckmans, P. A., Lurie, P. M., Manaster, J., and Vamecq, G.,** Mode of action of chemotherapy *in vivo* on human acute leukemia. II. Vincristine, *Eur. J. Cancer,* 9, 613, 1973.

92. **Huber, H., Huber, Ch., Michlmayr, G., Asamer, H., and Braunsteiner, H.,** In-vitro-Proliferation leukämischer Blasten und Ansprechen auf Daunorubidomyzin/Cytosin-Arabinosid, *Schweiz. Med. Wochenschr.,* 101, 1785, 1971.

93. **Kremer, W. B., Vogler, W. R., and Chan, Y.-K.,** An attempt at synchronization of marrow cells in acute leukemia, *Cancer,* 37, 390, 1976.

94. **Lampkin, B. C., McWilliams, N. B., Mauer, A. M., Flessa, H. C., Hake, D. A., and Fisher, V.,** Manipulation of the mitotic cycle in the treatment of acute myelogenous leukaemia, *Br. J. Haematol.,* 32, 29, 1976.

95. **Moore, M. and Robinson, W. A.,** Granulopoietic activity of urine and cells from patients with chronic granulocytic leukemia, *Proc. Soc. Exp. Biol. Med.,* 146, 499, 1974.

96. **Moore, M. A. S., Williams, N., and Metcalf, D.,** *In vitro* colony formation and leukemic human hematopoietic cells: interaction between colony-forming and colony-stimulating cells, *J. Natl. Cancer Inst.,* 50, 591, 1973.

97. **Goldman, J. M., Th'ng, K. H., and Lowenthal, R. M.,** *In vitro* colony forming cells and colony stimulating factor in chronic granulocytic leukaemia, *Br. J. Cancer,* 30, 1, 1974.

98. **Moberg, C., Olofsson, T., and Olsson, I.,** Granulopoiesis in chronic myeloid leukaemia, *Scand. J. Haematol.,* 12, 381, 1974.

99. **Böyum, A., Lövhaug, D., and Boecker, W. R.,** Regulation of bone marrow cell growth in diffusion chambers: the effect of adding normal and leukemic (CML) polymorphonuclear granulocytes, *Blood,* 48, 383k, 1976.

100. **Berthier, R., Douady, F., Marcille, G., Sotto, J. J., Schaerer, R., and Hollard, D.,** Etude des cellules formant des clones et des agrégats (CFCA) "in vitro" du sang et de la moelle de sujets atteints de leucemie myéloide chronique, *Nouv. Rev. Fr. Hematol.,* 15, 365, 1975.

101. **Berthier, R., Douady, F., and Hollard, D.,** Cellular factors regulating granulopoiesis in myeloid leukemia, *Blood Cells,* 3, 461, 1977.

102. **Kuroyanagi, T. and Saito, M.,** Proliferative capacity of leukemic cells studied with tritiated thymidine *in vitro, Tohoku J. Exp. Med.,* 80, 168, 1962.

103. **Brandt, L.,** Difference in uptake of tritiated thymidine by myelocytes from bone marrow and spleen in chronic myeloid leukemia, *Scand. J. Haematol.,* 11, 23, 1973.

104. **Stryckmans, P. A., Manaster, J., Peltzer, T., Socquet, M., and Vamecq, G.,** Cell proliferation in chronic myeloid leukemia under discontinuous treatment from diagnosis to blast crisis, in *Recent Results in Cancer Research,* Vol. 30, Mathe, G., Ed., Springer-Verlag, New York, 1970, 156.

105. **Clarkson, B., Ota, K., O'Connor, A., and Karnofsky, D. A.,** Production of granulocytes by the spleen in chronic granulocytic leukemia, *J. Clin. Invest.,* 42, 924, 1963.

106. **Stryckmans, P. A.,** Current concepts in chronic myelogenous leukemia, *Semin. Hematol.,* 11, 101, 1963.

107. **Vincent, P. C., Cronkite, E. P., Greenberg, M. L., Kirsten, C., Schiffer, L. M., and Stryckmans, P. A.,** Leukocyte kinetics in chronic myeloid leukemia. I. DNA synthesis time in blood and marrow myelocytes, *Blood,* 33, 843, 1969.

108. **Brandt, L.,** Differences in the proliferative activity of myelocytes from bone marrow, spleen and peripheral blood in chronic myeloid leukemia, *Scand. J. Haematol.,* 6, 105, 1969.

109. **Baccarani, M. and Killmann, S.-A.,** Cytokinetic studies in chronic myeloid leukaemia: evidence for early presence of abnormal myeloblasts, *Scand. J. Haematol.,* 9, 283, 1972.

110. **Sjörgren, U. and Brandt, L.,** Different composition and mitotic activity of the haemopoietic tissue in bone marrow, spleen and liver in chronic myeloid leukaemia, *Acta Haematol.,* 55, 73, 1976.

111. **Sjörgren, U. and Brandt, L.,** Composition and mitotic activity of the erythroid part of the bone marrow in chronic myeloid leukaemia, *Scand. J. Haematol.,* 12, 18, 1974.

112. **Sjörgren, U. and Brandt, L.,** Differences in morphology and mitotic activity between intra- and extra-medullary erythropoietic tissue in chronic myeloid leukaemia, *Scand. J. Haematol.,* 13, 116, 1974.

113. **Mitelman, F., Nilsson, P. G., and Brandt, L.,** Abnormal clones resembling those seen in blast crisis arising in the spleen in chronic myelocytic leukemia, *J. Natl. Cancer Inst.,* 54, 1319, 1975.

114. **Hossfeld, D. K., Bremer, K., Meusers, P., Wenderhorst, E., and Reis, H. E.,** Extramedullary manifestation of the blastic phase of chronic myelocytic leukemia: a chromosome study, *Z. Krebsforsch. Klin. Onkol.,* 84, 49, 1975.

115. **Gomez, G., Hossfeld, D. K., and Sokal, J. E.,** Removal of abnormal clone of leukaemic cells by splenectomy, *Br. Med. J.,* 2, 421, 1975.

116. **Athens, J. W., Raab, S. O., Haab, O. P., Boggs, D. R., Ashenbrucker, H., Cartwright, G. E., and Wintrobe, M. M.,** Leukokinetic studies. X. Blood granulocyte kinetics in chronic myelocytic leukemia, *J. Clin. Invest.,* 44, 765, 1965.

117. **Galbraith, P. R.,** Granulocyte kinetic studies in chronic myelogenous leukemia, *Natl. Cancer Inst. Monogr.,* 30, 121, 1969.

118. Uchida, T., Leukokinetic studies in peripheral blood. II. Granulocytic kinetics in chronic myelocytic leukemia, *Acta Haematol. Jpn.*, 34, 186, 1971.
119. Senn, H. J. and Jungi, W. F., Neutrophil migration in health and disease, *Semin. Hematol.*, 12, 27, 1975.
120. Duvall, C. P. and Perry, S., The use of 51-chromium in the study of leukocyte kinetics in chronic myelocytic leukemia, *J. Lab. Clin. Med.*, 71, 614, 1968.
121. Scott, J. L., McMillan, R., Davidson, J. G., and Marino, J. V., Leukocyte labeling with ^{51}chromium. II. Leukocyte kinetics in chronic myelocytic leukemia, *Blood*, 38, 162, 1971.
122. Moxley, J. H., Perry, S., Weiss, G. H., and Zelen, M., Return of leukocytes to the bone marrow in chronic myelogenous leukemia, *Nature* (London), 280, 1281, 1965.
123. Chikkappa, G. and Galbraith, P. R., Studies on the exchange of leukocytes between blood and bone marrow in chronic myelogenous leukemia, *Can. Med. Assoc. J.*, 97, 64, 1967.
124. Perry, S., Moxley, J. H., Weiss, G. H., and Zelen, M., Studies of leukocyte kinetics by liquid scintillation counting in normal individuals and in patients with chronic myelocytic leukemia, *J. Clin. Invest.*, 45, 1388, 1966.
125. Marsh, J. C. and Perry, S., The granulocyte response to endotoxin in patients with hematologic disorders, *Blood*, 23, 581, 1964.
126. Vallejos, C. S., McCredie, K. B., Brittin, G. M., and Freireich, E. J., Biological effects of repeated leukapheresis of patients with chronic myelogenous leukemia, *Blood*, 42, 925, 1973.
127. Gatti, R. A., Robinson, W. A., Deinard, A. S., Nesbit, M., McCullough, J., Ballow, M., and Good, R. A., Cyclic leukocytosis in chronic myelogenous leukemia: new perspectives on pathogenesis and therapy, *Blood*, 41, 771, 1973.
128. Kennedy, B. J., Cyclic leukocyte oscillations in chronic myelogenous leukemia during hydroxyurea therapy, *Blood*, 35, 751, 1970.
129. Vodopick, H., Rupp, E. M., Edwards, C. L., Goswitz, F. A., and Beuchamp, J. J., Spontaneous cyclic leukocytosis and thrombocytosis in chronic granulocytic leukemia, *N. Engl. J. Med.*, 286, 284, 1972.
130. Shadduck, R. K., Winkelstein, A., and Nunna, N. G., Cyclic leukemic cell production in CML, *Cancer*, 29, 399, 1972.
131. Morley, A. A., Baikie, A. G., and Galton, D. A. G., Cyclic leukocytosis as evidence for retention of normal homeostatic control in chronic granulocytic leukemia, *Lancet*, 2, 1320, 1967.
132. Chikkappa, G., Borner, G., Burlington, H., Chanana, A. D., Cronkite, E. P., Öhl, S., Pavelec, M., and Robertson, J. S., Periodic oscillation of blood leukocytes, platelets and reticulocytes in a patient with chronic myelocytic leukemia, *Blood*, 47, 1023, 1976.
133. Wheldon, T. E., Kirk, J., and Finlay, H. J., Cyclic granulopoiesis in chronic granulocytic leukemia: a simulation study, *Blood*, 43, 379, 1974.
134. Baccarani, M., Santucci, A. M., Tura, S., and Killmann, S. A., Arabinosyl cytosine in chronic myeloid leukemia: evidence for high cytokinetic sensitivity of myeloblasts, *Scand. J. Haematol.*, 16, 335, 1976.
135. Schiffer, L. M., Kinetics of chronic lymphocytic leukemia, *Ser. Haematol.*, 1(3), 3, 1968.
136. Rubini, J. R., Bond, V. P., Keller, S., Fliedner, T. M., and Cronkite, E. P., DNA synthesis in circulating blood leukocytes labeled *in vitro* with H^3-thymidine, *J. Lab. Clin. Med.*, 58, 751, 1961.
137. Bond, V. P., Fliedner, T. M., Cronkite, E. P., Rubini, J. R., Brecher, G., and Schork, P. K., Proliferative potentials of bone marrow and blood cells studied by in vitro uptake of H^3-thymidine, *Acta Haematol.*, 21, 1, 1959.
138. Zimmerman, T. S., Godwin, H. A., and Perry, S., Studies of leukocyte kinetics in chronic lymphocytic leukemia, *Blood*, 31, 277, 1968.
139. Winkelstein, A. and Craddock, C. G., Comparative response of normal human thymus and lymph node cells to phytohemagglutinin in culture, *Blood*, 29, 594, 1967.
140. Christensen, B. C. and Ottesen, J., The age of leukocytes in the blood stream of patients with chronic lymphatic leukemia, *Acta Haematol.*, 13, 289, 1955.
141. Theml, H., Trepel, F., Schick, P., Kaboth, W., and Begemann, H., Kinetics of lymphocytes in chronic lymphocytic leukemia: studies using continuous ^{3}H-thymidine infusion in two patients, *Blood*, 42, 623, 1973.
142. Bierman, H. R., Byron, R. L., Jr., Kelly, K. H., Gilfillan, R. S., White, L. P., Freeman, N. E., and Petrakis, N. L., The characteristics of thoracic duct lymph in man, *J. Clin. Invest.*, 32, 637, 1953.
143. Binet, J. L., Logeais, Y., Villeneuve, B., Mathey, J., and Bernard, J., Examen de la lymphe au cours de la léucemie lymphöide chronique, *Nouv. Rev. Fr. Hematol.*, 6, 568, 1966.
144. Bremer, K., Schreml, W., and Flad, H. D., Chronic lymphoid leukemia: concentration of normal lymphocytes in the lymph, *Biomed. Express* (Paris), 21, 361, 1974.
145. Stryckmans, P. A., Chanana, A. D., Cronkite, E. P., Greenberg, M. L., and Schiffer, L. M., Studies on lymphocytes. IX. The survival of autotransfused labeled lymphocytes in chronic lymphocytic leukemia, *Eur. J. Cancer*, 4, 241, 1968.
146. Scott, J. L., McMillan, R., Marino, J. V., and Davidson, J. G., Leukocyte labeling with ^{51}chromium. IV. The kinetics of chronic lymphocytic leukemic lymphocytes, *Blood*, 41, 155, 1973.
147. Bremer, K., Wack, O., and Schick, P., Impaired recirculation of autotransfused blood lymphocytes via thoracic duct lymph in patients with chronic lymphoid leukemia, *Biomedicine*, 18, 393, 1973.
148. Cuttner, J., Cronkite, E. P., Kesse, M., and Fliedner, T. M., Behavior of autotransfused in vitro H^3-cytidine (H^3-CTR)-labeled lymphocytes in chronic lymphocytic leukemia, *J. Clin. Invest.*, 43, 1236, 1964.

149. Manaster, J., Frühling, J., and Stryckmans, P., Kinetics of lymphocytes in chronic lymphocytic leukemia. I. Equilibrium between blood and a "readily accessible pool," *Blood,* 41, 425, 1973.

150. Höcker, P., Pittermann, E., Gobets, M., Harst, B., Gazda, M., and Stracher, A., Therapeutische, funktionelle und kinetische Aspekte der Leukopheresetherapie chronischer lymphatischer Leukämien, *Blut,* 28, 396, 1974.

151. Schiffer, L. M., Chanana, A. D., Cronkite, E. P., Greenberg, M. L., Rai, K., Stryckmans, P., and Vincent, P., L'irradiation extra-corporelle du sang dans la leucémie lymphoïde chronique, *Nouv. Rev. Fr. Hematol.,* 8, 691, 1968.

152. Andersen, V., Weeke, E., and Killmann, S. A., Extracorporeal irradiation of the blood: clinical applications, *Strahlentherapie,* 148, 603, 1974.

153. Bazerbashi, M. B., Reeve, J., and Chanarin, I., Studies in chronic lymphocytic leukemia — the kinetics of ^{51}Cr-labeled lymphocytes, *Scand. J. Haematol.,* 20, 37, 1978.

154. Spivak, J. L. and Perry, S., Lymphocyte kinetics in chronic lymphocytic leukemia, *Br. J. Haematol.,* 18, 511, 1970.

155. Hersey, P., The separation and [51]chromium labeling of human lymphocytes with *in vivo* studies of survival and migration, *Blood,* 38, 360, 1971.

156. Pfisterer, H., Nennhuber, J., Bolland, H., and Stich, W., Lymphocytenabbau nach in-vitro-Markierung mit $Na_2{}^{51}CrO_4$. II. Untersuchungen bei chronischer lymphatischer Leukämie, *Klin. Wochenscher.,* 45, 1073, 1967.

157. Goswitz, F. A., Vodopick, H., and Clevenger, M., Blood lymphocyte kinetics in patients with chronic lymphocytic leukemia (CLL), *J. Nucl. Med.,* 10, 404, 1969.

158. Pfisterer, H., Bolland, H., Nennhuber, J., and Stich, W., Lymphocytenabbau nach in-vitro-Markierung mit $Na_2{}^{51}CrO_4$. I. Methode und Ergebnisse bei Normalpersonen, *Klin. Wochenschr.,* 45, 995, 1967.

159. Scott, J. L., Davidson, J. G., Marino, J. V., and McMillan, R., Leukocyte labeling with [51]chromium. III. The kinetics of normal lymphocytes, *Blood,* 40, 276, 1972.

Chapter 8
MOLECULAR GENESIS OF HUMAN LEUKEMIA

S. S. Agarwal and L. A. Loeb

TABLE OF CONTENTS

I. INTRODUCTION

Malignant change, like inflammation, is a pathological process which can be brought about by a variety of agents. The resulting clinical manifestations are, to a large extent, determined by the cell and tissue of origin. Thus, a variety of agents can produce very similar clinico-pathological pictures. In order to devise rational approaches for the treatment of malignancy, it is important to understand the unifying mechanisms underlying neoplastic change. For this purpose, in this chapter the different forms of human leukemia are considered together to analyze molecular mechanisms involved in the initiation and progression of this disease.

Studies on the leukemic cell provide several advantages over those on cells from solid tumors: (1) it is possible to obtain relatively large amounts of leukemic cells by leukapheresis. (2) These cells can be cultured in vitro as single-cell suspensions. (3) Different types of cells from the peripheral blood and bone marrow can be separated into homogeneous subpopulations,[1-3] making it possible to carry out biochemical and cytological analyses of one type of cell or of cells in different stages of differentiation. (4) An additional advantage of studying leukemic cells may be the opportunity of being able to compare malignant cells with normal proliferating counterparts. For example, as a control for acute lymphatic leukemic cells, normal dividing lymphocytes can be obtained by stimulating peripheral blood lymphocytes in culture with mitogenic agents. (5) Also, in vitro techniques have become available in recent years for studying differentiation of normal hemopoietic and leukemic cells.[4-7]

The purpose of this chapter is to consider recent molecular studies on human leukemic cells that relate directly to current theories of carcino-

TABLE 1

Somatic Mutation as the Basis for Malignancy

Evidence for	Evidence against
Agents causing malignancy interact with DNA, e.g., chemical carcinogens and radiation.	Also interact with RNA and protein; induce latent viruses; suppress host immune responses.
Oncogenic viruses are integrated into host DNA.	All cells with integrated oncogenic viruses are not malignant.
Most chemical carcinogens are mutagens.	Not all mutagens are carcinogens.
Malignant phenotype is permanent and heritable at the cellular level.	Does not exclude stable epigenetic changes. Reversal of the neoplastic state to a normal or quasinormal state has been reported.
Malignancy is frequently characterized by chromosomal aberrations.	May be an epiphenomenon. Significant number of neoplasms in early stages do not exhibit any karyotypic abnormality.
Defective DNA repair in patients of Xeroderma pigmentosum is associated with malignancy.	May be a unique example.
Single autosomal dominant lesions are associated with malignancy, e.g., retinoblastoma, familial polyposis of the colon, and bilateral medullary carcinoma of thyroid. Certain autosomal recessive mutations predispose to malignancy, e.g., Bloom's syndrome, Fanconi's anemia, and ataxia telangiectasia.	Both dominant and recessive mutations could make individuals susceptible to neoplastic change rather than causing it by themselves.

genesis. Our main effort is to focus attention on clinical studies that have helped in understanding molecular mechanisms of carcinogenesis.

II. MOLECULAR THEORIES OF CARCINOGENESIS

Current theories on the origin of malignancy can be divided into two broad groups. One hypothesis relates to somatic mutations, and the other, for lack of a more precise designation, can be considered under the vague title of aberrant differentiation.

A. Somatic Mutation Hypothesis

According to the somatic mutation hypothesis, cancer arises as a consequence of permanent changes in the genome of normal somatic cells. Such a mutated cell is presumed to possess a proliferative advantage over adjoining normal cells. By continuous proliferation, this cell gives rise to a clone of cells that is clinically observed as a tumor. Since these cells escape the normal host mechanisms which control growth and differentiation, the emerging tumor consists predominantly of undifferentiated cells. The ability to infiltrate locally and to spread to distant sites is also a characteristic of malignant cells. It is not known how many mutations are needed to initiate the process; whether they are recessive or dominant; whether they involve structural genes or regulator genes; or whether they represent addition of information, deletion of information, or alteration of existing information. Theoretically, mutations can occur spontaneously during DNA replication or DNA repair and have been shown to be brought about by exogenous or endogenous agents including chemicals, viruses, and radiation. However, direct proof of the occurrence of mutations in cancer cells is lacking.

The somatic mutation hypothesis was proposed by Boveri[8] at the turn of this century, long before the establishment of DNA as the genetic material, although the role of chromosomes as the carriers of Mendelian units of inheritance was becoming clear at that time. On the basis of his studies on chromosomes in dispermic sea urchin embryos, Boveri postulated that the general basis of malignant change must be an abnormality in chromatin.[8] Since then, the overriding evidence that malignancy is inherited at the cellular level has been the driving force behind the theory of somatic mutation. However, for every strong argument supporting this theory an equally strong counterargument can also be raised (see Table 1). Changes in base sequences in DNA are presumably beyond present means of resolution.[9-11] Short of that, one of the critical tests for the somatic mutation hypothesis is the demonstration that malignancy arises from a single cell. Evidence for and against a clonal origin in particular types of leukemia is considered below.

1. Clonal Origin of Leukemic Cells

The somatic mutation hypothesis presupposes that cancer arises in a single cell. On the basis of age-related mortality from all cancers in humans, it has been calculated that at least two and probably as many as five to six events occur during oncogenesis.[12-16] Assuming that the rate of mutations leading to cancer is the same as that for other genetic targets in eucaryotic cells, i.e., on the order of 10^{-5} to 10^{-6} per gene locus per generation,[17] it is exceedingly unlikely that the required number of somatic mutations can concurrently accumulate in more than one cell. Thus, statistical probability would predict that if somatic mutations are the cause of malignancy, malignancy must arise from a single cell.

The evidence for the clonal origin of malignancy in humans is most convincing for leukemia. In this disease it has been possible to obtain malignant cells free from contaminating nonmalignant stromal cells and to study their cytological and biochemical uniformity. The association of the Philadelphia chromosome (Phl) with chronic myeloid leukemia (CML) is well established.[18-21] The Phl chromosome is found in 85 to 90% of patients with CML, and in these patients it is demonstrable in essentially all dividing cells of the bone marrow. This chromosome is present not only in cells of the myelogenous series but in precursors of erythrocytes and megakaryocytes as well. However, it is not present in peripheral lymphocytes stimulated to divide with phytohemagglutinin or in cultured skin fibroblasts.[22,23] Furthermore, the Phl chromosome persists in the bone marrow cells during clinical remission, relapse and terminal blast crisis.[24] Evidence that the Phl chromosome is acquired and not inherited has come from studies on identical twins.[25,26] It was not found in the bone marrow cells of the normal co-twin where the index patient with CML was positive for Phl chromosome. Thus, the presence of this readily identifiable chromosomal marker in all the malignant cells and their progenitors throughout the course of the disease strongly supports a clonal origin of CML. However, if one considers the Phl chromosome to be a manifestation of viral transformation, one cannot categorically exclude the possibility of a particular virus simultaneously affecting the majority of stem cells. Evidence for or against this possibility rests on studies with known genetic mosaics in which the mosaic system is clearly defined in the subject prior to the onset of the disease.[27,28] One can then ask whether all the leukemic cells contain the genetic marker characteristic of only one of the mosaic cells.

Two case reports of the occurrence of Phl chromosome in sex chromosome mosaics appear in the literature.[29,30] However, the data from these studies is insufficient either to establish or to refute the clonal origin of the Phl chromosome. Tough et al.[29] reported a patient of CML who was an XY/XXY mosaic in the cells from the peripheral blood. The Phl chromosome was found in both the XY and XXY cells. Skin fibroblasts from this patient were only of the XXY type. It cannot be said whether the appearance of Phl chromosome predated or postdated the development of mosaicism. If there was no mosaicism in the hemopoeitic cells at the time of formation of Phl chromosome, the data would be compatible with a clonal orgin — the second subline having evolved by the loss of one X chromosome during tumor progression. On the other hand, if the mosaicism was present before the formation of Phl chromosome, it would suggest that the event leading to the development of Phl chromosome occurred in at least two different cells. In the second case, reported by Fitzgerald et al.,[30] Phl chromosome was found only in the XY cells, and all the XXY cells were negative for this marker. This case provides strong evidence in favor of the clonal origin of the Phl chromosome. However, there was one Phl-positive subline (46 XY, C+, G-, G-, t(GqGq)+, Phl) which could, at least theoretically, have evolved from Phl-positive XXY cells. Experiments to determine whether the extra C chromosome is an X chromosome were not carried out in this study.

More definitive evidence in favor of clonal origin of CML is provided by studies of Fialkow and colleagues on patients who were known to be mosaics for the enzyme glucose-6-phosphate dehydrogenase (G-6-PD).[31] The gene for the G-6-PD is located on the X chromosome, and the expression of the gene has been shown to follow Lyon's hypothesis. This hypothesis states that in females, one of the two X chromosomes is inactivated on a random basis during early embryonic life, and the progeny of these cells maintain the respective distribution of the inactive X chromosome (Figure

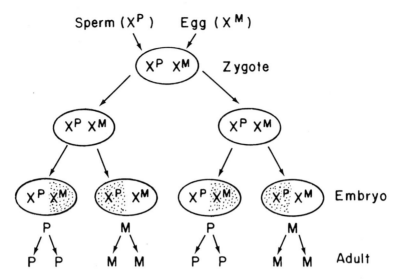

FIGURE 1.   Diagrammatic representation of the inactive-X hypothesis. One of the two X chromosomes in the female zygote is inherited from the mother (X^M) and the other is of paternal origin (X^P). At some time early in embryogenesis, the two X chromosomes begin to behave differently in each somatic cell. Only one of these is genetically active, while the other is inactive (the shaded X chromosome). The initial choice as to which X chromosome is to be inactive in a given cell is probably random; however, once made, it is fixed not only for that cell, but for all its descendants. Thus, the adult female is a mosaic of two cell types — those with an active X^M and those with an active X^P. (From Fialkow, P. J., in *Genetic Concepts and Neoplasia*, Williams & Wilkins, Baltimore, Md., 1970, 112. With permission.)

1). Thus, in female subjects who are heterozygotes for the normal and a variant G-6-PD enzyme, approximately half of the cells would contain only the normal enzyme and the other half only the variant enzyme. Such individuals are mosaics for the G-6-PD enzyme from very early life. In mosaic tissues, cells with each type of enzyme are equally represented.[32] African populations are particularly suitable for the study of G-6-PD mosaicism, since they have a high incidence of the A variant of G-6-PD which is readily identifiable by electrophoresis.[33] With this system one should be able to determine whether a particular cancer arose from a single cell or from many cells. If neoplasia arose from a single cell, all tumor cells would contain only one type of the G-6-PD enzyme, while if neoplasia arose from multiple cells, the tumor would probably contain both of the G-6-PD enzymes present in that individual. In a study of three female patients with CML who were known to be heterozygotes for A and B types of G-6-PD, the extracts from the red cells and granulocytes were found to have only one type of the G-6-PD enzyme (Type A).[31] Later, the same

group reported an additional case in which the red cells and granulocytes had only the B type of the enzyme.[34] These studies have now been extended to four more patients, and the single-enzyme phenotypes are seen not only in granulocytes and erythrocytes, but also in platelets and cultured monocytes.[147] Of the latter, three were typed as B and one as A type of G-6-PD. The likelihood that prior to the onset of leukemia all eight patients have no mosaicism in bone marrow cells while having both types of the G-6-PD enzyme in skin fibroblasts is remote. Although it can always be argued that the basic neoplastic change was multicellular in nature but conferred upon one of the variants a selective proliferative advantage,[35] these studies do demonstrate that in patients with CML all of the bone marrow cells of the erythrocytic, myelocytic, and megakaryocytic series can be derived from a single cell. It should be remembered that in normal heterozygote individuals both variants are present in approximately equal amounts. In the leukemic patients, the presence of only one variant of G-6-PD enzyme in red blood cells, granulocytes, and platelets is in accordance with the findings of Phl chromosome. Unfortunately, studies on lymphocytes could not be carried out from these patients. The lymphocytes would have been expected to have both types of enzymes and could have served as a built-in control.

Another X-linked character that has been studied in CML patients is blood group Xg^a. Fialkow and colleagues[36] studied 11 female patients with CML who were determined to be heterozygous at Xg locus (Xg^a/Xg) on the basis of family studies. All 11 patients were found to be of Xg^a type. Similar results were obtained by Lawler and Sanger.[37] It should be recalled that if the disease were of clonal origin, 50% of the heterozygous patients would be expected to be Xg^a and the other 50% to be Xg because of the random inactivation of the X chromosome. However, these results are not necessarily contradictory to those of the G-6-PD studies, since it is likely that the inactiviation of the X chromosome may not encompass the Xg locus.[38]

Surface immunoglobulin studies in patients with chronic lymphatic leukemia also suggest the possibility of an unicellular origin of the disease.[39-41] Similar studies need to be extended to other forms of leukemia and to preleukemic states.[42,43]

There is some evidence against a clonal origin of malignancy in at least one form of leukemia. In two patients with acute lymphoblastic leukemia (ALL), the relapse of the disease following successful allogenic bone marrow transplant was cytogenetically traced to donor cells (*vide infra*).[44,45] This suggests that the disease might be transmitted horizontally by a putative virus present in the luekemic individuals. The concept of horizontal transmission and the appearance of leukemia in the donor cells argues strongly against a clonal origin of ALL in this rather unique situation. Also, the kinetics of proliferation of leukemic cells in these patients during relapse, as judged by bone marrow and peripheral blood analyses, suggests that the initiation of relapse occurred in many cells simultaneously.

While discussing the concept of the clonal origin of malignancy, mention must be made that during tumor progression new clones of cells may continuously evolve. This implies that the tumor, as it clinically presents, could be heterogeneous with regard to genetic markers. In fact, in patients with CML, secondary chromosomal abnormalities

do appear during the course of the disease.[21] Nevertheless, the Phl chromosome continues to remain demonstrable in such subclones.

2. Role of Oncogenic Viruses

The demonstration that the virus-induced "malignant transformation" in culture is mediated through the insertion of viral genome into the host's genetic material is often cited as evidence supporting the somatic mutation hypothesis. In order to analyze this point, we will first summarize the evidence in favor of viral etiology in human leukemia and will then examine its relationship to the somatic mutation hypothesis.

Virus-like particles have been reported for many years to be present in human leukemic cells and in human plasma.[46] However, it had not been possible to establish that the particles observed under the electron microscope were "true viruses." The finding by Temin and Mizutani[47] and by Baltimore[48] that animal RNA tumor viruses contain an unique enzyme, "reverse transcriptase," has stimulated the search for human cancer viruses by trying to detect similar enzymes in human malignant cells.[49,50] Assays for enzyme activity are inherently more sensitive than observations by electron microscopy and thus provide a powerful tool to search for the "footprints" of a putative virus. In addition, efforts have been focused on trying to determine whether nucleic acids and proteins related to the oncogenic viruses could be identified in human leukemic cells. These studies are of added importance, since the production of complete virus seems to be a rare event in malignant cells. The evidence that has accumulated for the presence of reverse transcriptase and other information indicative of an RNA tumor virus in human leukemic cells is summarized in Table 2.[51-75] From this table it appears that there is considerable likelihood for the presence of a putative virus-like particle in cells from patients with leukemia. However, it must be stressed that these studies provide only indirect evidence for the presence of a putative etiologic agent, and by themselves cannot establish any causal relationship.

It has not been conclusively established that such particles are absent in normal cells. In most instances, the amount of normal blood cells used for comparison is not detailed or is quite limited. It is also possible that the viral information in normal cells is repressed[76] and is present in only a

TABLE 2

Selected Recent Evidence Supporting a Viral Etiology of Human Leukemia

Evidence	Comment	Reference
Presence of reverse transcriptase (RT)		
A DNA polymerase in the nucleic acid-free cell lysates that copied rat liver RNA was found in leukemic cells	3 patients of acute lymphoblastic leukemia – all positive. PHA-stimulated lymphocytes from 48 normal volunteers were all negative	51
RNAase-sensitive, endogenous DNA polymerase associated with particles containing 70S (or 35S) RNA. The DNA product hybridized with RLV RNA but not to MMTV RNA	ALL 6, AML 13, CLL 1, CML 3; 95% positive. 9 normal volunteers and 9 patients with high leukocyte counts were all considered negative	52
The particles have density of 1.16—1.18, and the endogenous product hybridizes to SiSV RNA and MuSV RNA	1 AML, 1 CML	53
An enzyme purified from postmitochondrial cytoplasmic pellet of mol wt 130,000 (or 70,000) copied heteropolymeric regions of AMV 70S RNA and RLV 70S RNA. Enzyme preferred poly rA·oligo dT over poly dA·oligo dT and efficiently copied poly rC·oligo dG	3 patients with acute leukemia	54—56
The above enzyme from the leukemic cells was specifically inhibited by A antisera prepared against purified polymerases from animal RNA tumor viruses	GaLV > SiSV > MLV. Almost no inhibition by antisera against FeLV, RD 114, and AMV	57, 58
Purification of a similar enzyme from spleen	1 CLL and 1 CML. 5 spleens from normals – all negative	59
Clinical studies	8 patients, including ALL, AML, and CML	60
RT was found in marrow cells during remission and relapse		
Particles containing RT in 2 patients, 2 and 4 months prior to the onset of clinical leukemia	1 patient developed AML and the other malignant histiocytosis	61
RT in peripheral blood leukocytes during remission	11 patients, including AML and ALL	62
Presence of Viral Nucleic Acids		
RNA		
Polysomal RNA obtained from white cells during active phase of the disease hybridizes with ^{3}H-DNA probe (cDNA) complementary to RLV RNA	ALL (9), CLL (2), AML (13), monocytic (3), 89% positive. Normal controls (33) including WBC, PHA-stimulated lymphocytes, lymphnodes, adult tissues, and fetal tissues were all negative	63

Note: RLV = Rauscher leukemia virus; MMTV = mouse mammary tumor virus, SiSV = simian sarcoma virus, MuSV = murine sarcoma virus, AMV = avian myeloblastosis virus, GaLV = Gibbon ape leukemia virus, MLV = murine leukemia virus, FeLV = feline leukemia virus, RD 114 = feline endogenous virus, SSAV = simian sarcoma-associated virus, ALL = acute lymphoblastic leukemia, AML = acute myeloblastic leukemia, CML = chronic myelo-

TABLE 2 (continued)

Selected Recent Evidence Supporting a Viral Etiology of Human Leukemia

Evidence	Comment	Reference
Poly-(A) containing RNA from leukemic cells hybridizes with cDNA endogenously synthesized on MuSV	22 of the 46 samples from all different types of leukemias were positive, 7 controls all negative	64
DNA product synthesized by endogenous reaction of particles (1.16—1.18 density) from human leukemic cells hybridizes with: (a) RNA from RLV but not MMTV; (b) RNA from SiSv, MuSV (and to some extent to MLV), but not to FeLV or AMV		52 53
DNA		
cDNA prepared as above hybridizes to sequences in DNA of leukemic WBC that are not present in normals	These sequences were shown to be complementary to RLV RNA	65, 66
Viral information present in leukemic patient but not in identical twin	2 pairs (AML)	67
Presence of viral structural proteins		
Cells from patients with acute leukemia contain P30 antigens specifically related to viruses of SSAV and GaLV group	Myelogenous (2), Histiocytic (1), Myelomonocytic (1), Unknown type (1)	68
Culture of virus particles		
Release of C-type particles from human cells cultured in arginine-deficient medium		69
Short-term release of particles into the culture medium from bone marrow cells which resemble oncornaviruses in density, biochemical properties (RT and 70S RNA) and morphology		70, 71
Sustained release of budding Type C virus from cultures of peripheral blood and bone marrow. Virus contains RT and P30 antigen related to SSAV and GaLV. The virus may be propagated in several cell types	1 patient with AML (HL-23)	72—74
Isolation of C-type oncornavirus from supernatants of bone marrow cells cultured with PHA for 3 days. Produced syncitia on cocultivation with XC cells and could replicate in human embryonic kidney cells	Lymphosarcoma progressing to lymphoblastic leukemia	75

few copies. Penner et al.[77] reported the presence of a DNA polymerase in phytohemagglutinin-(PHA)-stimulated normal human lymphocytes that could copy an RNA template. Unfortunately, the total synthesis was very limited, and studies on homology between the DNA product and the RNA template were not detailed. Bobrow et al.[78] reported evidence in PHA-stimulated normal lymphocytes for limited addition of deoxynucleotides onto polyribonucleotide initiators. They conclude that even though the reaction is RNA dependent, it is not RNA directed like that of a viral reverse transcriptase.

The physical and biochemical properties of virus-like particles observed in leukemic cells are similar to those of Type C RNA tumor viruses of animal origin. In particular, the particles seem to be most closely related to Type C virus particles isolated from subhuman primates. The similarity of the particle cultured from peripheral blood and bone marrow cells of a patient with AML[72,73] to simian sarcoma-associated virus is so close that it will be exceedingly difficult to unambiguously demonstrate that the putative human particle is distinct from that obtained from the subhuman primate. Since we are trying to identify a human virus that may be a causative agent of leukemia, one cannot readily fulfill Koch's postulates by injecting it into the host of origin. It will be necessary to demonstrate that cells from most leukemic patients, and not normal volunteers, contain information for this virus (provirus). Most importantly, it will be necessary to carry out seroepidemiologic studies to establish that the virus is causally associated with leukemia in humans.

Important clinical evidence in support of the viral etiology of human leukemia has come from two case studies. In 1971, Fialkow and colleagues[44] reported the case of a 16-year-old girl with ALL who suffered from the recurrence of the disease following successful transplantation with the bone marrow from her HL-A matched brother (Figure 2). The patient was given 1000 rad (midline tissue dose) total body radiation and was infused with 14.6×10^9 nucleated marrow cells on the next day (Day 0). Serial peripheral blood and bone marrow studies showed that up to Day 52 there was no evidence of relapse of the disease. However, on the 76th day, 80% of the bone marrow cells and about half of the peripheral blood cells were lymphoblasts. By the 80th day,

the peripheral blood count rapidly rose to about $50,000/mm^3$, and the patient died on Day 102. Cytogenetic studies of the marrow and peripheral blood cells without culture revealed that 100% of the cells on Days 76 and 79 were of XY karyotype. On the basis of careful analysis, it was concluded that the relapse occurred in the donor cells. The donor himself was completely normal up to 6 months after the donation of the marrow cells. One deficiency in this report was that the chromosomes of the recipient before the transplantation were not studied. A similar case of the recurrence of the disease in engrafted marrow cells was reported by Thomas et al.,[45] where it was established that the recipient was of XX karyotype. Several explanations were proposed for these observations, but one of the most plausible hypotheses is that the donor cells were infected by an oncogenic virus derived from host cells. The latter could have been induced by X-irradiation. Even though we are unaware of further similar reports in the literature, these studies in themselves raise several important questions. One is in relation to the clonal origin of malignancy. The other is in relation to the possibility of horizontal transmission, although it can be argued that close proximity of cells is essential. Finally, the possibility that continued presence of the virus may play a role in the progression of the disease must be considered in a therapeutic context (*vide infra*).

It is not clear whether the integration of viral DNA into an eukaryotic genome can be considered within the concept of the somatic mutation hypothesis. In favor is the argument that the introduction of a viral genome represents a permanent and inheritible change in the somatic cell which segregates with each cellular generation. The thought that it does not represent a point mutation, since there is the addition of several thousand nucleotide pairs from the viral genome, simply reflects the constraints of the definition of mutation rather than emphasis on the functional consequences to the cell. However, closer scrutiny of the phenomenon of viral integration indicates many possible differences from a somatic mutation. Most importantly, viral infection and subsequent integration of the viral genome can occur simultaneously in a large number of cells, while a somatic mutation is considered to be a rare and isolated event. Furthermore, infection by viruses can spread horizontally to neighboring cells, resulting in recruitment, and finally, there is always the

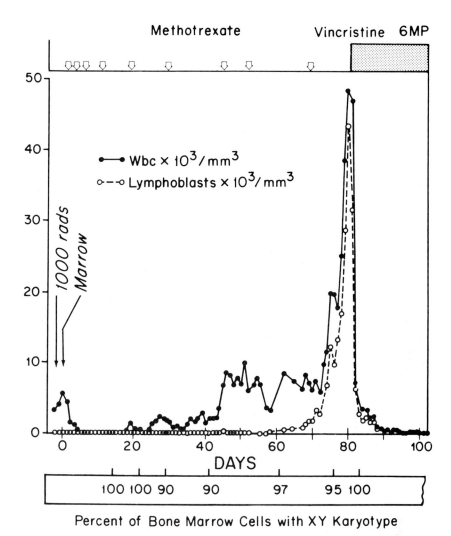

FIGURE 2. Peripheral WBC and lymphoblast counts and chemotherapy after marrow grafting. 6 MP = 6-mercaptopurine. (From Fialkow, P. J., Thomas, E. D., Bryant, J. I., and Neiman, P. E., *Lancet*, 1, 251, 1971. With permission.)

possibility of infecting germ cells causing subsequent vertical transmission of the viral genome.[76,79] It should also be noted that the number of proviruses in most tumor cells and the uniqueness of their sites of integration have not yet been defined. Some recent studies on the fidelity of DNA synthesis indicate the speculative possibility that the virus might be involved in initiating somatic mutations, but through an entirely different mechanism. To consider this point in detail, recent evidence on the involvement of DNA polymerases in the fidelity of DNA synthesis is reviewed below.

3. Fidelity of DNA Replication

The idea of DNA having a double-helical structure as formulated by Crick and Watson implies that the selection of nucleotides during DNA replication is guided by the specificity of hydrogen bonding between complementary base pairs.[80] This model assumes that DNA polymerases, the enzymes that copy DNA, act as a "zipper" and simply connect prealigned nucleotides into phosphodiester linkage. However, the difference in free energy between complementary (Watson-Crick base pairs) and noncomplementary (incorrect) base pairs is only 1 to 3 kcal and is insufficient to guarantee the requirements for the fidelity of DNA replication in living organisms.[81,82] In fact, the difference in free energy between complementary and noncomplementary base pairs is only sufficient to account for an

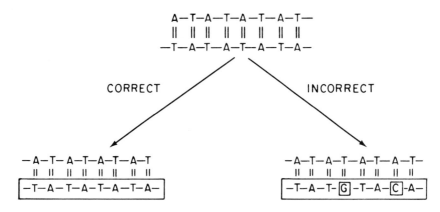

FIGURE 3.   Diagrammatic representation of the assay for infidelity of DNA synthesis.

accuracy in base selection of 1 in 10 to 1 in 100 nucleotides.

The first evidence for the involvement of DNA polymerases in base selection came from studies of Speyer[83] and Speyer et al.[84] with mutants of bacteriophage T_4. Speyer found that mutants affecting the DNA polymerase locus had an increased mutation frequency throughout their genome.[83] Subsequently, studies on purified DNA polymerases from mutant phages revealed that enzymes obtained from phages which had a high mutation rate made frequent mistakes in copying polynucleotides in vitro.[85,86] Conversely, enzymes obtained from phages with a low mutation rate made few mistakes in vitro. The differences in the accuracy of DNA synthesis by the enzymes obtained from mutants have been shown to be correlated, in part, with the presence of a $3' \rightarrow 5'$ exonuclease function that is part of the prokaryotic enzyme itself.[87-89] Those enzymes that make many mistakes have reduced amounts of exonuclease activity and vice versa.

In contrast to prokaryotic DNA polymerases, enzymes isolated from animal cells have no demonstrable exonucleolytic activity.[90] However, fragmentary evidence indicates that these enzymes can copy polynucleotides in vitro with few errors, indicating that the $3' \rightarrow 5'$ exonuclease ("proofreading") function is not essential for accurate DNA synthesis.[90,91] The high fidelity of purified eukaryotic DNA polymerases in vitro indicates that these enzymes function in base selection by themselves.

We and others have proposed that errors in DNA synthesis are causally related to malignant alterations.[81,92,93] We have begun to inquire whether malignant changes are brought about by

errors in the synthesis of DNA. A comparison was carried out between the ability of nucleic acid-free extracts of normal PHA-stimulated human lymphocytes and lymphocytes from patients with acute lymphatic leukemia to copy accurately the sequence of poly (d[A-T]) template.[94] As shown in Figure 3, the template consists of alternating residues of deoxythymidylate and deoxyadenylate. If this template is exactly copied, the newly synthesized strand would contain an A opposite every T and a T opposite every A. Erroneous base pairing would be manifested by the insertion of G and C as diagramed. Using this template and extracts from normal and leukemic lymphocytes, we measured the frequency of noncomplementary nucleotide incorporation into the product. Results of the initial study are shown in Table 3. Nucleic acid-free extracts of lymphocytes from patients with acute leukemia exhibited an error rate averaging about tenfold greater than the identical extracts from normal PHA-stimulated lymphocytes.

In these assays, one measures the incorporation of an exceedingly small fraction of a noncomplementary radioactive substrate of very high specific activity. Therefore, a large number of control experiments were carried out to show that the incorporated radioactivity indeed represents single-base substitutions linked in phosphodiester bonds. First, the purity of the template was established by showing that different DNA polymerases copy the same template with different error rates. Secondly, the purity of the labeled added noncomplementary nucleotide was established by chromatography and by showing that incorporation was dependent on the presence of complementary nucleotide. Proof that the reaction

TABLE 3

Incorporation of dCTP with poly (d [A-T])

Enzyme source	Correct nucleotide incorporation (pmol)	Incorrect nucleotide incorporation (pmol)	Frequency of misincorporation
Normal lymphocytes			
Donor			
1	439	0.092	1/4800
2	51	0.025	1/1990
3	221	0.064	1/3460
4	335	0.056	1/5980
5	309	< 0.01	< 1/30,900
6	382	0.091	1/4200
Acute lymphatic leukemia			
Patient			
1	53	0.11	1/480
2	108	0.43	1/250
3	189	0.35	1/540
4	58	0.069	1/850

Adapted from Springgate, C. F. and Loeb, L. A., *Proc. Natl. Acad. Sci. U.S.A.*, 70, 245, 1973. With permission.

TABLE 4

Reaction Requirements for Correct and Incorrect Nucleotide Incorporation with poly (d [A-T])

	% Incorporation			
	Normal		Acute leukemic	
Reaction mixture	Correct dTTP	Incorrect dCTP	Correct dTTP	Incorrect dCTP
Complete	100 (330 pmol)	100 (0.06 pmol)	100 (150 pmol)	100 (0.30 pmol)
Minus enzyme	0	0	0	0
Minus poly (d[A-T])	0.05	16 ± 7	0.05	20 ± 4
Minus Mg^{++}	0	0	0	0
Minus dATP and dTTP	—	13 ± 11	0	12
Heated enzyme	0	0	0	0

Note: Results given as mean ± standard error of mean (SEM).

Adapted from Springgate, C. F. and Loeb, L. A., *Proc. Natl. Acad. Sci. U.S.A.*, 70, 245, 1973. With permission.

was catalyzed by a polymerase was indicated by the requirements for both complementary and noncomplementary nucleotides. All incorporation was abolished by deletion of either the complementary nucleotide, magnesium, template, or the nucleic acid-free extract (Table 4). The product of the reaction was analyzed on sucrose and cesium sulfate gradients to demonstrate that the noncomplementary radioactivity is present in poly (d[A-T]). Digestion of the reaction product with a nuclease that works in reverse to polymerase, snake venom phosphodiesterase, clearly established that the noncomplementary nucleotide is incorporated evenly throughout the product.

Recovery of the label in the form of dCMP demonstrated that the noncomplementary nucleotide was present in phosphodiester linkage.

Three explanations have been considered to account for the infidelity of DNA synthesis by the leukemic extracts. First, the greater number of apparent errors may result from a terminal transferase that is uniquely present in acute leukemic lymphocytes.[95] In fact, recent studies have shown that such an enzyme is present in these cells.[96-100] A hypothesis on the mutagenic role of this enzyme in antibody formation has also been proposed.[101] Recently Saffhill and Chaudhri,[102] while confirming the infidelity of DNA synthesis by mouse spleen leukemic extracts, have shown that a terminal transferase copurifies with DNA polymerase up to the step of purification on a phosphocellulose column. Further purification on Sephadex® G-200 column results in the separation of terminal transferase and DNA polymerase with a concomitant decrease in mistakes. It would be interesting to examine whether these experiments are applicable to human leukemic cells. Evidence against the role of terminal transferase is the fact that in studies on cells from humans, the noncomplementary nucleotides were shown to be evenly distributed throughout the polynucleotide product. Furthermore, the dependence of noncomplementary nucleotide incorporation on complementary nucleotide is exactly the opposite from what one would predict with a terminal transferase reaction in which the complementary nucleotide would compete with the noncomplementary nucleotide and thus reduce the incorporation of the latter.

A second explanation for the high frequency of errors during DNA replication is that altered DNA polymerases are present in leukemic cells and that these enzymes accumulate during malignant progression. If this is indeed the case, purification of the DNA polymerases from leukemic cells might yield information concerning the presence of an altered enzyme. However, it should be pointed out that altered DNA polymerases may have different chromatographic properties and might be lost during purification. In this context, studies on the heat stability of the DNA polymerases in normal and leukemic cells might provide information as to whether the enzyme present in leukemic cells is altered.

The third explanation is that in leukemic cells there is a viral DNA polymerase that has an abnormally high frequency of noncomplementary nucleotide incorporation. This interpretation is open to immediate experimental attack, for one can ask what is the frequency of misincorporation by DNA polymerases from known animal RNA tumor viruses. Since the latter enzymes can be obtained from a variety of viruses in homogeneous form, detailed analysis of the infidelity of DNA synthesis by these enzymes has been carried out. We found that the DNA polymerase from avian myeloblastosis virus produced a surprisingly large number of errors in copying a variety of polynucleotide templates.[103,104] For example, with poly rA as a template, as many as 1 dCMP for every 400 to 600 dTMP were incorporated into the poly-dT product. Chemical analysis of the product indicated that the incorrectly base-paired nucleotides were randomly distributed. Similar studies indicated that DNA polymerases from Rauscher leukemia virus,[105] Rous sarcoma virus, and mammary tumor virus had similar rates of misincorporation.[148] It is now important to determine whether a viral polymerase which is faulty in base selection is present in human leukemic cells. If so, infidelity in copying polynucleotide templates might be an important assay for the presence of a viral polymerase in human leukemic cells. However, irrespective of the cause, the increased infidelity points to the possibility of a higher mutation rate in leukemic cells.

The hypothetical role of a mutagenic DNA polymerase in the pathogenesis of malignancy is shown in Figure 4. In this model one must assume that many of the manifestations of malignant transformation observed in culture are not sufficient to ensure tumorigenesis. A number of these changes are easily reversible and thus not within the concept of a somatic mutation hypothesis. In fact, it has recently been demonstrated that established sublines of human cells transformed by SV40 failed to form tumors when inoculated into athymic nude mice, while bonafide neoplastic cells invariably were tumorigenic.[106] Thus, the morphologic changes that occur during malignant transformation in culture are not sufficient for or are only coincidentally related to the neoplastic state. Furthermore, this model assumes that once mutations are initiated by a viral DNA polymerase, many cellular proteins are synthesized incorrectly, including DNA polymerases and other enzymes functioning in base selection. A similar model for the initiation of malignancy can be constructed for

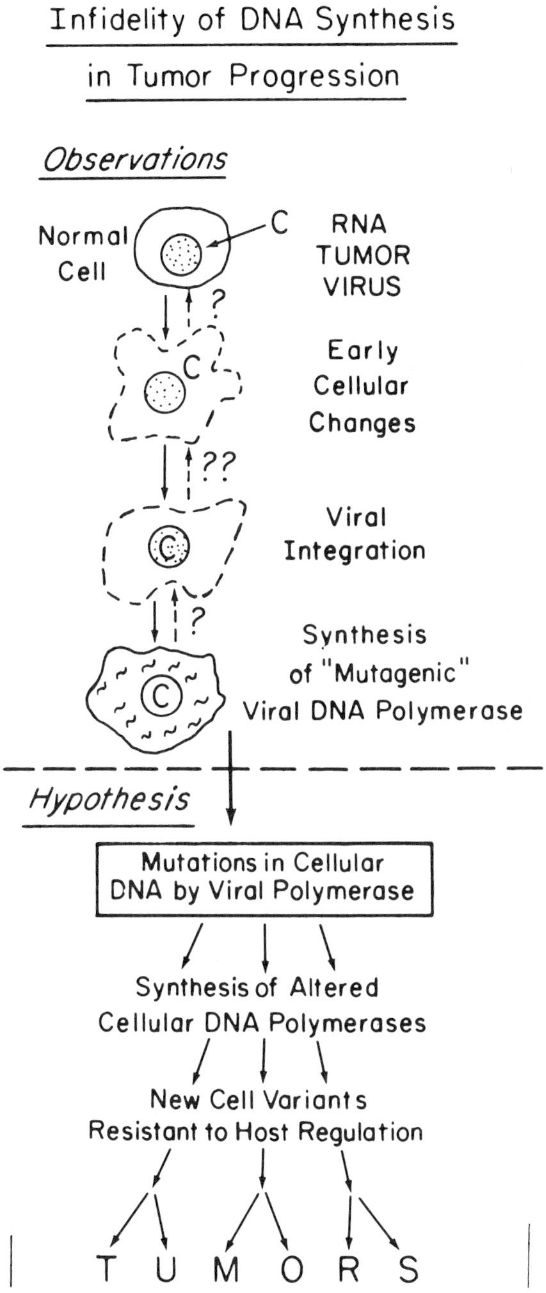

Infidelity of DNA Synthesis

in Tumor Progression

Observations

FIGURE 4. A proposed model for the role of infidelity of DNA synthesis in the initiation and progression of malignancy.

any mutagenic agent. As a secondary event, further production of errors in DNA synthesis by these altered enzymes brings about a cascading of mutations during malignant progression.

Other evidences listed in favor of somatic mutation hypothesis are not analyzed in detail,

since the studies on leukemic cells do not directly contribute to these arguments.

B. Aberrant Differentiation

The second major category of theories of carcinogenesis is based on the assumption that malignancy is the result of alteration in gene expression.[107-111] In fact, the counterarguments considered in Table 1 against the theory of somatic mutation can be rephrased into arguments supporting a theory of aberrant differentiation. In molecular terms, an abnormality in differentiation implies a quantitative and/or qualitative change in the expression of genes that control the processes of cell division and maturation. The underlying assumption is that there is no change in the base sequence of DNA; the change is in the control mechanisms for the synthesis of particular RNAs and/or their translation into specific proteins. This implies alterations at the level of cellular control mechanisms involving postulated inducers and repressors of gene expression. It should be mentioned that the expression of a putative viral (or nonviral) endogenous oncogene could itself be due to the loss of regulatory controls.[76,79] Furthermore, as was pointed out above, a somatic mutation could involve a regulatory gene, and, thus, the two major concepts of carcinogenesis need not be mutually exclusive.

The concept of aberrant differentiation as the determinant of malignant change assumes that the emergence of a stable phenotype, viz. malignancy, does not require a change in the genome per se. It is based on analogy with normal development: the fertilized egg can differentiate into highly specialized tissues and organs which differ markedly from each other, yet their cells are presumed to carry the same genetic information. This morphologic and functional variability remains constant in successive cellular progeny in these tissues. The understanding of these processes in eukaryotes is only beginning to emerge.[112] However, by analogy to bacterial systems,[113] differentiation is attributed to the expression of a unique set of genes in each tissue. Some proponents of the theory of aberrant differentiation consider that two fundamental changes in malignant cells, continued proliferation and lack of maturation, indicate reversion to an embryonic phenotype. It is implied that this results from the loss of regulators for the expression of genes. This hypothesis is supported by the fact that malignant cells often reexpress fetal antigens[114] and may even become ectopic sites for the production of hormones,[115] expressing those genes which were permanently switched off in these tissues.

The underlying hope in this concept is that malignant cells may be capable of differentiating into normal, functionally mature cells under appropriate conditions. In fact, at least some human tumors do show spontaneous regression.[116-118] This concept of the reversibility of malignancy at the cellular level has been tested in many experimental systems.[119-122] The recent demonstration in allophenic mice, by Mintz and Illmensee, that teratoma cells are capable of differentiating into normal adult tissues is most convincing.[123] Obviously, such sophisticated single-cell analyses cannot be applied to human beings. Nevertheless, in vitro studies have been carried out with leukemic leukocytes.[124-129] It has been shown that the cells from the peripheral blood as well as from the bone marrow of patients with AML and CML can give rise to in vitro myeloid colonies. The extent of differentiation toward normality in the structure and function of cells in these colonies is under study. These studies suggest that the primary defect in leukemia might not be in the cell itself. It is either the lack of required factor(s) or the presence of inhibitor(s) which results in the failure of leukemic blast cells to further differentiate. It can be postulated that failure in differentiation disrupts the feedback regulatory mechanisms resulting in uncontrolled proliferation of precursor cells. If this were true, it could be possible to theoretically "cure" the disease. However, it should be mentioned that the concept of aberrant differentiation does not necessarily guarantee reversibility. Changes in gene expression can proceed by interwoven pathways, the sum of which may not be easily reversible.

III. IMPLICATIONS FOR THERAPY

A. Therapy Based on Somatic Mutation Hypothesis

If permanent change in the genome is responsible for the initiation and progression of a carcinogenic process, the only recourse for successful treatment of malignant disease is to eradicate all malignant cells. In fact, this appears to be the goal of contemporary chemotherapy[130] and most proposed protocols of immunotherapy.[131] This concept is supported by the clinical observation

that the prolongation of life in leukemia, particularly ALL, is related to the success of induction and maintenance of remission. Some long-term survivors in ALL indicate that the treatment can be successful in permanently eradicating all leukemic cells.[132] However, a number of observations including karyotype analysis,[133-135] in vitro soft-agar colony assays,[136] studies on leukemia-related antigens,[137,138] and recent studies on viral markers like reverse transcriptase[62] indicate that even in patients with well-consolidated remission the normal-looking cells are not necessarily nonneoplastic. Relapse is an all too frequent phenomenon. It is attributed to the emergence of resistant cells, and the failure of treatment is blamed on the limitations of present-day methodologies. It may be interesting to ponder whether these failures do, in fact, indicate the limitations of the concept of the somatic mutation hypothesis.

B. Therapy Based on Viral Etiology

The optimism generated by the viral etiology of human leukemia perhaps stems from the general success in the containment of many viral infections. If one can identify the causative agent, one may develop a suitable vaccine. However, such optimism needs to be tempered at least to some extent. For all we know, it is possible that the putative virus may not behave like an ordinary virus. The integration of the viral genome into the host's genetic material, the latency of the infection, and the biological behavior of the virus pose substantial conceptual problems. Nevertheless, a start has been made. It has been possible to immunize certain strains of mice against mouse mammary tumor virus (MMTV) and other tumor viruses, and the studies are being extended to humans.[139,140] In cats, the leukemia virus has been shown to spread horizontally.[141] The search for the putative viral agent in human leukemic cells has been rewarding. Thus, the possibility of preventing the disease cannot be discounted.

A viral etiology for human leukemia also presents a possible macromolecular target for chemotherapeutic attack. A number of proteins, most prominently the viral reverse transcriptase, are clearly required for the replication of animal tumor viruses. Considerable evidence indicates the presence of such enzymes in leukemic cells. It may be argued that once the viral genome is integrated with the host's DNA and the malignant disease process has been initiated, it is futile to prevent viral replication. However, the bone marrow transplantation studies, in which it was demonstrated that the donor cells become leukemic, beg the question of whether the virus is not only required for the initiation of the disease but is also required for its maintenance. Thus, the idea of interfering with viral replication, which superficially seems very naive, may be of considerable importance. Although the mechanism of DNA replication by the polymerases present in RNA tumor virus appears to be exceedingly similar to that of normal cellular DNA polymerases, a number of substances, such as rifamycin derivatives, have been found that preferentially inactivate viral DNA polymerases over cellular DNA polymerases.[142] The use of these agents in the treatment of experimental leukemias is already in progress.

C. Therapy Based on Infidelity of DNA Synthesis

The concept of infidelity of DNA synthesis in the pathogenesis of malignancy implies progressive accumulation of random mutations.[81] The need to eradicate all malignant cells may be similar to if not greater than that indicated by a somatic mutation hypothesis. However, the idea that malignancy is mediated by enzymes that are altered in base recognition might afford a modality for chemotherapeutic attack. One can ask whether altered DNA polymerases are more susceptible to particular chemotherapeutic agents, but since the alterations in these enzymes might also be random, each chemotherapeutic agent might have to be evaluated by individual in vitro behavior of leukemic cells. One of the interesting leads related to this framework is the finding that leukemic cells contain a lower zinc content than do normal cells.[143] It has been demonstrated recently that DNA polymerases are zinc metalloenzymes.[144] One can ask whether agents that effectively chelate zinc would have preferentially detrimental effect on the leukemic cells compared to normal cells.[145] In this respect, it is interesting to point out that the viral reverse transcriptase is also a zinc metalloenzyme.[146]

D. Therapy Based on the Theory of Aberrant Differentiation

Although the concept of aberrant differentiation offers the maximum hope of being able to reverse the malignant disease process, it may not necessarily be so. First, little is known about the control of RNA transcription and protein synthesis as related to growth and division in normal eukaryotic cells. There is a prerequisite for the attainment of a large body of fundamental knowledge before one can use this approach on a rational basis. Second, it can be argued that during aberrant differentiation the regulatory pathways may become progressively altered, and it may be difficult if not impossible to reverse the process. However, the search for various factors that influence the in vitro differentiation of leukemic leukocytes offers the promise of finding some agent that can influence the course of this disease.

IV. EPILOGUE

In this chapter, we have considered human leukemia as a single pathological entity. This oversimplification permitted us to consider leukemia within the framework of general theories of carcinogenesis. We recognize the possibility that distinct clinical and morphologic forms of leukemia may also be etiopathogenetically distinct entities. Thus, even though the evidence in favor of a clonal origin for CML appears convincing, it does not preclude the possibility that AML and ALL are of multiclonal origin. Similarly, the discussion of the somatic mutation hypothesis and theories of aberrant differentiation under separate headings does not imply that the two mechanisms may not operate together. In this regard, models can be constructed relating mutagenicity to differentiation. The main purpose of this somewhat artificial dichotomy was to analyze the implications of the mechanisms of carcinogenesis to therapeutic approaches.

ACKNOWLEDGMENTS

This study was supported by grants from the National Institutes of Health (CA-11524, CA-06551, CA-15139) and by the National Science Foundation (BMS73-06751), by grants to the Institute for Cancer Research from the National Institutes of Health (CA-06927, RR-05539), and by an appropriation from the Commonwealth of Pennsylvania.

REFERENCES

1. **Boyum, A.,** Separation of leukocytes from blood and bone marrow, *Scand. J. Clin. Lab. Invest.,* 21 (Suppl. 97), 31, 1968.
2. **Miller, R. G. and Phillips, R. A.,** Separation of cells by velocity sedimentation, *J. Cell Physiol.,* 73, 191, 1969.
3. **Shortman, K.,** Separation methods for lymphocyte populations, in *Contemp. Top. Mol. Immunol.,* 3, 161, 1974.
4. **Pluznik, D. H. and Sachs, L.,** The cloning of normal "mast" cells in tissue culture, *J. Cell. Comp. Physiol.,* 66, 319, 1965.
5. **Bradley, T. R. and Metcalf, D.,** The growth of mouse bone marrow cells *in vitro, Aust. J. Exp. Biol. Med. Sci.,* 44, 287, 1966.
6. **McCulloch, E. A.,** Granulopoiesis in cultures of human haemopoietic cells, *Clin. Haemotol.,* 4, 509, 1975.
7. **Fibach, E., Gerassi, E., and Sachs, L.,** Induction of colony formation *in vitro* by human lymphocytes, *Nature,* 259, 127, 1976.
8. **Boveri, T.,** *The Origin of Malignant Tumors,* Williams & Wilkins, Baltimore, Md., 1929.
9. **Gavosto, F., Maraini, G., and Pileri, A.,** Nucleic acids and protein metabolism in acute leukemia cells, *Blood,* 16, 1555, 1960.
10. Proceedings of the symposium on nucleic acid metabolism in normal and leukemic cells, Munich, 1970, *Acta Haematol.,* 45, 133, 1971.
11. **Polli, E. E.,** Human leukemia, nucleic acids and viruses, hypothesis and perspectives, *Acta Haematol.,* 49, 257, 1973.
12. **Armitage, P. and Dole, R.,** The age distribution of cancer and a multistage theory of carcinogenesis, *Br. J. Cancer,* 8, 1, 1954.
13. **Armitage, P. and Doll, R.,** A two-stage theory of carcinogenesis in relation to distribution of cancer, *Br. J. Cancer,* 11, 161, 1957.
14. **Ashley, D. J. B.,** The two-hit and multiple-hit theories of carcinogenesis, *Br. J. Cancer,* 23, 313, 1969.
15. **Knudson, A. G.,** Mutation and cancer: statistical study of retinoblastoma, *Proc. Natl. Acad. Sci. U.S.A.,* 68, 820, 1971.
16. **Cairns, J.,** The cancer problem, *Sci. Am.,* 233, 64, 1975.
17. **Propping, P.,** Comparison of point mutation rates in different species with human mutation rates, *Humangenetik,* 16, 43, 1972.
18. **Nowell, P. C. and Hungerford, D. A.,** A minute chromosome in human chronic granulocytic leukemia, *Science,* 132, 1497, 1960.
19. **Beck, W. S.,** Chromosomal patterns in myelocytic leukemia. *N. Engl. J. Med.,* 289, 220, 1973.
20. **Hayata, I., Sakurai, M., Kakati, S. K., and Sandberg, A. A.,** Chromosomes and causation of human cancer and leukemia. XVI. Banding studies of chronic myelocytic leukemia, including five unusual Ph[1] translocations, *Cancer,* 36, 1177, 1975.
21. **Meisner, L. F.,** Cytogenetic analysis in leukemia, *CRC Crit. Rev. Clin. Lab. Sci.,* 6, 157, 1975.
22. **Maniatis, A. K., Amsel, S., Mitus, W. J., and Coleman, N.,** Chromosome pattern of bone marrow fibroblasts in patients with chronic granulocytic leukemia, *Nature,* 222, 1278, 1969.
23. **Whang, J., Frei, E., Tjio, J. H., Carbone, P. P., and Brecher, G.,** The distribution of the Philadelphia chromosome in patients with chronic myelogenous leukemia, *Blood,* 22, 664, 1963.
24. **Carnellos, G. P., DeVitta, V. T., Whang-Peng, J., and Carbone, P. P.,** Haematologic and cytogenetic remission of blast transformation in chronic granulocytic leukemia, *Blood,* 38, 671, 1971.
25. **Dougan, L., Scott, I. D., and Woodliff, H. J.,** A pair of twins, one of whom has chronic granulocytic leukemia, *J. Med. Genet.,* 3, 217, 1966.
26. **Goh, K., Swisher, S., and Herman, E.,** Chronic myelocytic leukemia and identical twins, *Arch. Intern. Med.,* 120, 214, 1967.
27. **Gartler, S. M.,** Utilization of mosaic systems in the study of the origin and progression of tumors, in *Chromosomes and Cancer,* German, J., Ed., John Wiley & Sons, New York, 1974, 313.
28. **Fialkow, P. J.,** Genetic marker studies, in *Genetic Concepts and Neoplasia,* Williams & Wilkins, Baltimore, Md., 1970, 112.
29. **Tough, I. M., Court-Brown, W. M., Baike, A. G., Buckton, K. E., Harnden, D. G., Jacobs, P. A., King, M. J., and McBride, J. A.,** Cytogenetic studies in chronic myeloid leukemia and acute leukemia associated with mongolism, *Lancet,* 1, 411, 1961.
30. **Fitzgerald, P. H., Pickering, A. F., and Eiby, J. R.,** Clonal origin of the Philadelphia chromosome and chronic myeloid leukemia. Evidence from a sex chromosome mosaic, *Br. J. Haematol.,* 21, 473, 1971.
31. **Fialkow, P. J., Gartler, S. M., and Yoshida, A.,** Clonal origin of chronic myelocytic leukemia in man, *Proc. Natl. Acad. Sci. U.S.A.,* 58, 1468, 1967.
32. **Davidson, R. G., Nitowsky, H. M., and Childs, B.,** Demonstration of two populations of cells in the human female heterozygous for glucose-6-phosphate dehydrogenase variants, *Proc. Natl. Acad. Sci., U.S.A.,* 50, 481, 1963.
33. **Kirkman, H. N.,** Glucose-6-phosphate dehydrogenase, *Adv. Hum. Genet.,* 2, 1, 1971.
34. **Barr, R. D. and Fialkow, P. J.,** Clonal origin of chronic myelocytic leukemia, *N. Engl. J. Med.,* 289, 307, 1973.

35. **Prehn, R. T.,** Analysis of antigenic heterogeneity with individual 3-methylcholanthrene-induced mouse sarcoma, *J. Natl. Cancer Inst.,* 45, 1039, 1970.
36. **Fialkow, P. J., Lisker, R., Giblett, E. R., and Zavala, C.,** Xg locus: failure to detect inactivation in females with chronic myelocytic leukemia, *Nature,* 226, 367, 1970.
37. **Lawler, S. D. and Sanger, R.,** Xg blood-groups and clonal origin theory of chronic myeloid leukemia, *Lancet,* 1, 584, 1970.
38. Editorial: Is Lyonization total in man, *Lancet,* 2, 29, 1970.
39. **Preud'homme, J. L. and Seligmann, M.,** Surface bound immunoglobulins as a cell marker in human lymphoproliferative disorders, *Blood,* 40, 777, 1972.
40. **Aisenberg, A. C., Bloch, K. J., and Long, J. C.,** Cell surface immunoglobulin in chromic lymphatic leukemia and allied disorders, *Am. J. Med.,* 55, 184, 1973.
41. **Piessens, W. F., Schur, P. H., Moloney, W. C., and Churchill, W. H.,** Lymphocyte surface immunoglobulin. Distribution and frequency in lymphoproliferative disease, *N. Engl. J. Med.,* 288, 176, 1973.
42. Editorial: Preleukemia, *Lancet,* 1, 1426, 1973.
43. **Pierre, R. V.,** Preleukemic stages, *Semin. Haematol.,* 11, 73, 1974.
44. **Fialkow, P. J., Thomas, E. D., Bryant, J. I., and Neiman, P. E.,** Leukemic transformation of engrafted human marrow cells *in vivo, Lancet,* 1, 251, 1971.
45. **Thomas, E. D., Bryant, J. I., Buckner, C. D., Clift, R. A., Fefer, A., Johnson, F. L., Neiman, P., Ramberg, R. E., and Strob, R.,** Leukemic transformation of engrafted human marrow cells *in vivo, Lancet,* 1, 1310, 1972.
46. **Dmochowski, L., Taylor, H. G., Grey, C. E., Dreyer, D. A., Sykes, J. A., Langford, P. L., Rogers, T., Schullenberger, C. C., and Howe, C. D.,** Viruses and mycoplasma (PPLO) in human leukemia, *Cancer,* 18, 1345, 1965.
47. **Temin, H. M. and Mizutani, S.,** RNA-dependent DNA polymerase in virions of Rous sarcoma virus, *Nature,* 226, 1211, 1970.
48. **Baltimore, D.,** Viral RNA-dependent DNA polymerase in virions of RNA tumor viruses, *Nature,* 226, 1209, 1970.
49. Editorial: Reverse transcriptase in acute leukemia, *Lancet,* 2, 542, 1973.
50. **Hehlmann, R., Baxt, W., Kufe, D., and Spiegelman, S.,** Molecular evidence for a viral etiology of human leukemias, lymphomas and sarcomas, *Am. J. Clin. Pathol.,* 60, 65, 1973.
51. **Gallo, R. C., Yang, S. S., and Ting, R. C.,** RNA-dependent DNA polymerase of human acute leukaemia cells, *Nature,* 228, 927, 1970.
52. **Baxt, W., Hehlmann, R., and Spiegelman, S.,** Human leukaemic cells contain reverse transcriptase associated with a high molecular weight virus-related RNA, *Nature (London) New Biol.,* 240, 72, 1972.
53. **Gallo, R. C., Miller, N. R., Saxinger, W. C., and Gillespie, D.,** Primate RNA tumor-like DNA synthesized endogenously by RNA-dependent DNA polymerase in virus-like particles from fresh human acute leukemic blood cells, *Proc. Natl. Acad. Sci. U.S.A.,* 70, 3219, 1973.
54. **Sarngadharan, M. G., Sarin, P. S., Reitz, M. S., and Gallo, R. C.,** Reverse transcriptase activity of human acute leukaemic cells: purification of enzyme, response to AMV 70S RNA, and characterization of DNA product, *Nature (London) New Biol.,* 240, 67, 1972.
55. **Bhattacharyrya, J., Xuma, M., Reitz, M., Sarin, J. S., and Gallo, R. C.,** Utilization of mammalian 70S RNA by a purified reverse transcriptase from human myelocytic leukemic cells, *Biochem. Biophys. Res. Commun.,* 54, 324, 1973.
56. **Mondal, H., Gallagher, R. E., and Gallo, R. C.,** RNA-directed DNA polymerase from human leukemic blood cells and from primate type-C virus producing cells: High and low molecular weight forms with variant biochemical and immunological properties, *Proc. Natl. Acad. Sci. U.S.A.,* 72, 1194, 1975.
57. **Todaro, G. J. and Gallo, R. C.,** Immunological relationship of DNA polymerase from human acute leukaemia cells and primate and mouse leukaemia virus reverse transcriptase, *Nature,* 244, 206, 1973.
58. **Gallagher, R. E., Todaro, H. J., Smith, R. G., Livingston, D. M., and Gallo, R. C.,** Relationship between RNA-directed DNA polymerase (reverse transcriptase) from human acute leukemic blood cells and primate type-C viruses, *Proc. Natl. Acad. Sci. U.S.A.,* 71, 1309, 1974.
59. **Witkin, S., Ohno, T., and Spiegelman, S.,** Purification of RNA-instructed DNA polymerase from human leukemic spleens, *Proc. Natl. Acad. Sci. U.S.A.,* 72, 4133, 1975.
60. **Mak, T. W., Aye, M. T., Messner, H., Sheinin, R., Till, J. E., and McCulloch, E. A.,** Reverse transcriptase activity: increase in marrow cultures from leukaemic patients in relapse and remission, *Br. J. Cancer,* 20, 433, 1974.
61. **Vosika, G. J., Krivit, W., Gerard, J. M., Coccia, P. F., Nesbit, M. E., Coalson, J. J., and Kennedy, B. J.,** Oncornavirus-like particles from cultured bone marrow cells preceding leukemia and malignant histiocytosis, *Proc. Natl. Acad. Sci. U.S.A.,* 72, 2804, 1975.
62. **Viola, M. V., Frazier, M., Wiernik, P. H., McCredie, K. B., and Spiegelman, S.,** Reverse transcriptase in leukocytes of leukemic patients in remission. *N. Engl. J. Med.,* 294, 75, 1976.
63. **Hehlmann, R., Kufe, D., and Spiegelman, S.,** RNA in human leukemic cells related to the RNA of a mouse leukemia virus, *Proc. Natl. Acad. Sci. U.S.A.,* 69, 435, 1972.
64. **Larsen, C. J., Marty, M., Hamelin, R., Feries, J., Boiron, M., and Tavitian, A.,** Search for nucleic acid sequences complementary to a murine onconaviral genome in poly (A) rich RNA of human leukemic cells, *Proc. Natl. Acad. Sci. U.S.A.,* 72, 4900, 1975.

65. **Baxt, W. G. and Spiegelman, S.,** Nuclear DNA sequences present in human leukemic cells and absent in normal leukocytes, *Proc. Natl. Acad. Sci. U.S.A.,* 69, 3737, 1972.

66. **Baxt, W. H.,** Sequences present in both human leukemic cell nuclear DNA and Rauscher leukemia virus, *Proc. Natl. Acad. Sci. U.S.A.,* 71, 2853, 1974.

67. **Baxt, W., Yates, J. W., Wallace, H. J., Jr., Holland, J. F., and Spiegelman, S.,** Leukemia-specific DNA sequences in leukocytes of the leukemic member of identical twins, *Proc. Natl. Acad. Sci. U.S.A.,* 70, 2629, 1973.

68. **Sherr, C. J. and Todaro, G. J.,** Primate type C virus p30 antigen in cells from humans with acute leukemia, *Science,* 187, 855, 1975.

69. **Kotler, M., Weinberg, E., Haspel, O., Olshevsky, U., and Becker, Y.,** Particles released from arginine deprived human leukemic cells, *Nature (London) New Biol.,* 244, 197, 1973.

70. **Mak, T. W., Manaster, J., Howatson, A. F., McCulloch, E. A., and Till, J. E.,** Particles with characteristics of leukoviruses in cultures of marrow cells from leukemic patients in remission and relapse, *Proc. Natl. Acad. Sci. U.S.A.,* 71, 4336, 1974.

71. **Mak, T. W., Kurtz, S., Manaster, J., and Housman, D.,** Viral-related information in oncornavirus-like particles isolated from cultures of marrow cells from leukemic patients in relapse and remission, *Proc. Natl. Acad. Sci. U.S.A.,* 72, 623, 1975.

72. **Gallagher, R. E. and Gallo, R. C.,** Type C RNA tumor virus isolated from cultured human acute myelogenous leukemia cells, *Science,* 187, 350, 1975.

73. **Teich, N. M., Weiss, R. A., Salahuddin, S. Z., Gallagher, R. E., Gillespie, D. H., and Gallo, R. C.,** Infective transmission and characterization of a C-type virus released by cultured human myeloid leukaemia cells, *Nature,* 256, 551, 1975.

74. **Gallagher, R. E., Salahuddin, S. Z., Hall, W. T., McCredie, K. B., and Gallo, R. C.,** Growth and differentiation in culture of leukemic leukocytes from patients with acute myelogenous leukemia and reidentification of type-C virus, *Proc. Natl. Acad. Sci. U.S.A.,* 72, 4137, 1975.

75. **Nooter, K., Aarssen, A. M., Bentvelzen, P., de Grott, F. G., and Van Pelt, F. G.,** Isolation of infectious C-type oncornavirus from human leukaemic bone marrow cells, *Nature,* 256, 595, 1975.

76. **Todaro, G. J. and Huebner, R. J.,** The viral oncogene hypothesis: new evidence *Proc. Natl. Acad. Sci. U.S.A.,* 69, 1009, 1972.

77. **Penner, P. E., Cohen, L. H., and Loeb, L. A.,** RNA-dependent DNA polymerase in human lymphocytes during gene activation by phytohemagglutinin, *Nature (London) New Biol.,* 232, 58, 1971.

78. **Bobrow, S. N., Smith, R. G., Reitz, M. S., and Gallo, R. C.,** Stimulated normal human lymphocytes contain a ribonuclease-sensitive DNA polymerase distinct from viral RNA directed DNA polymerase, *Proc. Natl. Acad. Sci. U.S.A.,* 69, 3228, 1972.

79. **Temin, H. M.,** On the origin of genes for neoplasia: G.H.A. Clowes Memorial Lecture, *Cancer Res.,* 34, 2835, 1974.

80. **Kornberg, A.,** *DNA Synthesis,* W. H. Freeman & Co., San Francisco, 1974.

81. **Loeb, L. A., Springgate, C. F., and Battula, N.,** Errors in DNA replication as a basis of malignant changes, *Cancer Res.,* 34, 2311, 1974.

82. **Mildvan, A. S.,** Mechanism of enzyme action, *Ann. Rev. Biochem.,* 43, 357, 1974.

83. **Speyer, J. F.,** Mutagenic DNA polymerase, *Biochem. Biophys. Res. Commun.,* 21, 6, 1965.

84. **Speyer, J. F., Karam, J. D., and Lenny, A. B.,** On the role of DNA polymerase in base selection, *Cold Spring Harbor Symp. Quant. Biol.,* 31, 693, 1966.

85. **Hall, Z. W. and Lehman, I. R.,** An *in vitro* transversion by a mutationally altered T_4-induced DNA polymerase, *J. Mol. Biol.,* 36, 321, 1968.

86. **Hershfield, M. S.,** On the role of deoxyribonucleic acid polymerase in determining mutation rates, *J. Biol. Chem.,* 248, 1417, 1973.

87. **Brutlag, D. and Kornberg, A.,** Enzymatic synthesis of deoxyribonucleic acid. XXXVI. A proof-reading function of 3'-5' exonuclease activity in DNA polymerases, *J. Biol. Chem.,* 247, 241, 1972.

88. **Muzyczka, N., Poland, R. L., and Bessman, M. J.,** Studies on the biochemical basis of spontaneous mutation. I. Comparison of DNA polymerases of mutator, antimutator and wild type strains of bacteriophage T_4, *J. Biol. Chem.,* 243, 627, 1968.

89. **Goulian, M., Lucas, Z. J., and Kornberg, A.,** Enzymatic synthesis of DNA XXV purification and properties of DNA polymerase induced by infection with phage T_4, *J. Biol. Chem.,* 243, 627, 1968.

90. **Loeb, L. A.,** Eukaryotic DNA polymerases, *The Enzyme,* 10, 173, 1974.

91. **Chang, L. M. S.,** Low molecular weight deoxyribonucleic acid polymerase from calf thymus chromatin. II. Initiation and fidelity of homopolymer replication, *J. Biol. Chem.,* 248, 6983, 1973.

92. **Burnet, F. M.,** A genetic interpretation of ageing (hypothesis), *Lancet,* 2, 480, 1973.

93. **Wheldon, T. E. and Kirk, J.,** An error cascade mechanism for tumor progression, *J. Theor. Biol.,* 42, 107, 1973.

94. **Springgate, C. F. and Loeb, L. A.,** Mutagenic DNA polymerase in human leukemic cells, *Proc. Natl. Acad. Sci. U.S.A.,* 70, 245, 1973.

95. **Srivastava, B. I. S.,** Fidelity of deoxyribonucleic acid polymerases from normal and leukemic human cells in polydeoxynucleotide replication, *Biochem. J.,* 141, 585, 1974.

96. **McCaffrey, R., Smoler, D. F., and Baltimore, D.,** Terminal deoxynucleotidyl transferase in a case of childhood acute lymphoblastic leukemia, *Proc. Natl. Acad. Sci. U.S.A.,* 70, 521, 1973.

97. Coleman, M. S., Hutton, J. J., de Simone, P., and Bollum, F. J., Terminal deoxynucleotidyl transferase in human leukemia, *Proc. Natl. Acad. Sci. U.S.A.,* 71, 4404, 1974.

98. Sarin, P. S. and Gallo, R. C., Terminal deoxynucleotidyl transferase in chronic myelogenous leukemia, *J. Biol. Chem.,* 249, 8051, 1974.

99. McCaffrey, R., Harrison, T. A., Parkman, R., and Baltimore, D., Terminal deoxynucleotidyl transferase activity in human leukemic cells and in normal thymocytes, *N. Engl. J. Med.,* 292, 775, 1975.

100. Sarin, P. S., Anderson, P. N., and Gallo, R. C., Terminal deoxynucleotidyl transferase activities in human blood leukocytes and lymphoblast cell lines, *Blood,* 47, 11, 1976.

101. Baltimore, D., Is terminal deoxynucleotidyl transferase a somatic mutagen in lymphocytes?, *Nature,* 248, 409, 1974.

102. Saffhill, R. and Chaudhri, L., The presence of terminal deoxynucleotidyl transferase in N-methyl-N-nitrosourea induced leukemia in BDF1 mice and its effect on the accuracy of the DNA polymerase, *Nucleic Acid Res.,* 3, 277, 1976.

103. Battula, N. and Loeb, L. A., The infidelity of avian myelobastosis virus deoxyribonucleic acid polymerase in polynucleotide replication, *J. Biol. Chem.,* 249, 4086, 1974.

104. Battula, N. and Loeb, L. A., On the fidelity of DNA replication. Characterization of polynucleotides with errors in base-pairing synthesized by avian myeloblastosis virus DNA polymerase, *J. Biol. Chem.,* 250, 4405, 1975.

105. Sirover, M. A. and Loeb, L. A., Infidelity of DNA synthesis: a general property of RNA tumor viruses, *Biochem. Biophys. Res. Commun.,* 61, 410, 1974.

106. Stiles, C. D., Desmond, W., Jr., Gato, G., and Saier, M. H., Jr., Failure of human cells transformed by simian virus 40 to form tumors in athymic nude mice, *Proc. Natl. Acad. Sci. U.S.A.,* 72, 4971, 1975.

107. Pitot, H. C. and Heidelberger, C., Metabolic regulatory circuits and carcinogens, *Cancer Res.,* 23, 1694, 1963.

108. Dustin, P., Jr., Cell differentiation and carcinogenesis. A critical review, *Cell Tissue Kinet.,* 5, 519, 1972.

109. Pierce, G. B., Neoplasms, differentiations and mutations, *Am. J. Pathol.,* 77, 103, 1974.

110. Pitot, H. C., Neoplasia: a somatic mutation or a heritable change in cytoplasmic membranes, *J. Natl. Cancer Inst.,* 53, 905, 1974.

111. Rubin, H., Carcinogenicity tests, *Science,* 191, 241, 1976.

112. Talwar, G. P., Ed., *Regulation of Growth and Differentiated Function in Eukaryotic Cells,* Raven Press, New York, 1975.

113. Epstein, W. and Beckwith, J. R., Regulation of gene expression, *Ann. Rev. Biochem.,* 37, 411, 1968.

114. Stonehill, E. M. and Bendich, A., Retrogenic expression: the reappearance of embryonal antigens in cancer cells, *Nature,* 228, 370, 1970.

115. Gellhorn, A., Ectopic hormone production in cancer and its implications for basic research on abnormal growth, *Adv. Int. Med.,* 15, 299, 1969.

116. Smithers, D. W., Maturation in human tumors, *Lancet,* 2, 949, 1969.

117. Everson, T. C. and Cole, W. H., *Spontaneous Regression of Cancer,* W. B. Saunders, Philadelphia, 1966.

118. Jensen, R. D. and Miller, R. W., Retinoblastoma: epidemiological characteristics, *N. Engl. J. Med.,* 285, 307, 1971.

119. Braun, A. C., A demonstration of the recovery of the crown-gall tumor cell with the use of complex tumors of single-cell origin, *Proc. Natl. Acad. Sci. U.S.A.,* 45, 932, 1959.

120. McKinnell, R. G., Deggins, B. A., and Labat, D. D., Transplantation of pluripotential nuclei from triploid frog tumors, *Science,* 165, 394, 1969.

121. Goldstein, M. N., Burdman, J. A., and Journey, L. J., Long-term tissue culture of neuroblastomas. II. Morphologic evidence for differentiation and maturation, *J. Natl. Cancer Inst.,* 32, 165, 1974.

122. MacPherson, I. A., Reversion in cells transformed by tumor viruses, *Proc. R. Soc. London Ser B.,* 177, 41, 1971.

123. Mintz, B. and Illmensee, K., Normal genetically mosaic mice produced from malignant teratocarcinoma cells, *Proc. Natl. Acad. Sci. U.S.A.* 72, 3585, 1975.

124. Golde, D. W. and Cline, M. W., Human preleukemia. Identification of a maturation defect, *N. Engl. J. Med.,* 288, 1083, 1973.

125. Paran, M., Sachs, L., and Barak, Y., *In vitro* induction of granulocyte differentiation in hematopoietic cells from leukemic and non-leukemic patients, *Proc. Natl. Acad. Sci. U.S.A.,* 67, 1542, 1970.

126. Greenberg, P. L., Nichols, W. C., and Schrier, S. L., Granulopoieses in acute myeloid leukemia and preleukemia, *N. Engl. J. Med.,* 284, 1225, 1971.

127. Robinson, W. A., Kurnick, J. E., and Pike, B. L., Colony growth of human leukemic peripheral blood cells *in vitro,* *Blood,* 38, 500, 1971.

128. Moore, M. A. S., Williams, N., and Metcalf, D., *In vitro* colony formation by normal and leukemic human hematopoietic cells: characterization of colony forming cells, *J. Natl. Cancer Inst.,* 50, 603, 1973.

129. Athens, J. W., Disorders of neutrophil proliferation of circulation; a pathophysiological review, *Clin. Haematol.,* 4, 553, 1975.

130. Frei, E., III, and Freireich, E. J., Progress and perspectives in the chemotherapy of acute leukemia, *Adv. Chemother.,* 2, 269, 1965.

131. Bluming, A. Z., Current status of clinical immunotherapy, *Cancer Chemother. Rep.,* 59, 901, 1975.

132. Simone, J., Aur, R. J. A., Hustu, H. O., and Pinkel, D., Total therapy, studies of acute lymphocytic leukemia in children: current results and prospects for cure, *Cancer,* 30, 1488, 1972.

133. Whang-Peng, J., Freireich, E. J., Oppenheim, J. J., Frei, E., and Tjio, J. H., Cytogenetic studies in 45 patients with acute lymphocytic leukemia, *J. Natl. Cancer Inst.,* 42, 881, 1969.

134. Duttera, M. J., Whang-Peng, J., Bull, J. M. C., and Carbone, P. P., Cytogenetically abnormal cells *in vitro* in acute leukaemia, *Lancet,* 1, 715, 1972.

135. Craddock, C. G. and Crandall, B. F., Remission in myeloblastic leukemia; clonal suppression or maturation, *Blood,* 42, 1013, 1973.

136. Bull, J. M., Duttera, M. J., Stashick, E. D., Northup, J., Henderson, E., and Carbone, P. P., Serial *in vitro* marrow culture in acute myelocytic leukemia, *Blood,* 42, 679, 1973.

137. Halterman, R. H., Leventhal, B. G., and Mann, D. L., An acute-leukemia antigen: correlation with clinical status, *N. Engl. J. Med.,* 287, 1272, 1972.

138. Gutterman, J. U., Mavligit, G., Burgess, M. A., McCredie, K. B., Hunger, C., Freireich, E. J., and Hersh, E. M., Immunodiagnosis of acute leukemia: detection of residual disease, *J. Natl. Cancer Inst.,* 53, 389, 1974.

139. Symposium: immunological control of virus associated tumors in man: prospects and problems, *Cancer Res.,* 36, 559, 1976.

140. Hersh, E. M., Gutterman, J. U., Mavligit, G., Gschwind, C. R., Freiireich, E. J., Levine, P. H., and Plata, E. J., Human immune response to active immunization with RLV, *J. Natl. Cancer Inst.,* 53, 317, 1974.

141. Hardy, W. D., Jr., Old, L., Mess, P., Essex, M., and Cotter, S. M., Horizontal transmission of feline leukemia virus: a field study, *Nature,* 244, 266, 1973.

142. Green, M., Gerard, G. F., RNA-directed DNA polymerase-properties and functions in oncogenic RNA viruses and cells, *Prog. Nucleic Acid. Res. Mol. Biol.,* 14, 187, 1974.

143. Vallee, B. L., Fluharty, R. G., and Gibson, J. G., 2nd *Acta Union Intern Contre Cancer* 6, 869, 1949.

144. Springgate, C. F., Mildvan, A. S., Abramson, R., Engle, J. L., and Loeb, L. A., *Escherichia coli* deoxyribonucleic acid polymerase I, a zinc metalloenzyme, *J. Biol. Chem.,* 248, 5987, 1973.

145. Mildvan, A. S., Sloan, D. L., Springgate, C. F., and Loeb, L. A., Magnetic resonance studies of the mechanism of DNA polymerase I from *E. coli,* in *Cancer Enzymology,* Schultz, J. and Ahmad, F., Eds., 8th Miami Winter Symposia, 1976, Academic Press, New York, in press.

146. Poiesz, B. J., Seal, G., and Loeb, L. A., Reverse transcriptase: correlation of zinc content with activity, *Proc. Natl. Acad. Sci. U.S.A.,* 71, 4892, 1974.

147. Fialkow, P. J., personal communication.

148. Weymouth, L., personal communication.

Chapter 9
CELL SURFACE MARKERS IN THE CHARACTERIZATION
OF HUMAN LYMPHORETICULAR DISEASES

Stephen Davis and Arnold D. Rubin

TABLE OF CONTENTS

I. INTRODUCTION

The cells comprising the lymphoreticular (LR) system are functionally and morphologically heterogeneous. The thymus-derived (T-cell) and bone marrow-derived (B-cell) lymphocyte are not only distinguishable functionally but can be identified by specific markers on their surfaces. The presence of synthesized surface immunoglobulin (Ig) and receptors for complement (C) and aggregated Ig (which adheres to cell surfaces by means of the Fc portion of Ig) are identifying features of B cells.[1] In man, the identification of T cells is facilitated by their ability to form rosettes with neuraminidase-treated sheep erythrocytes.[2] Small percentages of activated T cells may also express Fc receptors. Recently, populations of lymphocytes having either multiple markers or no detectable markers ("null cells") have been described. These cells cannot be precisely classified as T or B, but a hypothetical role of these cells as lymphoid precursor cells has been advanced.[3] Monocytes and histiocytes also bear C receptors and can absorb Ig to their surface via Fc receptors, but are believed to be distinguishable from lymphoid cells under appropriate in vitro conditions by a receptor for cytophilic antibody (IgGEA).[4] Recent studies have shown that

neoplastic LR cells also possess cell surface receptors. On the basis of these distinguishing characteristics it is suggested that the lineage of normal and neoplastic cells might be determined and used as a classification for LR diseases. This chapter will attempt to correlate the results obtained from studies which use these markers into a scheme which pathogenetically characterizes LR malignancies. It must be stressed, however, that extrapolation of data obtained from normal cells to malignant tissue may be invalid since neoplasia may, in part, represent a dedifferentiated state.

II. CELLULAR INTERACTIONS WITHIN THE LYMPHORETICULAR SYSTEM

Figure 1 depicts the synthesized conclusions from interrelated studies and represents the role of monocyte-histiocyte (M-H) cells and lymphocytes in immunity. The initial encounter with an immunogen leads to a chain of metabolic and cellular events concerned with capture and processing of the immunogen, followed by cellular information transfer, proliferation, and differentiation.

The M-H cells are highly specialized to carry out the functions of ingestion and destruction of

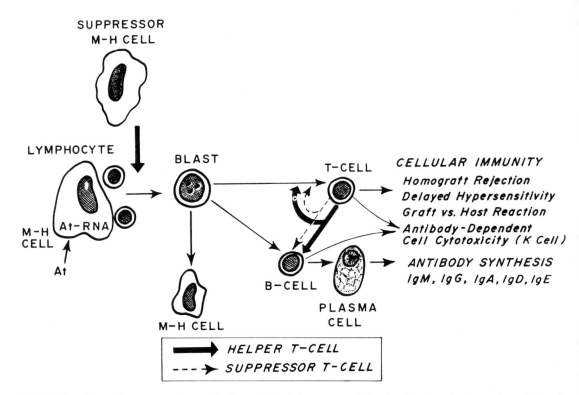

FIGURE 1. Schematic representation of the cellular interactions within the lymphoreticular system. M-H cell, monocyte-histocyte cell; At, antigen.

all particulate matter including bacteria, damaged autologous cells, and macromolecules. The ingestion is known to be facilitated by antibody and complement coating of the particle. Immunogenic substances may require processing by M-H cells. Following initial processing, there appears to be transfer of antigen to lymphoid cells in the form of antigen-RNA complexes or as antigen fragments. Evidence in support of the M-H-dependent lymphocyte response comes from studies which show that if antigen encounters a lymphocyte directly, inhibition of immune responsiveness (tolerance) results. Sensitization induces a mitotic response which is morphologically characterized by a metabolically active blast cell. Sensitized lymphocytes, in addition, may recruit additional M-H cells and lymphocytes to participate in the immune reaction by the release of nonspecific soluble macromolecules (lymphokines), e.g., migration inhibitory factor and blastogenic factor.

Thymus-derived cells are differentiated lymphocytes responsible for cell-mediated immunity, which includes graft vs. host reaction, delayed hypersensitivity reactions, and homograft rejec-

tion. Bone marrow-derived lymphocytes, on specific antigen contact, are induced to proliferate into memory cells or differentiate into mature plasma cells which are committed with regard to class and specificity of the antibody the plasma cell secretes. Those lymphocytes responsible for antibody-dependent cytotoxicity are termed K cells. They lack the ability to secrete Ig or form rosettes; however, they possess Fc receptors. Whether these cells represent T or B lymphocytes remains unsettled. It is now believed that T cells and M-H cells are intimately involved in the regulation of the immune process. Nude (athymic) mice immunized with immunogens induce multiplication of specific antigen-binding cells; however, there is no associated antibody production. These data suggest that a population of T cells (helper T cell) is more important in triggering terminal differentiation of B lymphocytes into antibody-producing cells than in triggering proliferation. Helper T cells also appear to be necessary for an adequate cell-mediated immune response.[5] The concept of suppressor cells regulating the immune response has recently been advanced. Several types of suppressor cells have been described. Thymic

(T)-derived suppressor cells appear to regulate B-cell activity in a classic feedback mechanism. Patients with systemic lupus erythematosus have a characteristic increase in antibody production to certain antigens. The hypergammaglobulinemia is believed by some investigators to result from a defect in suppressor T cells. Recent data from Broder et al.[6] suggest that the depressed levels of polyclonal Ig seen in patients with multiple myeloma is secondary to M-H cell suppression of antibody production. Similar results have been reported in animal models.[7]

Regardless of the mechanisms involved, one can readily accept that there is an interaction between the M-H cells of the reticuloendothelial system and lymphocytes and that the immune reaction by its very nature requires a controlled proliferation and differentiation.

In our current state of knowledge, we can explore concepts that abnormal immunologic interaction is manifested by the LR malignancies. Several models can be constructed. One might consider LR malignancies as manifestations of unbalanced growth occurring as a result of abnormal interactions between M-H cells and lymphocytes. In the normal mechanism, as was previously discussed, lymphocyte sensitization and subsequent proliferation depend on an interaction with M-H cells from which processed antigenic information is recieved. Cooper et al.[8] have suggested that in the Wiskott-Aldrich syndrome, M-H hyperplasia results from a prolonged bombardment with toxic polysaccharides which are not neutralized immunologically due to inability of these patients' lymphoid cells to recognize polysaccharide antigens. Such a hypothesis could explain LR malignancies which occur in children who survive the early phase of this disorder. Gleichman et al.[9] induced primary LR tumors by innoculation of parental spleen cells into H-2-incompatible F_1 hybrid mice. The gene types of the tumors formed in this graft vs. host reaction showed that LR malignancy can develop from host as well as donor cells. This further supports the concept of lymphomagenesis as a consequence of persistent stimulation by antigen. The high incidence of LR malignancies in human kidney recipients might also be attributed to persistent stimulation.

Certain viral infections have been implicated in the etiology of LR disorders. The Chediak-Higashi syndrome represents an inborn deficiency in phagocytic activity.[10] The development of lymphoma is well known in these patients. It is possible that a deficiency in host resistence leads to infection with an oncogenic virus. There is also evidence from animal studies that the thymus may play a role in the development of viral-induced LR disorders. In some animal lymphoma models, thymectomy will eliminate the subsequent development of viral tumor production.[11]

The hypo-agammaglobulinemias may be predicted on the failure of lymphocytes to differentiate into plasma cells. This failure of terminal differentiation must affect the prior lymphocyte stages of maturation or, alternatively, ineffective T-B interactions. Perhaps this failure of differentiation into plasma cells is related to the LR malignancies which subsequently develop in many patients. Dameshek labeled chronic lymphocytic leukemia (CLL) as an accumulative disease, implying that small lymphocytes lose their ability to proliferate and differentiate normally, and that the disease results from an abnormal accumulation of small lymphocytes. Thus, generalized arrest of lymphocyte differentiation might be expected to disrupt all manifestations of immunity.

Of the three models outlined, the first implies the appearance of isolated groups of M-H cells and lymphocytes proliferating out of control. The second might manifest itself either as a generalized infection of lymphocytes or as one infected cell giving rise to an expanding clone which could then disseminate. The last involves a generalized LR disorder resulting from an accumulation of cells which cannot undergo normal differentiation. These possibilities raise certain pathogenetic distinctions which may carry important therapeutic ramifications.

III. THEORETICAL DIFFERENTIATION OF THE LYMPHORETICULAR SYSTEM BASED ON CELL SURFACE MARKERS

The scheme depicted in Figure 2 introduces a hypothetical concept of lymphoid cell differentiation and its relationship to the monocytic-histiocytic series. This proposed differentiation scheme is based on the concept of progressive and regressive changes in surface alloantigens, a process

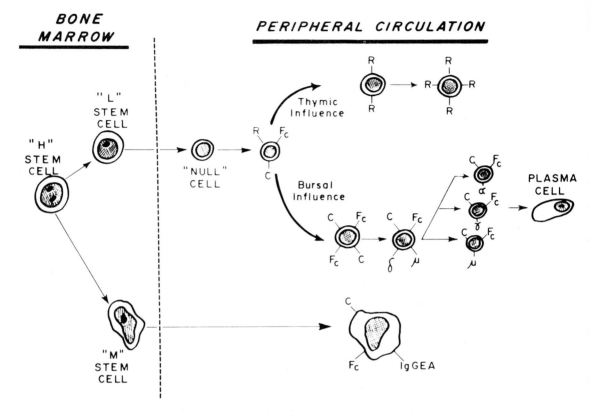

FIGURE 2.   Theoretical differentiation of the lymphoreticular system based on cell surface markers. "H," hemopoietic; "L," lymphoid; "M," monocytoid; R, receptor for sheep red blood cells; F_c, receptor for the F_c portion of immunoglobulin; C, receptor for complement; IgGEA, receptor for cytophilic antibody; δ IgD; μ, IgM; γ, IgG; α, IgA.

which has been well documented in mice.[12] In man, all mature blood cells are believed to arise from a common precursor cell. The first step in the maturation of this pluripotential stem cell is the production of a series of committed bone marrow stem cells, "L" (lymphoid), and "M" (monocytoid) stem cells. It is not known if "M" stem cells bear surface receptors, but it appears that bone marrow "L" stem cells bear no detectable markers.[13] The morphologic stages of development following the "M" stem cell are the monoblast, promonocyte, and mature monocyte. The relationship of the monocyte to the histiocyte has not been clearly delineated, but the histiocyte is believed to be a tissue-fixed monocytoid cell. Cell surface receptors have only been characterized on the mature monocytic-histiocytic cell. As shown in Figure 2, these cells bear for C, IgGEA, and Fc receptors. It is important to note that Ig is found on M-H cells; it differs from that found on lymphocytes in that it is absorbed to the cell surface via the Fc receptor and not secreted into in vitro culture media, and that it is not regenerated following membrane stripping with proteolytic

enzymes. The ability to synthesize surface Ig is clearly the hallmark of B lymphocytes.

The next step in the maturation of the "L"stem cell is the production of a circulating null cell, i.e., a morphologically recognizable lymphocyte with no detectable surface markers. The transition of "L" stem cells to circulating null cells has not been documented experimentally; however, the finding that null cells form lymphoid colonies in vitro suggests that they represent a lymphocyte precursor cell with the ability to develop into T or B cells.[14] Examination of the peripheral blood of healthy individuals has consistently revealed a distinct population of small lymphocytes (2 to 13.5%) bearing no detectable surface markers.

Continued differentiation of the null cell would result in a cell capable of expressing both T- and B-cell markers. Combined phase and fluorescent microscopy have shown SRBC rosettes and Fc or C receptors simultaneously on from 2 to 6% of individual lymphocytes of normal patients. Maturing lymphocytes subsequently fall under the influence of the central lymphoid organs. Cells destined for the T-cell compartment migrate to the thymus and undergo alterations both in functional capacity and in cell surface markers. B cells mature in a fashion similar to T cells by developing from a multiple marker cell into cells endowed only with receptors for aggregated Ig and C. Surface Ig is the last marker to be acquired. Recent studies have suggested that Ig determinants also develop in a sequential fashion with IgM (μ) appearing first, closely followed by IgD (δ), IgG (γ), and IgA (α), respectively. Terminal differentiation beyond this stage of the lymphocyte to a plasma cell occurs with the loss of B-cell surface determinants.

IV. CELL SURFACE MARKERS ON MALIGNANT LYMPHORETICULAR CELLS

Histiocytic medullary reticulosis (HMR) is considered the prototype of a malignant M-H cell proliferation. Functionally, the neoplastic cells found in the spleen and bone marrow retain their ability to phagocytize, suggesting retention of some normal M-H cell characteristics. Jaffe et al.[15] studied cell surface markers, in frozen sections and in cell suspensions, on spleen and lymph node cells in a case of HMR. In cell suspensions, 53% of cells bound Ig GEA (control:7%), whereas only 19% (control:41%) of cells demonstrate lymphocyte markers, confirming the reduced lymphocytic and increased M-H populations observed histologically. In frozen section preparations, the malignant cells seen histologically bound only IgG EA.

Leukemic reticuloendotheliosis ("hairy cell leukemia," LRE) is a clinical entity in which the origin of the malignant cell remains controversial. By a variety of techniques LRE cells have been shown to share characteristics with lymphocytes or monocytes or to express characteristics of both. Jaffe et al.[15] studied the spleen of LRE patients and have shown that these neoplastic cells bear the receptor for IgGEA but lack lymphocytic markers. Using indirect immunofluorescence, we have detected small amounts of Ig on LRE cells in two of five cases. The Ig in these cases was monospecific IgM which regenerated following removal of the Ig by proteolytic enzymes, a property unique to B lymphocytes. Similarly, Fu et al.[16] have found that although LRE cells have phagocytic properties, they demonstrate surface IgD, IgM, and Fc and C receptors, suggesting a monoclonal B-cell proliferation. The circulating mononuclear cells ("hairy" cells) of a case of LRE we

studied responded to phytohemagglutinin in vitro, a property believed to reside exclusively with lymphocytes;[17] however, PHA responsiveness cannot be found in all cases of LRE. Based on available data, it appears best to consider LRE as a disease in which the origin of the neoplastic cell cannot be clearly delineated. Perhaps these data suggest two pathogenetically different diseases with similar clinical presentations. We have found that surface markers in LRE have no prognostic significance, nor do they influence the response to splenectomy of chemotherapy.

Acute lymphoblastic leukemia (ALL) is a heterogeneous disease in regard to clinical presentation, response to chemotherapy, and prognosis. Many investigators report a poorer prognosis in those patients who present at an age of less than one or more than ten; with a mediastinal mass; or with central nervous system involvement, and WBC count greater than 50,000/mm^3. Despite this heterogeneity in clinical findings, lymphoblasts in each case appear morphologically indistinguishable. Cell surface marker studies have shown that in most cases of ALL (75%) the lymphoblasts have no differentiative markers (null cells). In most of the remaining cases of ALL the lymphoblasts were of T-cell origin (formed rosettes with SRBC), whereas a small number have B-cell characteristics. The finding of lymphoblasts which are B, T, and "null" cells suggests that the clinical heterogeneity of ALL may be related to the extent of differentiation of lymphocyte (Figure 2). Most cases of ALL may arise from a bone marrow-derived null cell, the others from cells differentiating toward mature T or B cells. Evidence in support of this concept has been reported by McCaffrey et al.[18] These investigators reported the presence of an enzyme, terminal deoxynucleotide transferase, in patients with ALL. This enzyme is only found in bone marrow cells (presumably prethymocytes) and thymocytes, but is absent from mature circulating T cells and all other mammalian tissue. Recently, "null" ALL lymphoblasts have been shown to have detectable HL-B alloantigens. These non-HL-A human alloantigens are believed to be selectively expressed on B lymphocytes. In the opinion of these authors, the majority of ALL lymphoblasts may be of B-cell origin, however, HL-B antigens are also present on M-H cells. From these data, Fu et al.[19] suggest that the ALL blast represents early bone marrow stem cells. The biologic implications of these findings in ALL remain conjectural; however, they are reported to have clinical significance. Borella and Sen[20] have suggested that patients with ALL fall into a poor-risk group if their lymphoblasts have the ability to bind SRBC (T cells). Since a mediastinal mass is commonly found in the patients of this poor-risk group, it is possible that many of these patients actually represent cases of childhood lymphoblastic lymphoma (CLSA), which is also presumed to be of T-cell origin.[21] Despite these data, analysis of large numbers of ALL cases suggest that age and WBC count at presentation carry the greatest prognostic significance; patients aged three to seven with WBC counts less than 10,000 have a $> 90\%$ 5-year survival, responding definitively to chemotherapy.

Based on studies on circulating lymphocyte surface markers, many investigators have classified CLL as a B-cell malignancy.[22] However, the existence of T-cell CLL has recently been demonstrated.[23] Work in our laboratories has pointed to a more fundamental abnormality in the pathogenesis of CLL. We have studied the response of purified circulating T and B cells from patients with CLL to mitogenic stimulation by PHA. Our results have shown the characteristic 3- and 5-day delay in proliferation, irrespective of whether the cells bore T- or B-cell markers on their surface or whether the patient was considered to have "T-cell predominant" and "B-cell predominant" CLL.[24] These findings suggested to us that both T and B cells are abnormal in CLL. We suggest that CLL involves a defect acquired early in the maturation of the lymphocyte. The defect would then be reflected in inadequate development of surface determinants which result eventually in failure of terminal differentiation and altered lymphocyte recirculation dynamics. This view is compatible with the clinical manifestations of impaired antibody synthesis and depressed cell-mediated immunity seen in the disease.

The Sezary syndrome is characterized by erythrodermia and generalized pruritis with an associated increase in large, abnormal cells in the skin and peripheral blood. Morphologic and ultrastructural studies have confirmed the lymphocytic origin of these Sezary cells. Recently, a small cell variant of the Sezary syndrome has been described which, by morphologic and clinical criteria, may be difficult to distinguish from "T-cell predominant" CLL cells.[25] Immunologic and morphologic

similarities also exist between the abnormal lymphocytes in Sezary syndrome and mycosis fungoides. Most of the tumor cells in mycosis fungoides represent T cells. In addition, Sezary syndrome may present in a form clinically indistinguishable from mycosis fungoides. Based on the above data, it is tempting to suggest that "T-cell predominant" CLL, Sezary syndrome, and mycosis fungoides may represent three manifestations of a single disease process.

Cell surface marker studies in cases of lymphoma have shown an age-dependent variation. A poorly differentiated diffuse lymphocytic lymphoma (PDDLL) in children (CLSA). The presence of an anterior mediastinal mass, infiltration of thymic-dependent areas of the LR system, and the ability of tumor cells to form rosettes support a T-cell origin. These findings are in contrast to data obtained from stem cell (Burkitt's) lymphoma of childhood. Of 35 African Burkitt's lymphoma biopsies, von Furth et al.[26] found 21 which secreted monoclonal IgM; similar results have been obtained in cases of nonendemic Burkitt's. Mann et al.[27] have suggested that the germinal centers of lymph nodes are selectively involved by tumor in cases of nonendemic Burkitt's lymphoma, implying that the B lymphocytes of normal germinal centers are the cells which have undergone malignant change. More work is needed before this hypothesis can be accepted.

Cases of adult nodular lymphoma (NL) have consistently shown C and secretory Ig on tumor cells. Based on these findings, it appears that the majority of NL cases represent B-cell malignancies which may, like Burkitt's lymphoma, originate from germinal center B cells.[28] Diffuse lymphoma in adults demonstrates a more varied pattern. The majority of cases of PDDLL in adults is of B-cell origin; however, T-cell PDDLL and "null"-cell PDDLL have been described. Although studies of surface markers in malignant lymphoma may offer an understanding of pathogenetic mechanisms, at the present time no clinical or prognostic significance has resulted from these studies.

Marker studies in pathologically diagnosed histiocytic lymphoma are inconsistent. Gajl-Peczalska et al.[29] were unable to detect any B- or T-cell markers on all six of their reported cases; however, they did not attempt to identify IgGEA receptors to determine a possible M-H origin of the tumor cells. Tumor cells in three cases of histiocytic lymphoma we have studied had detectable secretory Ig without IgGEA receptors suggesting a B-cell lineage; four additional cases failed to demonstrate lymphocyte or M-H specific markers. The variability of these findings does not allow us to clearly postulate the origin of the "histiocytic lymphoma" cell. Newer techniques are obviously required before the exact origin of the "histiocytic" lymphoma cell is determined.

The recent advances in immunobiology described in this chapter have focused on the LR system as functional unit and have documented some important facts regarding the biologic significance of normal LR-cell proliferation and differentiation based on surface markers. The question of whether surface markers will have biologic and clinical applicability in relation to LR neoplasms must await further studies.

REFERENCES

1. **Raff, M. C.,** Two distinct populations of peripheral lymphocytes distinguishable by immunofluorescence, *Immunology,* 19, 637, 1970.
2. **Weiner, M. S., Bianco, C., and Nussenzweig, V.,** Enhanced binding of neuraminidase-treated sheep erythrocytes to human T lymphocytes, *Blood,* 42, 939, 1973.
3. **Davis, S.,** Hypothesis: differentiation to the human lymphoid system based on cell surface markers, *Blood,* 45, 871, 1975.
4. **Jaffe, E. S., Shevach, E., Frank, M. M., and Green, I.,** Leukemic reticuloendotheliosis: presence of a receptor for cytophilic antibody, *Am. J. Med.,* 57, 108, 1974.
5. **Davis, S., Shearer, G. M., Mozes, E., and Sela, M.,** Genetic control of the murine cell-mediated immune response in vivo II H-2 linked responsiveness to the synthetic polypeptide poly(tyr, glu)-poly (DL-Ala)-poly(Lys), *J. Immunol.,* 115, 1530, 1975.
6. **Broder, S., Humphrey, R., Durm, M., Blackman, M., Meade, B., Goldman, C., Strober, W., and Waldmann, T.,** Impaired synthesis of polyclonal immunoglobulins by circulating lymphocytes from patients with multiple myeloma, *N. Engl. J. Med.,* 293, 887, 1975.
7. **Kirchner, H., Holden, H. T., and Herberman, R.,** Splenic suppressor macrophages induced in mice by injection of C. parvum, *J. Immunol.,* 115, 1212, 1975.
8. **Cooper, M. D., Chase, H. P., Lowman, J. T., Krivit, W., and Good, R. A.,** Wiskott-Aldrich Syndrome: An immunologic deficiency disease involving the afferent limb, *Am. J. Med.,* 44, 499, 1968.
9. **Gleichman, E., Gleichman, H., Schwartz, R. S., Weinblatt, A., and Armstrong, M. Y. K.,** Immunologic induction of malignant lymphoma: identification of donor and host tumors in the GVH model, *J. Natl. Cancer Inst.,* 54, 107, 1975.
10. **Padgett, G. A., Reiguam, C. W., Gorham, J. R., Henson, J. B., and O'Mary, C. C.,** Comparative studies of the Chediak-Higashi syndrome, *Am. J. Pathol.,* 51, 553, 1967.
11. **Miller, J. F.,** Analysis of the thymus influence in leukemogenesis, *Nature,* 191, 248, 1961.
12. **Raff, M. C.,** Surface antigenic markers for distinguishing T and B lymphocytes in mice, *Transplant. Rev.,* 6, 52, 1971.
13. **Borella, L. and Sen, L.,** The distribution of lymphocytes with T and B cell surface markers in human bone marrow, *J. Immunol.,* 112, 836, 1974.
14. **Geha, R. A., Rosen, F. S., and Merles, E.,** Identification and characterization of subpopulations of lymphocytes in human peripheral blood after fractionation on discontinuous gradients of albumin, *J. Clin. Invest.,* 52, 1726, 1973.
15. **Jaffe, G. S., Shevach, G. M., Sussman, E. H., Frank, M. M., Green, I., and Berard, C. W.,** Membrane receptor sites for the identification of lymphoreticular cells in benign and malignant conditions, *Br. J. Cancer,* 31, 107, 1975.
16. **Fu, S. M., Winchester, R. J., Rai, K. R., and Kunkel, H. G.,** Hairy cell leukemia: proliferation of a cell with phagocytic and B lymphocyte properties, *Scand. J. Immunol.,* 3, 847, 1974.
17. **Rubin, A. D., Havemann, K., and Dameshek, W.,** Studies in chronic reticulolymphocytic leukemia: further studies of the proliferative abnormality of the blood lymphocyte, *Blood,* 33, 313, 1969.
18. **McCaffrey, R., Smoler, D. F., and Baltimore, D.,** Terminal deoxynucleotidyl transferase in a case of childhood acute lymphoblastic leukemia, *Proc. Natl. Acad. Sci. U.S.A.,* 70, 521, 1973.
19. **Fu, S. M., Winchester, R. J., and Kunkel, H. G.,** The occurrence of the HL-B alloantigens on the cells of unclassified acute lymphoblastic leukemias, *J. Exp. Med.,* 142, 1335, 1975.
20. **Sen, L. and Borella, L.,** Clinical importance of lymphoblasts with T markers in childhood acute leukemia, *N. Engl. J. Med.,* 292, 828, 1975.

21.   **Kaplan, J., Mastrangelo, R., and Peterson, W. D.,** Childhood lymphoblastic lymphoma, a cancer of thymus-derived lymphocytes, *Cancer Res.,* 34, 521, 1974.
22.   **Aisenberg, A. C. and Block, K. J.,** Immunoglobulins on the surface of neoplastic lymphocytes, *N. Engl. J. Med.,* 287, 272, 1972.
23.   **Dickler, H. B., Siegal, F. P., Bentwich, Z. H., and Kunkel, H. G.,** Lymphocyte binding of aggregated IgG and surface Ig staining in CLL, *Clin. Exp. Immunol.,* 14, 97, 1973.
24.   **Schultz, E. F., Davis, S., and Rubin, A. D.,** Further characterization of the circulating cell in CLL, *Blood,* 48, 223, 1976.
25.   **Edelson, R. L., Kirkpatrick, C. H., Shevagh, E. M., Schein, P. S., Smith, R. W., Green, I., and Lutzner, M.,** Preferential antaneous infiltration of neoplastic thymus-derived lymphocytes, *Ann. Int. Med.,* 80, 685, 1974.
26.   **Von Furth, R., Gorter, H., Nadkarni, J. S. et al:** Synthesis of immunoglobulins by biopsied tissues and cell lines from Burkitt's lymphoma, *Immunology,* 22, 847, 1972.
27.   **Mann, R. B., Jaffe, E. S., Braylan, R. C., Nanba, K., Frank, M. M., Zeigler, J. H., and Berard, C. W.,** Non-endemic Burkitt's lymphoma: a B-cell tumor related to germinal centers, *N. Engl. J. Med.,* 295, 685, 1976.
28.   **Jaffe, E. S., Shevach, E. M., Frank, M. M., Berard, C. W., and Green, I.,** Nodular lymphoma — evidence for origin from follicular B lymphocytes, *N. Engl. J. Med.,* 290, 813, 1974.
29.   **Gajl-Peczalska, K. J., Bloomfield, C. D., Coccia, P. F., Sosin, H., Brunning, R. D., and Kersey, J. H.,** B and T cell lymphomas, Analysis of blood and lymph nodes in 87 patients, *Am. J. Med.,* 59, 674, 1975.

Chapter 10

BIOSYNTHESIS OF IMMUNOGLOBULINS IN MYELOMA, MACROGLOBULINEMIA, HEAVY-CHAIN DISEASES, AND AGAMMAGLOBULINEMIA*

Joel N. Buxbaum

TABLE OF CONTENTS

I. INTRODUCTION

Current concepts of lymphoid differentiation accept a major dichotomous development of lymphocytes from a single stem cell.[1] Thymus-derived (or -dependent) cells (T cells) and bone marrow-derived cells (B cells) comprise the two primary classes of lymphocytes. The B-lymphocyte line is ultimately responsible for immunoglobulin synthesis. Several authors have offered possible schemes of B-lymphocyte differentiation based on various lines of evidence including repopulation experiments, studies of cell surface markers, and responses to mitogens.[2,3] Other investigators have attempted to demonstrate that both human and murine B-cell tumors can be compared to different stages in B-cell develop-ment.[4,5] If the tumors represent frozen stages in the B-cell maturational process, they can be studied for insight into the normal process by which the B cell recognizes and responds to antigen.

The differentiation of antibody-forming cells demands that a cell, which has the genetic capacity for synthesizing an immunoglobulin molecule with a particular specificity, express that specificity on its surface prior to exposure to antigen. On seeing its antigen, the sensitive clone both proliferates and differentiates. Hence, one can find B cells with and without surface immunoglobulin and plasma cells which synthesize and secrete most, if not all, of their immunoglobulin as glycosylated, disulfide-linked (H_2L_2) or $(H_2L_2)_n$ molecules.

To become a mature secreting plasma cell, a

*The studies from the author's laboratory cited in this review were supported by grants from the National Cancer Institute (CA 12152) and a Veteran's Administration Research and Education Associateship and Clinical Investigatorship.

naive B lymphocyte must derepress the genetic information for constant and variable regions of both chains, then link either each V and C gene or their RNA transcripts to form single units. The linkage may occur in a preprogrammed manner or after a discrete stimulus. It may take place only in the embryo or in the mature immunologically competent animal. Sufficient data are not yet available to determine which of these is the case. Present evidence indicates that linkage at the DNA level is more likely. The messages must be translated and the protein product transported either to the surface of the cell as receptor, or to the exterior as functional antibody.

Proliferative disorders of the B-lymphocyte-plasma cell system have provided considerable information about these cells and their secreted products. Chronic lymphocytic leukemia cells have served as prototypes for the assay and the study of surface Igs, the receptor for the third component of complement, and the receptor for the immune complexes (Fc receptor). Monoclonal proteins obtained from patients with macroglobulinemia and multiple myeloma have allowed detailed analysis of the chemical structure of immunoglobulins, while cells obtained from these patients have served as isolated systems in which the processes of Ig synthesis, assembly, and secretion could be analyzed. Developmental disorders of Ig synthesis have also proven useful in the formation of our concepts of human immunodifferentiation. In fact, numerous animal experiments involving lymphoid organ extirpation were stimulated by the so-called "experiments of nature" seen in human immunologic deficiency states.

The basic structure of all immunoglobulins (Igs) consists of four polypeptide chains. There are two identical heavy chains and two identical light chains in any given molecule. The heavy chains are specific for each class of Igs (γ = IgG, α = IgA, μ = IgM, δ = IgD, ϵ = IgE) whilst the two light chain classes (K and λ) are found in all the Ig classes, usually in a ratio of 2:1. This is not yet established for normal IgD. IgD myelomas seem to have a K:λ of 1:10 to 1:20 in different series. Spleen cells which stain for cytoplasmic IgD also have a K/λ ratio of 1:10 to 1:20.

Each chain can be structurally divided into two segments: the constant region, which is responsible for its properties as a member of its class, and the variable, which contains the chemical structure responsible for antibody specificity. Serologic and primary structural analyses of large numbers of monoclonal proteins coupled with population studies of the distribution of genetic markers associated with different Ig classes and subclasses have suggested that each of these regions is coded by a separate gene. The individual gene segments are probably linked at the DNA level.[7] This genetic phenomenon represents an outstanding departure from the Lederberg dictum that "one gene codes for one polypeptide chain." The interpretation of the sequence data is dependent upon the assumption that the pathway from DNA to RNA to protein is intact and is analogous to that in *Escherichia coli.*

Most analyses of the process of Ig synthesis assembly and secretion have been carried out in four experimental systems: the hyperimmunized rabbit, the immunized mouse, murine plasmacytomas synthesizing and secreting all the classes of Igs, and cells obtained from humans with myeloma, macroglobulinemia, lymphomas, or agammaglobulinemia.

Igs are not synthesized throughout the cell cycle. A large number of experiments using synchronized human lymphoid lines and murine myeloma cells which are constitutive for Ig production have indicated that Igs are synthesized during the late G_1 and S phases of the cell cycle.[8-10] At least one cell line also synthesizes Ig in part of G_2.[11] The significance of the periodic synthesis is uncertain at this point; however, it has been noted that normal murine spleen cells can secrete anti-sheep erythrocyte antibody (IgM) without going through a phase of DNA synthesis.[12]

The basic features of synthesis in a cell producing Ig for export involve transcription of the appropriate genomic areas to yield mRNAs for heavy and light chains using the appropriate RNA polymerases. The messages for heavy and light chains are transcribed separately from DNA on different chromosomes.[13] It is not clear if they are under coordinate control at the transcriptional level. The mRNAs are longer than necessary to code for polypeptides the exact size of heavy and light chains.[14,15] Like most mammalian messages, there is an untranslated tract of polyadenylic acid at the 3' end of the molecule.[16] The 5' end of the molecule displays the so-called "cap" structure containing a terminal methylated guanosine residue.[17]

When the mRNA has been processed and

transported from the nucleus to the cytoplasm, it is translated on polyribosomes.[18,19] This appears to take place predominantly on membrane-bound polyribosomes, but some studies have suggested that a portion of Ig synthesis occurs on free polysomes.[20,21] The heavy chains are synthesized on larger polysomes than the light chains.[18,19] Both chains are synthesized as polypeptides which are 20 to 25 amino acids longer than the final secreted product.[14,22,23] These residues appear to be removed by an enzyme which is associated with the endoplasmic reticulum. The removal may be universal in the processing of all proteins made for secretion.

All heavy chains and some light chains are glycosylated.[25] Glycosylation of many proteins takes place via a dolichol intermediate. The so-called "core sugars" are assembled into an oligo-saccaride-lipid complex which transfers the sugars *en bloc* to the polypeptide chain.[113] The more distal sugars are then added to the chain in a stepwise fashion. Although early experiments suggested that the individual sugars were added sequentially by a series of glycosyltransferases with the first sugar attached to the asparagine of a ASN-X-$_{SER}^{THR}$ sequence, more recent data indicate that glycosylation of immunoglobulins also follows the dolichol pathway.[26,113] The initial attachment to either ASP or SER takes place while the polypeptide is still nascent on the ribosome.[27] Additional sugars are added either in the Golgi apparatus or the cisternae, while the final glycosyl moieties, fucose and sialic acid, are added as the protein leaves the cell.[28,29] It is still uncertain whether glycosylation is a prerequisite for secretion or whether it merely accompanies the secretory process temporally.[30] The latter seems more likely, since light chains can be released from the cell without the benefit of added sugar, and a recent report suggests that the same may be true for secretion of some heavy chains.[31]

Although it only takes 30 sec for the cell to synthesize a light chain and 60 sec for a gamma chain, it takes about 20 min for the newly synthesized molecules to get out of the cell.[19] This allows time for both assembly and glyco-sylation to take place. In IgM-secreting cells, despite the additional assembly steps, the secretory rate appears to be the same.[32,33]

In normal immune cells, heavy- and light-chain synthesis is balanced, or a small excess of light chains is produced.[34] This is reflected in the excretion of small amounts of free kappa and lambda light chains in normal urine.[35,36] The extent of the excess of light-chain production is not known, since free light chains are both digested and excreted by the normal kidney.[37] Turnover studies have suggested that excess light chains are synthesized at the rate of 8 to 18 mg/kg/day in normal humans.[38] In the same study, IgG was produced at rates of 35 to 62 mg/kg/day. However, labeling experiments carried out with bone marrow cells from patients with polyclonal hyperglobulinemia have revealed almost balanced synthesis (Figure 1).

If one considers the sequence of disulfide bond formation between chains, there are a finite number of ways to assemble H_2L_2.

$$H + L \longrightarrow HL$$
$$HL + HL \longrightarrow H_2L_2 \tag{1}$$

$$H + L \longrightarrow HL$$
$$HL + H \longrightarrow H_2L$$
$$H_2L + L \longrightarrow H_2L_2 \tag{2}$$

$$H + H \longrightarrow H_2$$
$$H_2 + L \longrightarrow H_2L$$
$$H_2L + L \longrightarrow H_2L_2 \tag{3}$$

$$H + H \longrightarrow H_2$$
$$L + L \longrightarrow L_2$$
$$H_2 + L_2 \longrightarrow (H_2)(L_2) \tag{4}$$

The formation of the initial L-L, H-L, or H-H disulfides probably occurs while one chain is still on the polysome, although it may not always be the case.[18,19] Most of the disulfide formation takes place within the cisternae of the endoplasmic reticulum. The sequence of disulfide bond formation is related to the number and position of the bonds between the heavy chains, a property of the particular subclass of IgG.[39] Recent data from several laboratories have indicated that the sequence of disulfide formation is determined by the primary structure of the molecule, since the same assembly intermediates are formed when the iso-

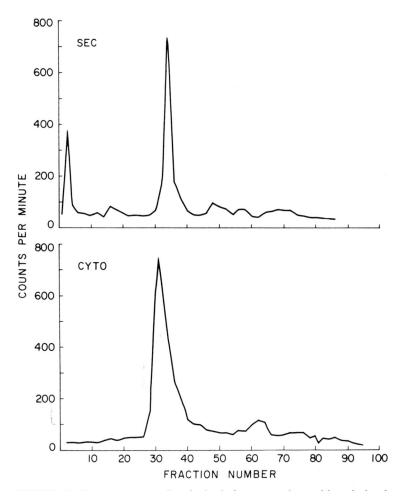

FIGURE 1. Bone marrow cells obtained from a patient with polyclonal hypergammaglobulinemia whose urine contained normal amounts of free kappa and lambda chains were incubated in short-term tissue culture for 4 hr with radioactive amino acids. The cells were removed and the supernatant medium treated as secreted material. The cell pellet was washed and lysed with a nonionic detergent which lyses cell membranes but leaves nuclear membranes intact. The detergent-treated cytoplasm (bottom panel) and the supernatant medium (top) were then precipitated with an antiserum directed against the light-chain-containing portion of the IgG molecule which reacted with both free and bound kappa and lambda chains. The precipitates were washed, dissolved in sodium dodecyl sulfate (SDS) (an anionic detergent which interrupts noncovalent molecular interactions without disturbing covalent linkages), and electrophoresed on SDS-containing polyacrylamide gels. The electrophoresis separates molecules on the basis of molecular weight. The largest molecules are furthest to the left. Marker proteins, H_2L_2, HL, H, and L were run on the same gels (not shown). The gels were then fractionated and the radioactivity per fraction counted. The cytoplasm contained a major peak of radioactivity corresponding to the H_2L_2 marker, which on reduction and alkylation with 2-mercaptoethanol and iodo-acetamide yielded heavy and light chains (not shown). A small peak probably containing a small amount of unbound light chain is seen between fractions 61 and 64. The secretions contained two peaks, one corresponding in mobility to that seen in the cytoplasm ($\gamma_2 L_2$), and a larger protein migrating to fraction 4, which represents 19S IgM.

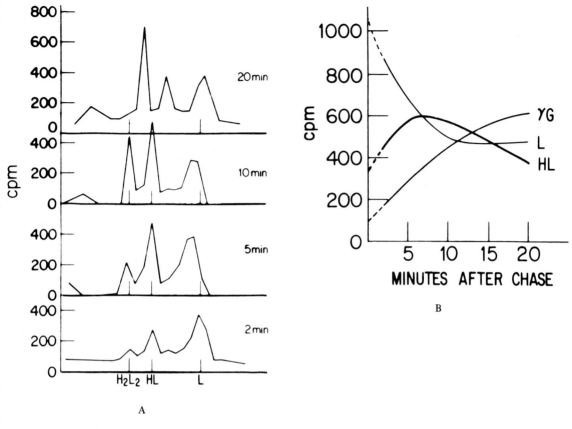

FIGURE 2. Bone marrow cells from a patient with an IgG-producing myeloma were incubated for 2 min with radioactive amino acids (pulse). At 2 min a large excess of unlabeled amino acids was added to the incubation mixture, allowing protein synthesis to continue but effectively stopping the incorporation of radioactive precursor by dilution (chase). Aliquots of cells were removed at the times indicated and treated as described in Figure 1. The electropherograms of the immunologically precipitated cytoplasms at various times after chase are shown in Figure 2A. A kinetic plot demonstrating the precursor nature of L and HL is shown in Figure 2B.

lated Igs are reduced and allowed to reoxidize in the test tube.[40,41] For at least one human IgG subclass (IgG_1), the rate of disulfide formation in vitro is similar to that seen inside the cell. The rate of reoxidation of IgG_4, however, is much slower. There is no comparative data available for the intracellular assembly of IgG_4, nor of any of the other human IgG subclasses.

A typical assembly experiment in human cells producing an IgG_1 protein is shown in Figure 2a. The patient produced an excess of light chains; however, it is clear from the kinetic plot that some of the L chains were precursors of HL and that both were precursors of H_2L_2 via the HL pathway (Figure 2b).

When a large series of mouse myeloma tumors was studied, it was evident that the major pathway of assembly was a property of the class of IgG produced by the tumor.[42] Since each of the murine classes also has a characteristic number and position of interchain disulfides, it is likely that it is the determining factor.[43,44]

Figure 3 shows a cytoplasmic sample from a patient with IgA myeloma which contains H_2L_2, H_2L, and HL. Without kinetic data (like that shown in Figure 2b), it was not possible to tell which of these were precursor intermediates and which were end-products.

The postribosomal assembly of IgA and IgM present additional problems to the cell. IgM exists in the serum as a pentamer of H_2L_2 subunits, while IgA proteins exist as monomers or dimers. The polymers, when isolated from serum, consist of four-chain monomers and an additional polypeptide with a molecular weight of 15,000, called J chain, which is presumed to serve a linkage

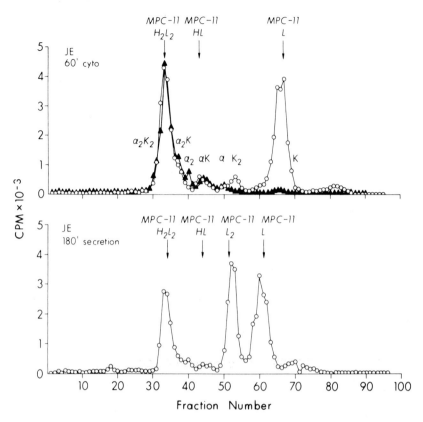

FIGURE 3. Electropherograms of immunologically precipitated cytoplasm and secreted material from labeled bone marrow cells obtained from a patient with an IgA myeloma. A variety of intracellular intermediates were seen including α, αK, α_2, and $\alpha_2 K$. ○——○ anti-light chain precipitate, △——△ anti-α chain precipitate.

function.[45,46] When IgA monomers obtained from the cytoplasm of murine myeloma cells were mixed in vitro with isolated J chain and a disulfide interchange enzyme, there was quantitative association to form dimers.[47] However, not all IgA-producing cells assemble their monomers into covalently bound dimers.[48]

Two observations have been made which suggest that polymerization is still not fully understood. The first indicates that some but not all IgG-synthesizing myelomas also synthesize the J chain.[49,108] The explanation for the cellular synthesis of a protein which is not necessary for assembly of its Ig is not apparent. The second is the heterogeneity of human cells producing both IgA and IgM with respect to the presence of intracellular covalently assembled polymers.[48,50] The latter could be explained by different concentrations of J chain present in different myeloma cell populations, with the amount of available J chain being a limiting factor. Recently, kinetic studies have demonstrated the intracellular incorporation of J chain into Ig polymers and suggest that the latter is true.[51]

When the secretory process is examined, there appears to be a characteristic relationship between the incorporation of radioactive precursors into intracellular material and the secretion of immunoglobulin. Most populations of marrow cells in which plasma cells are prominent reach intracellular equilibrium of labeled material by 4 hr. The amount of labeled Ig secreted exceeds the intracellular level at about the same time (Figure 4). In nonsecreting cell populations, the extracellular label never exceeds the intracellular label. This is true no matter what the nature of the final intracellular Ig product.

II. MYELOMA

In multiple myeloma, chain synthesis may be balanced or unbalanced (Table 1). When bone

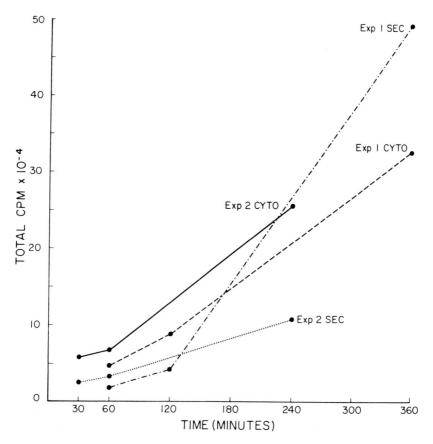

FIGURE 4. Bone marrow cells obtained from a patient whose serum and urine contained free λ chains were incubated as described in Figure 1. Experiment 1 was carried out before therapy had reduced the plasma cell content (30%) of the marrow. Experiment 2 was performed when there were fewer than 1% plasma cells present. The amount of radioactive precursor incorporated into protein per aliquot of cells was determined by trichloroacetic acid precipitation. Experiment 1 demonstrates linear incorporation of precursor into cytoplasmic proteins through the 6-hr incubation period. By 180 min the radioactivity in the secretions exceeds that found intracellularly, indicating that the bulk of the protein synthesized during this period is made for secretion. This is the typical pattern seen in cells secreting large amounts of immunoglobulins. Experiment 2 shows a similar experiment in a predominantly nonsecreting cell population. The amount of labeled secreted material never exceeds the amount of labeled cytoplasmic protein, although the kinetics of incorporation are virtually identical, since the slopes of incorporation into cytoplasmic proteins in Experiments 1 and 2 are the same.

marrow cells from patients with myeloma are labeled in short-term culture, only 20 to 25% of patients with IgG and 10 to 15% with IgA myeloma proteins exhibit balanced synthesis of H and L chains.[48,52] About 20% of myelomas are characterized by the production of light chains only.[53] In general, monomers (L) are the dominant intracellular form, while the dimer (L_2) is the major extracellular molecular species. Exceptions to this occur with moderate frequency. Very rarely, light-chain polymers larger than dimers

have been seen.[54,55] One case has been noted in which disulfide-linked polymers were found intracellularly.[109]

Hence, in human myeloma cells the kinetics of synthesis and secretion have been established. A variety of intermediates have been seen, and some questions have been raised concerning the formation of higher molecular weight polymers.

One group of myeloma patients which has not been adequately investigated is the 1% of patients classified as nonsecretors. This appears to be a

TABLE 1

Molecular Structure of Proteins in Myeloma

	Serum protein	Urine Protein
IgG	$\gamma_2 K_2$	0, K, or K_2
	$\gamma_2 K_2$ + K or K_2	0, K, or K_2
	$\gamma_2 \lambda_2$	0, λ, or λ_2
	$\gamma_2 \lambda_2$ + λ or λ_2	0, λ, or λ_2
IgA	$\alpha_2 K_2 \pm (\alpha_2 K_2)_n$	0, K, or K_2
	$\alpha_2 K_2 \pm (\alpha_2 K_2)_n$ + K or K_2	0, K, or K_2
	$\alpha_2 \lambda_2 \pm (\alpha_2 \lambda_2)_n$	0, λ, or λ_2
	$\alpha_2 \lambda_2 \pm (\alpha_2 \lambda_2)_n$ + λ or λ_2	0, λ, or λ_2
K or λ	0	K or K_2, λ or λ_2
	K, K_2, or K_4[a]	K or K_2
	λ, λ_2, or λ_4[a]	λ or λ_2
HCD	γ_2	0 or γ_2
	$\alpha_2 \ldots (\alpha_2)_2$	0
	μ_{10}	0 or K or λ
Normal	$\gamma_2 K_2 + \gamma_2 \lambda_2$ (2:1)	K, K_2, λ, λ_2 K:λ = 2:1
	$\alpha_2 K_2 + \alpha_2 \lambda_2$ (2:1)	K, K_2, λ, λ_2 K:λ = 2:1
	$(\alpha_2 K_2)_2 + (\alpha_2 \lambda_2)_2$	

[a]Free light chains are found in the serum in significant amounts in the presence of severe renal disease or when present in a highly polymerized form.[35-37,54,55]

heterogeneous group, some of which have an abnormality of the rough endoplasmic reticulum which is necessary for the normal synthesis of large amounts of Igs.[56] Immunofluorescent studies on these patients reveal no intracellular fluorescence. Cells from another group of patients whose serum and urine contained no detectable monoclonal protein have demonstrated peculiar immunofluorescent patterns, suggesting either unusual or deficient antigenicity of their intracellular Ig chains.[57,58] When biosynthetic studies were carried out with cells obtained from several of these patients, they incorporated radioactivity into immunoglobulin at a much lower rate than cells from the usual myeloma.[110] Each appeared to synthesize and secrete excess light chains of normal size and antigenicity. Some cell populations also synthesized other molecules with Ig antigenic determinants with unusual molecular weights, hence uncertain molecular configurations. It could not be determined if these represented structurally aberrant heavy chains or heavy chains without carbohydrate. Thus, it appears that some of these tumor cell populations synthesize nothing; others synthesize and secrete small amounts of free light chains and other molecules in vitro. Either they fail to do this in vivo, which is unlikely, or the amounts produced are too small to detect by conventional methods. Small amounts of free light chains and other Ig fragments are catabolized by the normal kidney and may not be seen either in the serum or urine.

There are no data available on the qualitative aspects of the synthesis, secretion, and assembly of IgE or IgD by myeloma cells. It is likely that their assembly processes will be similar to those noted for IgG.

III. MACROGLOBULINEMIA

In patients with Waldenström's macroglobulinemia, the marrow contains a pleiomorphic lymphoplasmacytic cell population which has been compared to that seen in the granulocytic series in the chronic myelogenous leukemia.[60] It usually contains small and medium-sized lymphocytes and plasma cells. Immunofluorescent studies have indicated that the lymphocytes synthesize and display monoclonal IgM on the cell surface, while the plasma cells have little or no surface IgM, and contain large amounts in the cytoplasm, presumably synthesized for secretion.

In the mouse, individual IgM-producing tumors are less pleiomorphic, but examination of five of these tumors revealed that some synthesize most of their IgM for insertion into the cell membrane, while others have little on the surface and secrete most of that which is synthesized.[5]

IgM synthesis has been studied extensively in cells obtained from macroglobulinemic humans and mice.[32,33,50] The basic features of synthesis from transcription to the assembly of H_2L_2 are probably identical to those of IgG. The assembly of the 8S subunits into 19S molecules and the relationship of the assembly process to secretion are still not clear.

The 8S subunits are assembled as rapidly as IgG or IgA via similar pathways. In about one fourth of the human macroglobulinemics and six of seven murine tumors studied, the subunit persisted as the major intracellular Ig. Little or no 19S polymer was seen inside the cell. In one mouse tumor and most human samples, the major intracellular IgM was the 19S polymer. In the former, it was not possible to demonstrate the progression of radioactively labeled subunits into and out of a rapidly turning over intracellular 19S pool. In the latter, one could easily see the progression of molecules from 8S monomers to 19S polymers.[61] There did appear to be some dilution of newly assembled μ_2L_2 molecules by the pool of 8S monomers which appears to be present. Hence, there was heterogeneity in assembly among human and mouse cells producing IgM. There also appeared to be a species difference in the major pathway of assembly.

There is little amino acid sequence data available to compare human and mouse IgM, but it does appear that all the murine IgMs examined to date lack a cysteine-containing peptide analogous to that containing the intersubunit bond in the human. When the cysteine-containing peptides of murine proteins which were not assembled intracellularly were compared with those that were, no differences were observed.[62,111]

Cells demonstrating both types of assembly patterns contain J chain. It has not been determined whether they have similar amounts of the putative joining peptide.

The phenomena described above raise several questions. Are cellular differences responsible for the assembly or lack of assembly in various IgM-producing cell populations, or does the difference in process merely reflect differences in the chemical structure of the different proteins? There are no chemical data available to suggest this in the human IgMs, and the few studies available in the mouse have not yet demonstrated a significant structural difference.

Are the 8S monomers of cells which do not contain intracellular 19S assembled inside the cell? If they are, what is the relationship between assembly and secretion? The inability to chase subunits into intracellular polymer is difficult to reconcile with an intracellular assembly process. The appearance of some subunits extracellularly plus the observation that some SH groups can be alkylated with ^{14}C-iodoacetamide as the IgM is released into the medium in vitro suggests that the process may take place extracellularly, perhaps with the subunits still fixed to the cell membrane.[112] This is not consistent with recent data obtained in mouse spleen cells indicating that IgM destined to be secreted as 19S polymer could not be labeled by the lactoperoxidase iodination procedure, i.e., it was not available to the enzyme at the cell surface.[72]

Why don't intracellular 8S monomers spontaneously polymerize intracellularly? Some experiments have demonstrated that intracellular subunits will polymerize if the cytoplasm is mildly reduced with dithiothreitol or 2-mercaptoethanol.[64] This observation, coupled with the experiments demonstrating subunit J-chain recombination in the presence of disulfide interchange enzyme, suggest that the intersubunit SH groups are blocked inside the cell and polymerization takes place only when disulfide interchange occurs as an active process.[51] Spleen cells obtained from immunized rabbits can be extracted to yield a substance which will cause IgM subunits obtained from concanavalin A stimulated (non-immune) rabbit spleen cells to sediment as 19S molecules on sucrose gradients.[65] It was not fully established that the polymerization was covalent; nonetheless, the results are comparable to those seen in the mouse system. The data also indicated that an inhibitor of polymerization was present both in spleen and liver. Hence, it may be that the polymerizing activity is induced in rabbit spleen during the course of immunization to a degree sufficient to overcome the inhibitor. The only objection to this hypothesis is the inconsistency between the rate of polymerization in vitro, which is slow, and that seen intracellularly, which must be very rapid. Additional experiments have also suggested that the subunits present in NP-40 (a nonionic detergent) cell lysates can polymerize under appropriate conditions without prior reduction or the addition of additional J chain or disulfide interchange enzyme.[112]

IV. HEAVY-CHAIN DISEASES

The most recently described of the immunoproliferative disorders associated with the presence of a monoclonal protein in the serum are the heavy-chain diseases (HCD). They comprise a group of conditions in which there is a predominantly lymphocytic proliferation and an apparently characteristic clinical picture for each of the three classes of immunoglobulin heavy chain.[66] Gamma heavy-chain disease is most commonly associated with a lymphomatous disorder with hepatosplenomegaly, anemia, and multiple infections.[67] Most cases of alpha heavy-chain disease have been seen in patients with the Mediterranean type of abdominal lymphoma with malabsorption. A few cases have been seen with nonmalignant pulmonary disease.[68] Mu heavy-chain proteins have been found in patients with atypical chronic lymphocytic leukemia.[69] The nature of the relationship between the type of HCD protein and the particular clinical syndrome is not clear. The cell populations synthesizing the various classes of HCD proteins generally reflect the cell populations normally responsible for the synthesis of nonmalignant intact Igs of the same class, i.e. lymphocytes synthesize IgM, gut-associated plasma cells synthesize IgA, and splenic and nodal lymphocytes produce IgG.

Investigation of the molecular pathology of the HCDs has indicated that the molecules in the serum and urine are incomplete heavy chains. Amino acid sequence analyses of many of these proteins have shown that most have internal deletions which start in the variable region and extend into the constant region either to a position just proximal to (from the amino terminus) or distal to the hinge region of the heavy chain. Some of the deletions appear to be N-terminal.[70]

The second defect, thus far seen only in alpha and gamma HCD, is the absence of light-chain synthesis in the cells synthesizing the deleted heavy chains. Mu chain disease cells frequently synthesize light chains which are not linked to the aberrant heavy chains.[71] A few cases have been described in which a γ-chain deletion has not included the cysteine which participates in the heavy-light disulfide. In these cases, the final cell product consists of an $H_2 L_2$ molecule in which the heavy chain is abnormal.[70]

Biosynthetic studies have been carried out with cells from several patients with γHCD, αHCD, and μ chain disease. None of the studies have indicated that a degradative process is primary in the generation of the short chains. Longer precursors were not seen in any instance, although in one case the serum protein was slightly smaller than that found intra- or extracellularly in vitro.[72-74] The in vitro studies have also indicated that the heavy-chain fragments polymerize in a manner similar to the intact proteins, even though the light chains are absent.

Certain questions have still not been answered concerning the molecular biology of the primary defect in these cells. The size of the heavy-chain messenger RNA has not been established. The size of the message will provide evidence as to the presence of a deletion at the DNA level or an area of missense which has resulted in a normal-sized mRNA. It has not yet been established whether light-chain mRNA is present in any of the cells which do not synthesize L-chain proteins. Some data have been presented that the latter occurs in at least one murine cell line.[75]

The precise relationship between the HCD proteins and normal Ig synthesis has not yet been established. Perhaps studies of these cells and proteins will provide insight into the mechanism of integration of the genomic information for variable and constant regions of Ig chains.

V. SURFACE Ig IN MACROGLOBULINEMIA AND MYELOMA

Readily detectable surface Ig is a primary identifying characteristic of normal peripheral B lymphocytes. In the human, when SIg is carefully analyzed, using the $(Fab')_2$ fragments of monospecific antisera as the fluoresceinated reagent after in vitro overnight incubation of the subject lymphocytes, 10 to 15% of normal peripheral lymphocytes carry readily detectable Ig. The majority of these display either IgM, IgD, or both.[59,76]

Since the first demonstration of Igs on the surface of some lymphocytes (SIg), it has been difficult for investigators to reach consensus on the presence of SIg on cells which secrete substantial amounts of Ig. A variety of techniques have been used to detect SIgs. Immunofluorescence, radioiodination, reversed immunocytoadherence, and the displacement type of radioimmunoassay have all been employed with sometimes conflicting results. It now seems certain that most, but not all, plasma cells have SIg.[77] Detection of surface staining and capping on some cells may require inhibition of protein synthesis in order to reduce the amount of protein secreted so that the assay system is not in antigen excess.

In the largest series of myeloma patients, SIg corresponding antigenically to the monoclonal serum protein was found on the marrow myeloma cells in 62% of the patients.[77] In the remaining 38% of patients, a variety of SIg patterns were noted, some of which were not consistent with our current understanding of Ig and SIg synthesis. In those cases, antigens of more than one heavy chain were found on single cells. If those observations are confirmed, further studies will be required to ascertain whether this is a normal phenomenon or one which is associated with malignancy or adaptation to culture.

An additional phenomenon which has been noted in myeloma has caused a considerable degree of controversy. In some patients (5 of 40 in one series), a fraction of the peripheral lymphocytes has been found to display SIg with the same heavy- and light-chain determinants as the monoclonal protein found in the serum.[78,79] Several explanations have been offered to account for these observations. The first interprets the stained cells as a circulating subset of the monoclonal population seen in the marrow. These may be either plasma cells or lymphocytes (in the manner hypothesized for macroglobulinemia).

A second interpretation implicates nonspecific binding of the circulating monoclonal protein via the B-cell Fc receptor. This cannot be totally responsible, since experiments in which the SIg is removed by in vitro trypsinization followed by incubation and resynthesis have revealed that the lymphocytes themselves synthesized the monoclonal protein.

The most radical suggestion offered to explain these observations invokes a transfer of information from the malignant myeloma cells to normal lymphocytes, converting their SIg to that of the malignant clone.[80] Several studies have now been reported in which RNA has been extracted from mouse myeloma cells and either injected into virgin mice or added to virgin spleen cells in vitro. In both cases, a significant proportion of the recipient lymphocytes are converted to possess surface Ig identical to the monoclonal protein synthesized by the tumor cells of the RNA donor.[81] These provocative observations must be confirmed and extended by other workers before the validity of the hypothesis can be judged.

In macroglobulinemia, the marrow and peripheral lymphocytes SIgs carry both the class and idiotypic specificities of the serum protein.[77] It is possible that the SIg of the peripheral lymphocytes reflect the same process as in myeloma (*vide supra*); however, there is little stimulus to hypothesize, since there is already evidence for monoclonal lymphocytic proliferation in the bone marrow.

As was previously stated, the lymphocyte population in the marrow is monoclonal but is heterogeneous in size and in the intracellular distribution of its IgM. The small lymphocytes show SIg, while the plasma cells show substantial cytoplasmic staining.

Mouse tumors synthesizing IgM have been likened to normal B lymphocytes frozen in maturation at different times after mitogen stimulation.[5] Several had the bulk of their IgM expressed on the cell surface, while several others synthesized most or all of their IgM for secretion. It was clear, however, that the same cell could do both. It is presently not known how the cell determines which molecules go to the surface for integration into the cell membrane and which are assembled for secretion. It is also possible that they are two entirely separate pools of molecules.[82]

Despite the ready availability of material for study, data concerning the details of synthesis of SIg are insufficient. Many studies have examined the kinetics of release (or shedding) of SIg into the culture medium in vitro, the time necessary to reexpress SIg after enzymatic digestion, and the nature of the SIg molecule itself by radioiodination or biosynthetic labeling followed by analysis on acrylamide gel electrophoresis.[83-86,90]

These studies have revealed that the cells which express monoclonal IgM on their surfaces do so as a $\mu_2 L_2$ subunit. There has been some discussion concerning the size of the molecule, since on gels it appears to be 20 to 30% greater in molecular weight than expected. The surface membrane-bound IgM will not polymerize to form the 19S polymer even after it is shed from the cell. It must, therefore, be qualitatively different from that which is synthesized for secretion either in its intrinsic structure or because it is bound to some other cell constituent. The latter would prevent it from behaving as an IgM subunit destined to be assembled into a secreted antibody. Studies on the human lymphoid line (Daudi) reveal that, despite the fact that its SIg is not truly a secretory protein, it is synthesized on membrane-bound polysomes and is glycosylated as if it were synthesized for secretion.[87] Some of the available experimental data in other systems suggest that there may be either a qualitative or kinetic difference in the terminal glycosylation of membrane-associated IgM, but it could not be established whether the observation was related to cause or effect.[5]

The data for turnover times are confusing. A cultured lymphoid line (8866) treated with puromycin shed its SIg with a half-life of about 45 min. However, in other lines, resynthesis experiments, either after antibody-induced modulation or enzymatic digestion, have revealed a resynthesis half-life of 3 to 9 hr; hence, there is a discrepancy using these two techniques.[87-90]

Examination of the turnover time of the SIgM in normal murine spleen cells has also resulted in discordant results; however, recent data in this system suggests that there may be two discrete pools of surface Ig each with a different half-line.[82] Perhaps the same situation prevails in human cells, accounting for the different results from different laboratories.

VI. REGULATION OF Ig SYNTHESIS IN MYELOMA AND MACROGLOBULINEMIA

Some patients and mice bearing Ig-producing tumors have been found to be immunologically deficient.[91-93] They cannot mount an adequate primary immune response to new antigens. This may be the reason for their frequent bacterial infections. Several hypotheses for the defect have been offered and rejected. It is not the consequence of cellular nutrient deficiency or crowding out of immunocompetent cells by tumor cells,

since it does not occur in other nonplasmacytic tumors with equal marrow involvement. The fractional catabolic rate of some classes of IgG increase with their increasing serum level, but this cannot totally account for the low levels of other classes of Ig or the insufficient IgM response to primary immunization.

Some data have been obtained in the murine plasmacytoma system which indicate that a humoral factor is produced either by the tumor cells or by normal cells in response to the tumor cells.[94,95] This factor is capable of inhibiting the primary immune response to sheep erythrocytes. Some workers have suggested that RNA from the myeloma cells is the humoral substance (*vide supra*).[81]

Recent observations in humans with myeloma are somewhat at odds with a humoral immunosuppressive agent.[96] Many patients with myeloma are unable to respond to stimulation with pokeweed mitogen (a B-cell mitogen). The normal response included both cell division and an increase in protein synthesis which was in large part IgM. When a cell population which adhered to plastic was isolated from the peripheral blood of some of these patients and mixed with normal lymphocytes capable of giving a positive response to pokeweed, it inhibited the normal cell's reaction. Since these experiments were carried out in a small number of patients, it may reflect a heterogeneity of suppressive mechanisms rather than a true contradiction of the other proposed mechanism. In either case, normal Ig synthesis is frequently suppressed in myeloma.

VII. AGAMMAGLOBULINEMIA – Ig SYNTHESIS

From the above, one can predict the circumstances under which Ig synthesis could be defective. The precursor B cells may be totally absent. They may be unable to synthesize the polypeptide chains. They may be able to synthesize but unable to secrete their Ig. Finally, B cells may be capable of performing all the steps necessary for the synthesis and secretion of Ig, yet are prevented from doing so by either a humoral or cellular suppressor or the lack of a necessary stimulator substance.

The primary humoral response to most antigens requires cooperation between T and B cells.[96,97] Hence, T cells can exert a positive regulatory effect on B-cell function. It is now also becoming evident that there are T cells which can exert negative control on humoral responses.[98] These suppressor cells seem to be a specific subset of T cells with characteristic surface antigens. It is not yet certain how they influence B cells, i.e., if suppression requires direct contact or is humorally mediated. Most of the present data favor a soluble mediator.

Patients with each of these types of humoral immunodeficiences have been described and investigated. In the majority of cases of infantile x-linked agammaglobulinemia, B-cell precursors are absent; hence, Ig-bearing lymphocytes are absent from the peripheral blood.[99] A small number of patients have been found to have normal or near-normal numbers of lymphocytes bearing the C_3 receptor, another B-cell marker, suggesting that in development the capacity of B cells to synthesize the C_3 receptor appears before the capacity to synthesize Ig. These cells do not respond to Pokeweed mitogen (PWM).[100]

Several categories of deficiency have been described in which circulating B lymphocytes are present.[101] These cells display SIg as well as other B-cell markers despite markedly reduced or absent serum Ig. They do not respond to mitogens. Patients with isolated IgA deficiency have normal numbers of circulating IgA-bearing lymphocytes, although they have little or no serum or secretory IgA.[102] When these cells are exposed to PWM, they can synthesize and secrete normal amounts of IgA into the medium. These cells appear to be blocked in the steps that allow final maturation into a secreting lymphocyte or plasma cell. Recently a patient has been described who had normal serum IgA but defective epithelial cell secretory component (SC) production.[103] Radio-labeling of intestinal biopsy cells of this patient revealed IgA synthesis to be intact, but secretion into the intestinal lumen was defective because of lack of attachment of SC. Unfortunately, cells of neither of these groups of patients have been effectively exploited experimentally to determine the precise nature of the molecular defects. The kinetics of synthesis after PWM would be particularly interesting in the IgA-deficient patients, since they must have the machinery available for normal IgA synthesis, and the induction process might be experimentally accessible.

The most interesting group of these patients is that falling into the heterogeneous category of common variable immunodeficiency (CVI). These patients may have normal, reduced, or increased numbers of SIg-bearing lymphocytes. They may or may not respond to a mitogenic factor released by normal thymocytes, and they may or may not suppress normal lymphocyte responses to PWM on cocultivation.[104] At this point, there is no single parameter which allows one to clearly distinguish different subsets of this population. Some of these individuals have circulating cells which are capable of suppressing the Ig-producing response of normal B cells to PWM.[105] These cells appear to be T cells, since they can be isolated by using unsensitized SRBCs to form "E" rosettes (a property of human T cells) and separating the rosette-forming cells by centrifugation. The separated population can then produce the suppressor phenomenon when incubated with normal peripheral blood lymphocytes from another individual. These T cells can thus negatively affect B-cell Ig synthesis.

If one measures spontaneous Ig synthesis in peripheral lymphocytes obtained from these patients, the rate of incorporation of radioactivity is very low compared to normal peripheral blood lymphocyte (PBL). One study purports to show a qualitative difference between these cells and normals, specifically a greater synthesis of IgM by the CVI cells with less secretion per unit time. The data supporting this contention are not convincing, particularly since the amounts of material synthesized are quite small and may be merely a reflection of the few normal B cells present.[106]

Recently, data have been presented suggesting that in at least one of these patients the Ig is not secreted because of a defect in glycosylation.[106,107] The authors imply that glycosylation of the Ig polypeptide chain is required for secretion. The experiments suggest that both glycosylation and secretion are faulty in the cells studied; however, there is no indication of a cause-and-effect relationship. Other investigators have convincingly demonstrated that glycosylation is not necessary for secretion in murine myeloma cells and their variants.[30,31]

Cells derived from agammaglobulinemic patients have yielded some interesting insights concerning possible mechanisms of regulation of cells synthesizing Igs, but still remain a relatively untapped source of potential information and excitement.

VIII. SUMMARY

Proliferative and developmental disorders of Ig-producing cells and their precursors have been extremely useful tools for the detailed analysis of the processes of Ig synthesis, assembly, and secretion. The ultimate relevance of these observations awaits their application to the analysis of normal cells under physiologic conditions. The techniques for these analyses are being developed during the study of the abnormal states, and the questions to be answered are becoming more sharply defined.

ACKNOWLEDGMENT

The author gratefully wishes to acknowledge the expert secretarial assistance of Ms. Linda Dezego.

REFERENCES

1. Greaves, M. F., Owen, J. J. T., and Raff, M. C., *T and B Lymphocytes, Origins, Properties and Roles in Immune Responses,* American Elsevier, New York, 1974.
2. Cooper, M. D. and Lawton, A. R., Development of T and B cells and their functional interactions, in *Immunodeficiency in Man and Animals,* Bergsma, D., Good, R. A., and Finstad, J., Eds., National Foundation and Sinauer Associates, Sunderland, Mass., 1975.
3. Möller, G., Ed., Separation of T and B lymphocyte subpopulations, *Transplant. Rev.,* 25, 1, 1975.
4. Salmon, S. E. and Seligmann, M., B-cell neoplasia in man, *Lancet,* ii, 1230, 1974.
5. Andersson, J., Buxbaum, J., Citronbaum, R., Douglas, S., Forni, L., Melchers, F., Pernis, B., and Stott, D., IgM producing tumors in the BALB/c mouse, a model for B-cell maturation, *J. Exp. Med.,* 140, 742, 1974.
6. Pernis, B., Governa, M., and Rowe, D. S., Light chain types in plasma cells that produce IgD, *Immunology,* 16, 685, 1969.
7. Dreyer, W. J., Gray, W. R., and Hood, L., The genetic molecular and cellular basis of antibody formation: some facts and a unifying hypothesis, *Cold Spring Harbor Symp. Quant. Biol.,* 32, 353, 1967.
8. Buell, D. N. and Fahey, J. L., Limited periods of gene expression in immunoglobulin-synthesizing cells, *Science,* 164, 1524, 1969.
9. Garatun-Tjeldsto, O., Pryme, I. F., Weltman, J. K., and Dowben, R. M., Synthesis and secretion of light-chain immunoglobulin in two successive cycles of synchronized plasma cells, *J. Cell Biol.,* 68, 232, 1976.
10. Cowan, N. J. and Milstein, C., Automatic monitoring of biochemical parameters in tissue culture. Studies on synchronously growing mouse myeloma cells, *Biochem. J.,* 128, 445, 1972.
11. Watanabe, S., Yagi, Y., and Pressman, D., Immunoglobulin production in synchronized cultures of human hematopoietic cell lines, *J. Immunol.,* 111, 797, 1973.
12. Sulitzeanu, D., Marbrook, J., and Haskill, J. S., Direct conversion of precursors into active PFC's *in vitro* without prior cell division, *Immunology,* 24, 707, 1973.
13. Martensson, L., Gm genes and γG molecules, in *Acta Univ. Lund. Sect. 2,* 3, 1, 1966.
14. Swan, D., Aviv, H., and Leder, P., Purification and properties of biologically active messenger RNA for a myeloma light chain, *Proc. Natl. Acad. Sci. U.S.A.,* 69, 1967, 1972.
15. Cowan, N. J. and Milstein, C., The translation *in vitro* of mRNA for immunoglobulin heavy chains, *Eur. J. Biochem.,* 36, 1, 1973.
16. Brownlee, G. G., Cartwright, E. M., Cowan, N. J., Jarvis, J. M., and Milstein, C., Purification and sequence of messenger RNA for immunoglobulin light chains, *Nature (London) New Biol.,* 224, 236, 1973.
17. Cory, S. and Adams, J. A., The modified 5' terminal sequences in messenger RNA of mouse myeloma cells, *J. Mol. Biol.,* 99, 519, 1975.
18. Shapiro, A. L., Scharff, M. D., Maizel, J. V., and Uhr, J. W., Polyribosomal synthesis and assembly of the H and L chains of gamma globulin, *Proc. Natl. Acad. Sci. U.S.A.,* 56, 216, 1966.
19. Askonas, B. A. and Williamson, A., Biosynthesis of immunoglobulins on polyribosomes and assembly of the IgG molecule, *Proc. R. Soc. London, Ser. B,* 166, 232, 1966.
20. Vassalli, P., Studies on cell free synthesis of rat immunoglobulins. I. A cell-free system for protein synthesis prepared from lymph-node microsomal vesilles, *Proc. Natl. Acad. Sci. U.S.A.,* 58, 2117, 1967.
21. Pryme, I. F., Garatun-Tjeldsto, O., Birckbichler, P. J., Weltman, J. K., and Dowben, R. M., Synthesis of immunoglobulins by membrane-bound polysomes and free polysomes from plasmacytoma cells, *Eur. J. Biochem.,* 33, 374, 1973.
22. Milstein, C., Brownlee, G. G., Harrison, T. M., and Mathews, M. B., A possible precursor of immunoglobulin light chains, *Nature (London) New Biol.,* 239, 117, 1972.

23. **Blobel, G. and Dobberstein, B.,** Transfer of proteins across membranes. I. Release of proteolytically processed and unprocessed nascent immunoglobulin light chains on membrane-bound polysomes of murine myeloma, *J. Cell Biol.,* 67, 835, 1975.

24. **Devillers, A., Thiery, A., Kindt, T., Scheele, G., and Blobel, G.,** Homology in amino terminal sequence of precursors to pancreatic secretory proteins, *Proc. Natl. Acad. Sci. U.S.A.,* 72, 5016, 1975.

25. **Abel, C. A., Spiegelberg, H. L., and Grey, H. M.,** The carbohydrate content of fragments and polypeptide chains of human γG myeloma proteins of different heavy chain subclasses, *Biochemistry,* 7, 1271, 1968.

26. **Schenkein, I. and Uhr, J. W.,** Glycosyl transferases for mouse IgG, *J. Immunol.,* 105, 271, 1970.

27. **Melchers, F. and Knopf, P. M.,** Biosynthesis of the carbohydrate portion of immunoglobulin chains: possible relation to secretion, *Cold Spring Harbor Symp. Quant. Biol.,* 32, 255, 1967.

28. **Parkhouse, R. M. E. and Melchers, F.,** Biosynthesis of the carbohydrate portions of immunoglobulin M, *Biochem. J.,* 125, 235, 1971.

29. **Zagury, D., Uhr, J. W., Jamieson, J. D., and Palade, G. E.,** Immunoglobulin synthesis and secretion. II. Radioautographic studies of sites of addition of carbohydrate moieties and intracellular transport, *J. Cell. Biol.,* 46, 52, 1970.

30. **Melchers, F.,** Biosynthesis, intracellular transport and secretion of immunoglobulins, effect of 2-deoxy glucose in tumor plasma cells producing and secreting immunoglobulin G, *Biochemistry,* 12, 1471, 1973.

31. **Weitzman, S. and Scharff, M. D.,** Mouse myeloma mutants blocked in the assembly, glycosylation and secretion of immunoglobulin, *J. Mol. Biol.,* 102, 237, 1976.

32. **Parkhouse, R. M. E. and Askonas, B. A.,** Immunoglobulin M synthesis, intracellular accumulation of 7S subunits, *Biochem. J.,* 115, 163, 1969.

33. **Buxbaum, J. and Scharff, M. D.,** The synthesis, assembly and secretion of gamma globulin by mouse myeloma cells. VI. Assembly of IgM proteins, *J. Exp. Med.,* 138, 278, 1973.

34. **Baumal, R. and Scharff, M. D.,** Synthesis, assembly and secretion of mouse immunoglobulin, *Transplant. Rev.,* 14, 163, 1973.

35. **Franklin, E. C.,** Physiochemical and immunologic studies of gamma globulins of normal urine, *J. Clin. Invest.,* 38, 2159, 1959.

36. **Stevenson, G. T.,** Detection in normal urine of protein resembling Bence-Jones protein, *J. Clin. Invest.,* 39, 1192, 1960.

37. **Wochner, R. D., Strober, W., and Waldmann, T. A.,** The role of the kidney in the catabolism of Bence-Jones proteins and immunoglobulin fragments, *J. Exp. Med.,* 126, 207, 1967.

38. **Waterhouse, C., Abraham, G., and Vaughan, J.,** The relationship between L-chain synthesis and γ-globulin production, *J. Clin. Invest.,* 52, 1067, 1973.

39. **Frangione, B., Milstein, C., and Pink, J. R. L.,** Structural studies of immunoglobulin G, *Nature,* 221, 145, 1969.

40. **Petersen, J. G. L. and Dorrington, K. J.,** An *in vitro* system for studying the kinetics of interchain disulfide bond formation in immunoglobulin G, *J. Biol. Chem.,* 249, 5633, 1974.

41. **Sears, D., Mohrer, J., and Beychock, S.,** A kinetic study *in vitro* of the reoxidation of interchain disulfide bonds in a human IgG₁ K correlation between sulfhydryl disappearance and intermediates in covalent assembly of H₂L₂, *Proc. Natl. Acad. Sci. U.S.A.,* 72, 353, 1975.

42. **Baumal, R., Potter, M., and Scharff, M. D.,** Synthesis, assembly and secretion of gamma globulin by mouse myeloma cells. III. Assembly of the three subclasses of IgG, *J. Exp. Med.,* 134, 1316, 1971.

43. **Depreval, C., Pink, J. R. L., and Milstein, C.,** Interchain bridges of mouse IgG 2A and IgG 2B, *Nature,* 221, 145, 1969.

44. **Svasti, J. and Milstein, C.,** Interchain bridges of mouse IgG 1, *Nature,* 228, 932, 1970.

45. **Halpern, M. S. and Koshland, M. E.,** Novel subunit in secretory IgA, *Nature,* 228, 1276, 1970.

46. **Mestecky, J., Zikan, J., and Butler, W. T.,** Immunoglobulin M and secretory immunoglobulin A: presence of a common polypeptide chain different from light chains, *Science,* 171, 1163, 1971.

47. **Della Corte, E. and Parkhouse, R. M. E.,** Biosynthesis of IgA and IgM requirement of J chain and a disulphide-exchanging enzyme for polymerization, *Biochem. J.,* 136, 597, 1973.

48. **Buxbaum, J., Zolla, S., Scharff, M. D., and Franklin, E. C.,** The synthesis and assembly of human immunoglobulins by malignant human plasmacytes. III. Heterogeneity in IgA polymer assembly, *Eur. J. Immunol.,* 4, 367, 1974.

49. **Kaji, H. and Parkhouse, R. M. E.,** Intracellular J chain in mouse plasmacytomas secreting IgA, IgM and IgG, *Nature,* 249, 45, 1974.

50. **Buxbaum, J., Zolla, S., Scharff, M. D., and Franklin, E. C.,** Synthesis and assembly of immunoglobulins by malignant human plasmacytes and lymphocytes. II. Heterogeneity of assembly in cells producing IgM proteins, *J. Exp. Med.,* 133, 1118, 1971.

51. **Parkhouse, R. M. E. and Della Corte, E.,** Biosynthesis of IgA and IgM. Control of polymerization by J Chain, *Biochem. J.,* 136, 607, 1973.

52. **Zolla, S., Buxbaum, J., Franklin, E. C., and Scharff, M. D.,** Synthesis and assembly of immunoglobulins by malignant human plasmacytes. I. Myelomas producing γ-chains and light chains, *J. Exp. Med.,* 132, 148, 1970.

53. **Stone, M. J. and Frenkel, E. P.,** The clinical spectrum of light chain myeloma. A study of 35 patients with special reference to the occurrence of amyloidosis, *Am. J. Med.,* 58, 601, 1975.

54. Grey, H. M. and Kohler, P. F., A case of tetramer Bence-Jones proteinemia, *Clin. Exp. Immunol.,* 3, 277, 1968.
55. Caggiano, V., Dominguez, C., Opfell, R. W., Kochwa, S., and Wasserman, C. R., Myeloma with closed tetrameric Bence-Jones Proteinemia, *Am. J. Med.,* 47, 978, 1969.
56. Gach, J., Simar, L., and Salmon, J., Multiple myeloma without M-type proteinemia, report of a case with immunologic and ultrastructure studies, *Am. J. Med.,* 50, 835, 1971.
57. Hurez, D., Preud'homme, J. L., and Seligmann, M., Intracellular monoclonal immunoglobulin in non-secretory human myeloma, *J. Immunol.,* 104, 263, 1970.
58. Preud'homme, J. L., Hurez, D., Danon, F., Brouet, J. C., and Seligmann, M., Intracytoplasmic and surface bound immunoglobulins in "nonsecretory" and Bence-Jones myeloma, *Clin. Exp. Immunol.,* 25, 428, 1976.
59. Van Boxel, J. A., Paul, W. E., Terry, W. D., and Green, I., IgD-bearing human lymphocytes, *J. Immunol.,* 109, 648, 1972.
60. Preud'homme, J. L. and Seligmann, M., Immunoglobulins on the surface of lymphoid cells in Waldenströms Macroglobulinemia, *J. Clin. Invest.,* 51, 701, 1972.
61. Stott, D. I., Biosynthesis and assembly of IgM. Addition of J chain to intracellular pools of 8S and 19S IgM, *Immunochemistry,* 13, 157, 1976.
62. Milstein, C. P., Richardson, N. E., Deversion, E. V., and Feinstein, A., Interchain disulphide bridges of mouse immunoglobulin M, *Biochem. J.,* 151, 615, 1975.
63. Melchers, F., Cone, R. E., Von Boehmer, H., and Sprent, J., Immunoglobulin turnover in B lymphocyte subpopulations, *Eur. J. Immunol.,* 5, 382, 1975.
64. Askonas, B. A. and Parkhouse, R. M. E., Assembly of immunoglobulin M. Blocked Thiol groups of intracellular 7S subunits, *Biochem. J.,* 123, 629, 1971.
65. Delamette, F., Marty, M. C., and Panijel, J., *In vitro* study of IgM polymerization, *Cell. Immunol.,* 19, 262, 1975.
66. Franklin, E. C., Lowenstein, J., Bigelow, B., and Meltzer, M., Heavy chain disease. A new disorder of serum γ-globulins, *Am. J. Med.,* 37, 332, 1964.
67. Bloch, K. J., Lee, L., Mills, J. A., and Haber, E., Gamma heavy chain disease. An expanding clinical and laboratory spectrum, *Am. J. Med.,* 55, 61, 1973.
68. Seligmann, M., Immunochemical, clinical and pathological features of α-chain disease, *Arch. Int. Med.,* 135, 78, 1975.
69. Franklin, E. C., μ-chain disease, *Arch. Int. Med.,* 135, 71, 1975.
70. Franklin, E. C. and Frangione, B., Structural variants of human and murine immunoglobulins, in *Contemporary Topics in Molecular Immunology,* Vol. 4, Inman, F. P., Ed., Plenum, 1975, 89.
71. Franklin, E. C., Frangione, B., and Prelli, F., The defect in μ heavy chain disease protein GL1, *J. Immunol.,* 116, 1194, 1976.
72. Ein, D., Buell, D. N., and Fahey, J. L., Biosynthetic and structural studies of heavy chain disease protein, *J. Clin. Invest.,* 48, 785, 1969.
73. Buxbaum, J. N. and Preud'homme, J. L., Alpha and gamma heavy chain diseases in man: Intracellular origin of the aberrant polypeptides, *J. Immunol.,* 109, 1131, 1972.
74. Buxbaum, J., Franklin, E. C., and Scharff, M. D., Immunoglobulin μ heavy chain disease: Intracellular origin of the μ chain fragment, *Science,* 169, 770, 1970.
75. Cowan, N. J., Secher, D. S., and Milstein, C., Intracellular immunoglobulin chain synthesis in non-secreting variants of a mouse myeloma. Detection of inactive light-chain messenger RNA, *J. Mol. Biol.,* 90, 691, 1974.
76. Winchester, R. J., Winfield, J. B., Siegal, F., Wernet, P., Bentwich, Z., and Kunkel, H., Analyses of lymphocytes from patients with rheumatoid arthritis and systemic lupus erythematosus, *J. Clin. Invest.,* 54, 1082, 1974.
77. Preud'homme, J. L., and Seligmann, M., Surface immunoglobulins on human lymphoid cells, in *Progress in Clinical Immunology,* Vol. 2, Schwartz, R. S., Ed., Grune and Stratton, New York, 1974, 128.
78. Lindström, F. D., Hardy, W. R., Eberle, W. J., and Williams, R. C., Multiple myeloma and benign monoclonal gammopathy. Differentiation by immunofluorescence of lymphocytes, *Ann. Int. Med.,* 78, 837, 1973.
79. Abdou, N. I. and Abdou, N. L., The monoclonal nature of lymphocytes in multiple myeloma. Effects of therapy, *Ann. Int. Med.,* 83, 42, 1975.
80. Chen, Y., Bhoopalam, N., Yakulis, V., and Heller, P., Changes in lymphocyte surface immunoglobulins in myeloma and the effect of an RNA containing plasma factor, *Ann. Int. Med.,* 83, 625, 1975.
81. Bhoopalam, N., Yakulis, V., Costea, N., and Heller, P., Surface immunoglobulins of circulating lymphocytes in mouse plasmacytoma. II. The influence of plasmacytoma RNA on surface immunoglobulins of lymphocytes, *Blood,* 39, 465, 1972.
82. Melchers, F. and Cone, R. E., Turnover of radioiodinated and of leucine-labeled immunoglobulin M in murine spleen lymphocytes, *Eur. J. Immunol.,* 5, 234, 1975.
83. Cone, R. E., Marchalonis, J. J., and Rolley, R. T., Lymphocyte membrane dynamics. Metabolic release of cell surface proteins, *J. Exp. Med.,* 134, 1373, 1971.
84. Baur, S., Vitetta, E. S., Sherr, C. J., Schenkein, I., and Uhr, J. W., Isolation of heavy and light chains of immunoglobulins from the surfaces of lymphoid cells, *J. Immunol.,* 106, 1133, 1971.
85. Sherr, L. J., Baur, S., Grundke, I., Zeligs, J., Zeligs, B., and Uhr, J. W., Cell surface immunoglobulin. III. Isolation and characterization of immunoglobulin from non-secretory human lymphoid cells, *J. Exp. Med.,* 135, 1392, 1972.

86. **Vitetta, E. S. and Uhr, J. W.,** Cell surface immunoglobulin. V. Release from murine splenic lymphocytes, *J. Exp. Med.,* 136, 676, 1972.

87. **Sherr, C. J. and Uhr, J. W.,** Immunoglobulin synthesis and secretion. VI. Synthesis and intracellular transport of immunoglobulin in nonsecretory lymphoma cells, *J. Exp. Med.,* 133, 901, 1971.

88. **Lerner, R. A., McConahey, P. J., Jansen, I., and Dixon, F. J.,** Synthesis of plasma membrane associated and secretory immunoglobulin in diploid lymphocytes, *J. Exp. Med.,* 135, 136, 1972.

89. **Hutteroth, T. H., Cleve, H., and Litwin, S. D.,** Modulation of membrane associated immunoglobulins of cultured human lymphoid cells by specific antibody, *J. Immunol.,* 110, 1325, 1973.

90. **Vitetta, E. S. and Uhr, J. W.,** Release of cell surface immunoglobulin by mouse splenic lymphocytes, *J. Immunol.,* 108, 577, 1972.

91. **Fahey, J. L., Scoggins, R., Utz, J. P., and Szwed, C. F.,** Infection antibody response and gamma globulin components in multiple myeloma and macroglobulinemia, *Am. J. Med.,* 35, 698, 1963.

92. **Cone, L. and Uhr, J. W.,** Immunological deficiency disorders associated with chronic lymphocytic leukemia and multiple myeloma, *J. Clin. Invest.,* 44, 1778, 1965.

93. **Zolla, S.,** The effect of plasmacytomas on the immune response of mice, *J. Immunol.,* 108, 1039, 1972.

94. **Tanapatchaiyapong, P. and Zolla, S.,** Humoral immunosuppressive substance in mice bearing plasmacytomas, *Science,* 186, 748, 1974.

95. **Broder, S., Humphrey, R., Durm, M., Blackman, M., Meade, B., Goldman, C., Strober, W., and Waldmann, T.,** Impaired synthesis of polyclonal (non-para-protein) immunoglobulins by circulating lymphocytes from patients with multiple myeloma, *N. Engl. J. Med.,* 293, 887, 1975.

96. **Barton, M. A. and Diener, E.,** A new perspective on B-cell triggering: control of the immune response by organizational changes in the lipid bilayer, *Transplant. Rev.,* 23, 1, 1975.

97. **Baker, P. J.,** Homeostatic control of antibody responses: A model based on the recognition of cell-associated antibody by regulatory T-cells, *Transplant. Rev.,* 26, 1, 1975.

98. **Gershon, R. K.,** A disquisition on suppressor T-cells, *Transplant. Rev.,* 26, 170, 1975.

99. **Schiff, R. I., Buckley, A. H., Gilbertsen, R. B., and Metzgar, R.,** Membrane receptors and in vitro responsiveness of lymphocytes in human immunodeficiency, *J. Immunol.,* 112, 376, 1974.

100. **Griscelli, C.,** T and B markers in immunodeficiencies, in *Immunodeficiency in Man and Animals,* Bergsma, D., Good, R. A., and Finstad, J., National Foundation and Sinauer Associates, Sunderland, Mass., 1975, 45.

101. **Cooper, M. D., Lawton, A. R., and Bockman, D. E.,** Agammaglobulinemia with B-lymphocytes: specific defect of lymphocyte differentiation, *Lancet,* ii, 791, 1971.

102. **Lawton, A. R., Royal, S. A., Self, K. S., and Cooper, M. D.,** IgA determinants on B-lymphocytes with deficiency of circulating IgA, *J. Lab. Clin. Med.,* 80, 26, 1972.

103. **Strober, W., Krakauer, R., Klaeveman, H. L., Reynolds, H. Y., and Nelson, D. L.,** Secretory component deficiency: A disorder of the IgA immune system, *N. Engl. J. Med.,* 294, 351, 1976.

104. **Geha, R. S., Schneeberger, E., Merler, E., and Rosen, T. S.,** Heterogeneity of acquired or common variable agammaglobulinemia, *N. Engl. J. Med.,* 291, 1, 1976.

105. **Waldmann, T. A., Broder, S., Blaese, R. M., Durm, M., Blackman, M., and Strober, W.,** Role of suppressor T cells in pathogenesis of common variable hypogamma globulinemia, *Lancet,* ii, 609, 1974.

106. **Choi, Y. S., Biggar, W. D., and Good, R. A.,** Biosynthesis and secretion of immunoglobulins by peripheral blood lymphocytes in severe hypogammaglobulinemia, *Lancet,* i, 1149, 1972.

107. **Ciccimarra, F., Rosen, F. S., Schneeberger, E., and Merler, E.,** Failure of heavy chain glycosylation of IgG in some patients with common variable agammaglobulinemia, *J. Clin. Invest.,* 57, 1386, 1971.

108. **Buxbaum, J. N.,** unpublished data.

109. **Buxbaum, J. N., Spiro, T., Hurley, M., and Chuba, J.,** unpublished data.

110. **Buxbaum, J. N. and Preud'homme, J. L.,** unpublished data.

111. **Buxbaum, J. N. and Frangione, B.,** unpublished data.

112. **Buxbaum, J. N.,** unpublished data.

113. **Waechter, C. J. and Lennarz, W. J.,** The role of polyprenol-linked sugars in glycoprotein synthesis, *Annu. Rev. Biochem.,* 45, 95, 1976.

Chapter 11
ANTIGENS ON HUMAN LEUKEMIC CELLS*

Marc E. Weksler

TABLE OF CONTENTS

I. INTRODUCTION

Leukemic cells escape the control mechanisms which limit the proliferation and survival of normal cells. Many of the metabolic adaptations observed in leukemic cells involve alterations at the cell surface.[1] Some of these changes can be recognized by the appearance of "new" antigenic determinants on leukemic cells. Study of the antigens carried by leukemic cells has given insight into the lineage of lymphocytic leukemia, has suggested genetic factors which may predispose to leukemia, has demonstrated the host's immune response to leukemic cells, and has offered a rationale for diagnostic and therapeutic approaches to leukemia. This chapter will summarize

*This investigation was supported by Grant CA 13339 and Research Career Development Award CA 32102, awarded by the National Cancer Institute, DHEW.

TABLE 1

Markers For Human Blood Mononuclear Leukocytes[2,16,69]

Characteristic	B Lymphocytes	T Lymphocytes	Monocytes
Rosette with sheep erythrocyte	−	+	−
Bind antibodies to human T lymphocytes	−	+	−
Receptor for measles virus	−	+	−
Bind antibodies to HL-B antigen	+	−	+
Receptor for Fc portion of immunoglobulin	+	−	+
Receptor for third component of complement	+	−	+
Receptor for aggregated immunoglobulin G	+	−	+
Receptor for Epstein-Barr virus	+	−	−
Surface membrane immunoglobulin	+[b]	−	−[a]

[a]Cytophilic immunoglobulin readily demonstrated.

[b]Not all the non-T lymphocytes have surface immunoglobulin. A third population (K cells) do not rosette with sheep erythrocytes and lack surface immunoglobulin, but have Fc receptors.

studies which have defined the antigenic array on human leukemic cells and the immune response these determinants engender. Finally, the prognostic significance of certain of these antigenic determinants and of the patient's response to these antigens will be discussed.

II. ANTIGENS FOUND ON NORMAL AND LEUKEMIC CELLS

A. Lymphoid Cell Surface Markers

The lymphocytic leukemias, like normal lymphocytes, can be categorized as being of B- or T-lymphocyte lineage. Although there are no morphological means to distinguish B from T lymphocytes, a number of surface markers can be used to identify B or T lymphocytes in the mononuclear leukocyte population of human blood (Table 1). Using these markers, virtually all normal blood lymphocytes can be identified as either B or T lymphocytes. Less than 5% of the lymphocytes have both B- and T-cell determinants or neither. Lymphocytes which carry neither T nor B determinants have been termed "null cells" and may represent lymphoid stem cells. In blood from healthy adults, B lymphocytes make up 20 to 25% and T lymphocytes 75 to 80% of the total lymphocyte population.[2] Malignant proliferation of B lymphocytes occurs in patients with chronic lymphatic leukemia (CLL), macroglobulinemia, hairy cell leukemia and lymphocytic lymphoma.[3,4] Neoplastic cells in patients with the Sezary syndrome and a group of patients with acute lymphoblastic leukemia (ALL) are derived from T lymphocytes (Table 2).[4]

TABLE 2

Lineage of Lymphoid Neoplasms[3,5,6]

I	B
Sezary syndrome	Myeloma (monoclonal)
CLL <2% of patients	Macroglobulinemia (monoclonal)
ALL 30% of patients	Hairy cell leukemia
	CLL (monoclonal)
	ALL 70% of patients
	Lymphocytic lymphoma

B. Chronic Lymphocytic Leukemia

The leukemic cells that proliferate in nearly all patients with CLL represent a monoclonal expansion of B lymphocytes. Most lymphocytes in these patients have easily demonstrated surface immunoglobulin and receptors for complement and aggregated immunoglobulin. When the peripheral blood lymphocyte count is over 10,000, most lymphocytes carry surface immunoglobulin, and the correlation between lymphocyte count and the number of B lymphocytes is clear. Seligmann and his colleagues[5] studied the lymphocytes from 96 patients with CLL. In 91 cases, monoclonal surface immunoglobulin was present. In two thirds of the cases, both mu and delta heavy chains and a single light chain determinant were present. Although most CLL cells carry the markers of normal B lymphocytes, in some cases the distribution of certain surface determinants is altered. Thus, lymphocytes from some patients with CLL lack surface immunoglobulin but carry other B lymphocyte markers: receptors for complement and the immunoglobulin F_c determinant.[6] In addition, Ross and his colleagues have reported that two to ten times as many CLL cells bind C3d as bind C3b, while normal lymphocytes bind more C3b than bind C3d.[7]

Lymphocytes from a small number of patients with clinically typical CLL lack surface immunoglobulin and receptors for complement and aggregated immunoglobulin but bind anti-T-lymphocyte antibody.[8,9] These leukemic lymphocytes appear to have a T-lymphocyte lineage. Despite the existence of such patients, over 98% of patients with CLL have an expansion of a single clone of B lymphocytes in the blood.[2]

C. Myeloma and Macroglobulinemia

In contrast to the rare secretion of immunoglobulin by the proliferating B lymphocytes in CLL, monoclonal immunoglobulin synthesis and secretion typifies myeloma and macroglobulinemia. Although clonal expansion of immunoglobulin-producing cells had been recognized in myeloma and macroglobulinemia, it is now known that a monoclonal proliferation of B lymphocytes also occurs in these diseases. Thus, 50% of lymphocytes in patients with macroglobulinemia have monoclonal surface immunoglobulin M identical to the serum monoclonal immunoglobulin.[4] This disease represents a proliferation of a clone of B lymphocytes with continuous morphologic transition from small lymphocytes to immunoglobulin M-secreting plasma cells. In view of the high number of lymphocytes bearing the monoclonal marker, the disorder might well be considered a leukemic process.[4] Similarly, it has been demonstrated recently that some, if not all, patients with myeloma have an expanded population of B lymphocytes bearing the same surface immunoglobulin as is secreted by the plasma cells that are the morphological hallmark of this disease.[4,10] It appears that CLL, macroglobulinemia, and myeloma are all syndromes resulting from the proliferation of a neoplastic clone of B lymphocytes. The diseases are distinguished by the morphological stage of B lymphocyte differentiation that predominates and by the secretion of an immunoglobulin product.

D. Sezary Syndrome

This syndrome is characterized by erythroderma, lymphadenopathy, and large atypical lymphoid cells circulating in the blood and infiltrating the skin. These atypical lymphoid cells have large convoluted nuclei and PAS-positive cytoplasmic vacuoles. The total white blood count may be elevated beyond 20,000 with the majority of the leukocytes being "Sezary cells."

Although the disease is generally considered a variant of mycosis fungoides, in cases with large numbers of circulating Sezary cells it resembles a leukemia. The atypical lymphocytes are derived from T lymphocytes. They rosette with sheep erythrocytes and lack both surface immunoglobulin and receptors for complement and aggregated immunoglobulin.[4]

E. Acute Lymphoblastic Leukemia

The origin of lymphoblasts in ALL has been more difficult to establish. Of patients with ALL, 20 to 35% have lymphoblasts which rosette with sheep erythrocytes, bind anti-T-lymphocyte antibody and clearly are derived from T lymphocytes. These patients usually have high leukocyte counts and thymic masses.[11] A very small number of patients with ALL have lymphoblasts carrying B lymphocyte markers.[12,13] These cells appear on morphological grounds to be related to Burkitt's lymphoma cells.[12] The majority (60 to 80%) of patients with ALL, however, have lymphoblasts which lack surface immunoglobulin, receptors for complement, and aggregated immunoglobulin, and do not rosette with sheep erythrocytes. Such lymphoblasts might have lost differentiated cell surface markers or have originated from a lymphoid stem cell which carries neither T- nor B-lymphocyte markers.

Recently, a new human alloantigen system, HL-B, has been defined.[14,15] This antigen system is selectively expressed on lymphoid cells of B lineage. Fu et al.[16] have found that lymphoblasts from four patients with ALL which lacked surface immunoglobulin and F_c and sheep erythrocyte receptors carried HL-B antigens. These investigators suggest that lymphoblasts from the majority of patients with ALL, which do not carry many of the B- or T-lymphocyte markers, can be identified by the HL-B antigen to be of B-lymphocyte lineage.

F. Histocompatibility Determinants

There is strong evidence that the susceptibility of mice to virus-induced leukemia is linked to the histocompatibility genes.[17,18] It is likely that the association between histocompatibility genes and susceptibility to leukemia relates to immune-response genes which are closely linked to the major histocompatibility complex. Evidence in support of this concept has been derived from the study of resistance to murine leukemia.[19] In this study, the capacity of mice to resist a transplantable murine leukemia depended on their capacity to make an immune response to a strong transplantable antigen (X.1), carried on the leukemia cells. The capacity to respond immunologically was shown to be a dominant genetic trait controlled by an H-2 linked immune-response gene. Furthermore, Zarling and his colleagues[20] have shown that mouse strains resistant to viral leukemia have natural cell-mediated immunity to viral antigens. Cell-mediated immunity to these viral antigens is lacking in strains susceptible to leukemia.

Although no virus has been demonstrated in any form of human leukemia, the viral etiology of human leukemia continues to be rigorously investigated. Recently, Gallagher and Gallo[21] and Teich et al.[22] have reported the isolation of a C-type particle from leukocytes of a patient with acute myeloblastic leukemia (AML). Mann and his colleagues[23] have offered evidence that the reactivity of an antiserum specific for leukocytes from patients with acute leukemia is lost following absorption with viral antigens. As susceptibility to viral leukemia in mice is so clearly linked to certain histocompatibility determinants, a search for an association between histocompatability antigens and susceptibility to human leukemia was undertaken by several groups. Thorsby and his colleagues[24] found that HLA-2 and HLA-12 occurred in higher frequency in patients with ALL than in the normal population. Subsequent studies have been contradictory. Some investigators found an increase in HLA-2 and HLA-12, or HLA-2 or a normal distribution of HLA antigens in patients with ALL.[17] The association of histocompatibility antigens with CLL or chronic myelocytic leukemia (CML)[17] is even less clear.

III. ANTIGENS ON LEUKEMIC CELLS IDENTIFIED BY SEROLOGICAL TECHNIQUES

A. Human Antibodies Reactive with Leukemic Cells

The clearest evidence for "new" antigens on leukemic cells is a specific immune response of the host to autochthonous leukemic cells. Although

autoantibodies of leukemic cells have been found in patients with leukemia, the specificity of the antigen system was not defined.[25,26] Of patients with acute or chronic leukemia, 50% were reported to have autoantibodies to leukemic cells using an immune adherence assay.[27] Although the presence of autoantibodies was not correlated with clinical prognosis, the titer of the autoantibody tended to increase during remission. Gutterman and his colleagues,[28] on the other hand, have reported that patients with AML who have autoantibodies that coat their leukemic cells have a favorable prognosis.

Two human autoantibodies have defined leukemia-associated antigens: gamma fetoprotein[29] and leukemia-associated nuclear antigen.[30] Gamma fetoprotein is a tumor-associated antigen found in leukemic and other neoplastic cells. This antigen was defined by the reactivity of serum from eight (one had leukemia) of 1518 cancer patients which reacted with an antigen present in normal fetal serum but absent from normal adult serum. This antigen in fetal serum had gamma electrophoretic mobility and was termed gamma fetoprotein. Gamma fetoprotein has been found in a variety of benign and malignant neoplasms but occurred in highest frequency in sarcomas (88%) and leukemias (82%). Gamma fetoprotein was present in cell extracts from 10 of 12 patients with ALL, from 2 of 3 patients with CLL, from 4 of 5 patients with AML, and from 7 of 8 patients with CML tested. Although gamma fetoprotein was not found in serum from 236 patients with non-neoplastic disease or 129 healthy subjects, it was present in 11% of 210 patients with cancer. Gamma fetoprotein was found in the serum of over 50% of the patients with ALL.

Klein and his colleagues[30] have recently reported the existence of a leukemia-associated nuclear antigen defined by human serum antibody. The capacity of serum antibody from a patient with AML to bind to the nuclei of autochthonous myeloblasts was revealed by a sensitive anti-complement immunofluorescent assay. Serum which reacted with this nuclear antigen was found in 73% of patients with AML, 35% of patients with ALL, 14% of patients with CML, and 19% of patients with CLL. The leukemia-associated nuclear antigen, however, was restricted to cells from 7 of 15 patients with AML. This leukemia-associated nuclear antigen has not been found in patients with ALL, CLL, or CML. One patient with CML in blast crisis had nuclear antigen. The leukemia-associated nuclear antigen was lost when patients with AML went into remission. These investigators also found that the leukemia-associated nuclear antigen is present in both a B and T human lymphoblastoid line and in lymphoblasts induced by incubating normal lymphocytes with phytohemagglutinin.

B. Antibodies Raised in Animals Reactive with Human Leukemic Cells

Leukemia-associated antigens have also been detected using antisera raised in experimental animals. Several laboratories have found that antisera from some rabbits immunized with membrane preparations from human B lymphoblastoid lines react with acute leukemic leukocytes. Mann and his colleagues[23] used a complement-mediated cytotoxic assay to measure the reactivity of antisera from rabbits immunized with a membrane extract from the "Raji" B lymphoblastoid line. Antisera from 3 of 24 rabbits reacted with blood leukocytes from all patients with ALL or AML tested and with leukocytes from two to three patients with CML in blast crisis. The antisera did not react with peripheral leukocytes from 947 normal individuals, normal bone marrow cells, or leukocytes from acute leukemic patients in remission.[23,31,32] Comparable results were obtained by Durantez and his colleagues[33] using antisera raised in rabbits immunized with a membrane preparation from another B lymphoblastoid line. Their antisera assayed by a lymphocyte-dependent antibody cytotoxicity assay reacted with leukocytes from patients with acute leukemia. Billing and Terasaki[34] raised antisera in rabbits with membrane preparation from yet another B lymphoblastoid line. This antisera had broader reactivity and was cytotoxic for leukocytes from patients with ALL, CLL, AML, and CML. Mann and his colleagues[23] have studied the reactivity of their antisera extensively. The reaction of the antisera with leukocytes from patients with acute leukemia correlated with the percentage of blasts in the bone marrow but not with the number of blasts in the peripheral blood. When patients entered bone marrow remission, the antisera no longer reacted with blood leukocytes. These antisera did not react with blood leukocytes from patients with CLL, CML, or infectious mononucleosis. Determinants which reacted with the antisera were determined by absorption

studies. These studies suggested that the antisera recognized a viral antigen. The antigen was present on human embryonic kidney cells infected with the Rauscher, the Kirsten, or the SV 40 virus, and on leukemic leukocytes. The non-virally infected kidney cell line did not inhibit the cytotoxicity of the antisera towards leukemic cells.

Greaves and his colleagues[35] have raised antisera in rabbits to ALL cells. The reaction of these antisera with leukocytes was detected by immunofluorescence. After absorption with various normal tissues and AML cells, the antisera reacted with leukocytes from 14 of 19 patients with ALL but not with normal leukocytes or leukocytes from patients with AML, CML, or CLL. In most cases, the staining of blood leukocytes was related to the number of lymphoblasts in the peripheral blood. However, in three patients with ALL, blood leukocytes were stained although lymphoblasts were absent from the peripheral blood. The diagnosis of ALL in these patients was made by examination of the bone marrow. When patients entered remission, the reactivity of the antisera toward blood leukocytes was lost or markedly reduced. Blood leukocytes from five patients with ALL did not react with the antisera. Among these five cases were the three patients in the entire group of 19 whose lymphoblasts had T lymphocyte markers. The authors concluded that their antisera may identify an antigenic determinant on ALL leukocytes of non-T-cell origin.

Mills and his colleagues[36] used rabbit antiserum to human thymus cells to identify lymphocytes from patients with ALL of T-cell lineage. The binding of this antiserum was measured by an indirect radiolabeling (^{125}I/goat antirabbit immunoglobulin) technique. The antithymus antiserum reacted with thymocytes, and normal and malignant T lymphocytes. After the antiserum was absorbed with normal blood leukocytes, reactivity with thymocytes and leukemic lymphocytes persisted, but all reactivity of the antisera with normal lymphocytes and bone marrow cells was eliminated. The absorbed antiserum did not react with leukocytes from patients with ALL in remission. Absorption of the antiserum with thymus cells abolished its reactivity toward leukemic cells. The authors conclude that thymus cells and leukemic lymphocytes share two antigenic determinants, one of which is also present on peripheral T lymphocytes. The antigen system proposed is reminiscent of the theta/TL system in

TABLE 3

Reactivity of Antisera with Leukemic Cells or Thymocytes

| | ALL | | | | | |
Antiserum	T	Non-T	AML	CLL	CML	Thymus
Rabbit anti-lymphoblastoid line	+	+	+	–	–	–
Rabbit anti-ALL cells	–	+	–	–	–	–
Rabbit anti-thymus cells	+	–	–	–	–	+
Mice anti-AML cells	–	–	+	–	–	N.D.
Human anti-myeloblast-associated nuclear antiserum	–	–	+	–	–	N.D.
Monkey anti-CLL cells	+	+	–	+	–	–
Monkey anti-CML cells	–	–	–	–	+	–
Monkey anti-AML cells	–	–	+	–	±	–
Human anti-gamma fetoprotein	+	+	+	+	+	–

Note: + = present, – = absent, N.D. = not done.

certain strains of mice.[37] In these strains, the theta antigen is found on thymus lymphocytes and all T-derived lymphocytes. The TL antigen is normally thymus specific but is also expressed on leukemic T lymphocytes. The existence of an antigen shared by thymus and leukemic cells has been suggested by other investigators using antisera prepared against human brain or leukemic cells.[38–40]

It has been difficult to raise antisera in rabbits with specificity for AML cells.[35] Baker and his colleagues[41] have developed antisera specific for AML or ALL by immunizing mice rendered tolerant to remission leukocytes with leukemic blasts from the same individuals. These antisera, after appropriate absorption, were cytotoxic for AML or ALL cells but not for normal leukocytes, bone marrow cells, or remission leukocytes from leukemic patients. As the absorbed antisera were specific for AML or ALL cells, the authors thought it unlikely that the reactivity of these antisera was directed toward species-specific, histocompatibility, differentiation, or cell cycle associated antigens.

Antisera to leukemic cells has also been raised in monkeys. Monkeys immunized with CML or CLL cells have yielded antisera which tend to react with myeloid or lymphoid leukemia, respectively, but do not distinguish acute from chronic forms. Thus, Metzgar and his colleagues[42,43] found that monkeys immunized with CLL cells produced antisera which after absorption recognize antigens common to all ALL and CLL cells tested. On the other hand, serum from monkeys immunized with

chronic myeloid leukemic cells reacted differently with AML and CML cells. The pattern of reactivity suggested that the antimyeloid leukemic antisera recognized determinants specific for AML or CML as well as other antigens present on both AML and CML cells. These antisera did not react with normal leukocytes, thymocytes, or cells from a patient with a leukemoid reaction. Table 3 summarizes the reactivity of human, rabbit, and monkey antisera that have been used to identify leukemia-associated antigens.

IV. ANTIGENS ON LEUKEMIC CELLS DEMONSTRATED BY CELL-MEDIATED IMMUNITY TO LEUKEMIC CELLS

In contrast to the small number of patients with cancer who have been shown to have antibodies to autochthonous tumor cells, a large number of patients with leukemia and other neoplasms have been shown to possess cellular immunity to autochthonous cancer cells.[44] Demonstration of cellular immunity to leukemic cells but not normal leukocytes has been used as evidence for the presence of leukemia-associated antigens. These studies have been greatly facilitated by the isolation of leukemic cells by continuous-flow centrifugation and their preservation in a viable state in liquid nitrogen. The availability of blast cells has permitted the measurement of cellular immunity to leukemic cells in patients during remission.

The first and apparently most direct demonstration of "new" antigens on leukemic cells was the capacity of leukemic cells, obtained during relapse, to stimulate the proliferation of autologous lymphocytes. Fridman and Kourilsky[45] showed that leukemic cells from six of nine patients with ALL and from one patient with AML stimulated thymidine incorporation by autologous lymphocytes. Viza and his colleagues[46] reported that leukemic cells from three of five patients with acute leukemia stimulated autologous lymphocyte proliferation and that this response was augmented following immunization with autologous leukemic cells. Since these observations, other investigators have corroborated the capacity of leukemic cells to stimulate the proliferation of autologous lymphocytes[45-50] and the augmentation of this response following immunization of leukemic patients with autologous or allogeneic leukemic cells.[46,49] Gutterman and his colleagues[28] studied the response of 35 patients with acute leukemia to autologous leukemic cells. Lymphocytes from 19 of 24 patients with AML and from 6 of 11 patients with ALL were stimulated by autologous leukemic cells. Patients with AML tended to have a greater proliferative response to autologous leukemic cells as compared to patients with ALL. In eight of nine patients with AML and one of five patients with ALL, the proliferative response of lymphocytes cultured with autochthonous leukemia cells was completely or partially inhibited by autologous serum. Paradoxically, this finding was associated with a favorable prognosis. In other studies, Gutterman and his colleagues[51] showed that soluble extracts from six out of seven leukemic cells stimulated autologous lymphocyte proliferation. This response was observed in four of five patients with AML, one patient with CML in blast crisis, and in one patient with ALL. As soluble histocompatibility antigens stimulate lymphocyte proliferation only after sensitization of the lymphocyte donor,[52] the authors propose that their results suggest prior sensitization of patients to leukemic antigens. This assay would then be an assay for specific tumor immunity. Gutterman et al.[53] have also reported that lymphocytes from patients with acute leukemia in remission may proliferate when cultured with autologous bone marrow cells also taken during remission. Such a response, they believe, can be used to detect residual leukemia in the bone marrow (see Section VII).

Leukemic cells have also been shown to stimulate proliferation of lymphocytes from identical twins and HLA-identical siblings. Han and Wang[54] reported that leukocytes (93% of which were lymphoblasts) from a patient with ALL in relapse stimulated the proliferation of lymphocytes from a normal identical twin. Leukocytes taken from the leukemic patient during remission did not stimulate the normal twin's lymphocytes. Fefer and his colleagues[55] reported that leukemic cells from two of three patients with ALL and one of five patients with AML stimulated the proliferation of lymphocytes from their identical twins. Cells from two of three leukemic patients stimulated lymphocytes from an unrelated donor more than did leukocytes from the normal twin. Finally, Bach et al.[56] and Santos and his colleagues[57] reported that leukocytes from a total of ten patients with acute leukemia stimulated lymphocytes from HLA-identical siblings. In these various studies, leukocytes from the normal twin or HLA-identical sibling were never found to stimulate the proliferation of lymphocytes from the leukemic patient.

V. SIGNIFICANCE OF IN VITRO LYMPHOCYTE REACTIONS TO LEUKEMIC CELLS

The capacity of leukemic cells to stimulate the proliferation of autologous lymphocytes has been taken as prima facie evidence of leukemia-associated antigens. This may not be correct. Kuntz et al.[60,61] have found that lymphoid cells obtained from normal subjects can also stimulate the proliferation of autologous lymphocytes. Thus, B lymphoblasts derived from normal subjects and maintained in continuous culture stimulated autologous lymphocyte proliferation.[58] Although nearly all such lymphoblasts carry the EB viral genome, this reaction does not depend upon the presence of the EB viral genome in the lymphoblast or upon immunity of the lymphocyte donor to the EB virus. Further, mitogen-induced lymphoblasts from subjects never infected with the EB virus stimulated autologous lymphocyte proliferation.[59] We had interpreted these experiments as demonstrating that a cell-cycle determinant expressed on the lymphoblast stimulated autologous lymphocyte proliferation and inferred that such a reaction might normally limit or prevent the proliferation of lymphoid cells seen in leukemia. Recently we have found a reaction to B lymphocytes isolated from human blood. B lymphocytes stimulate the proliferation of autologous T cells in culture.[60] For this reason, we are more cautious in attributing the reaction between leukemia cells and autologous lymphocytes to leukemia-associated antigens. However, it remains possible that this reaction may be an important defense against lymphocytic leukemia. This interpretation is suggested by our finding that lymphocytes from patients with CLL are not stimulated to proliferate by autologous B lymphocytes.[61] The reaction of lymphocytes in culture with autologous leukemic cells is probably important, but the determinants that stimulate autologous lymphocyte proliferation are not restricted to leukemic cells.

VI. ANTIGENS ON LEUKEMIC CELLS DEMONSTRATED BY DELAYED CUTANEOUS HYPERSENSITIVITY

Delayed cutaneous hypersensitivity is another means for measuring cell-mediated immunity. Cutaneous reactivity to autochthonous tumor cell extracts has been found in patients with Burkitt's lymphoma and malignant melanoma.[62,63] Char and his colleagues[64] tested cutaneous reactivity to recall antigens and to membrane extracts of leukemic blasts in 78 patients with acute leukemia. Normal reactivity to recall antigens was found during both relapse and remission. (Impaired skin reactivity had been previously reported.)[57,65,66] The response to autologous blast extracts was impaired during relapse as compared to remission. Thus, in ALL, one of five patients tested with blast extract in relapse had a positive reaction, while in remission 20 of 44 patients had a positive reaction. Patients with a negative skin reaction in relapse often developed positive reactions on entering remission. No cutaneous reactivity to extracts of remission leukocytes was observed. The specificity of the cutaneous response to blast extracts was tested using a variety of allogeneic cell extracts; 27% of ALL patients reacted to allogeneic lymphoblast extracts, but none responded to extracts from normal or remission leukocytes or from myeloblasts. Similarly, 57% of

patients with AML reacted to myeloblast extracts, but none reacted to extracts from normal or remission leukocytes or from lymphoblasts. The percentage of patients with ALL who developed a positive skin reaction to blast extract was not increased by immunization with allogeneic lymphoblasts.

Lymphocyte-mediated cytotoxicity is another assay that has been used to detect cell-mediated immunity to leukemia-associated antigens. Leventhal and her colleagues[48] showed that lymphocytes from 8 of 16 patients with acute leukemia were cytotoxic to autochthonous leukemic blasts. Rosenberg and his colleagues[67] measured lymphocyte-mediated cytotoxicity toward leukocytes from identical twins, one of whom had acute leukemia. Only one of ten twin pairs studied had blast cells in the peripheral blood. Attacking lymphocytes were obtained from the normal twin, family members, and unrelated individuals. Three of the normal twins had lymphocytes which were cytotoxic for leukocytes from the leukemic sibling. None of the leukemic patients had lymphocytes which were cytotoxic for leukocytes from the normal twin. Lymphocytes from 20 individuals (family members and unrelated persons) when tested against leukocytes from both twins were cytotoxic for leukocytes from the leukemic but not the normal twin. This pattern of reactivity was found with seven of the ten twin pairs studied. Lymphocytes from eight persons were cytotoxic for cells from both twins, and lymphocytes from 51 individuals were not cytotoxic for leukocytes from either twin. No lymphocytes tested were cytotoxic for the normal and not for the leukemic twin. The authors conclude that in seven pairs of twins, cytotoxicity detected against cells from the leukemic but not the normal twin indicated the presence of leukemia-associated antigens. Rosenberg et al.[67] feel that this discordant pattern of cytotoxicity cannot be attributed to increased sensitivity of leukemic leukocytes to cytotoxic attack. As this cytotoxic reaction occured with leukocytes from leukemic patients in remission as well as in relapse, the putative leukemia- associated antigens were not limited to leukemia blasts.

VII. CLINICAL SIGNIFICANCE OF ANTIGENS IN LEUKEMIC CELLS AND THE IMMUNE RESPONSE OF LEUKEMIC PATIENTS

Antigens on leukemic cells and the immune reactivity of patients with leukemia may predict the future course of the disease. T- and B-lymphocytic leukemia differ in clinical manifestations and natural history. Approximately one third of patients with ALL have lymphoblasts which rosette with sheep erythrocytes and bind anti-T-cell antibody. These patients tend to be older males with high leukocyte counts and thymic enlargement. The disease is more aggressive and more difficult to manage.[11] Similarly, the less frequent T-cell CLL (estimated at 2% of the total number of patients with CLL) may be distinguished by clinical manifestations from B-cell CLL. In T-cell CLL, splenomegaly and hepatomegaly occur without lymphadenopathy. Furthermore, these patients have skin lesions which on biopsy reveal lymphocytic infiltration. Whether the clinical course of T-cell CLL differs significantly from B-cell CLL is not yet apparent.[8]

The immune reactivity of patients with acute leukemia has been correlated with prognosis. Patients with active cutaneous reaction to recall antigens have an increased likelihood of entering remission.[64,65,68] Cutaneous reactions to blast extracts also appeared to be related to duration of remission.[64] Loss of cutaneous reactivity or failure to develop cutaneous reactivity during remission was found to be a poor prognostic sign. Similarly, in vitro manifestations of immunity have been correlated with prognosis in ALL. Gutterman and his colleagues[28] have reported that patients whose lymphocytes proliferated vigorously when cultured with leukemia antigens, whose serum altered (either inhibited or augmented) this proliferative response, and whose leukemic cells had bound immunoglobulin had more favorable progress than patients who did not show these reactions. Not only did the reactive patients have a greater chance of entering remission, but remission was better sustained. As had been observed with skin reactivity, appearance of or persistence of a positive in vitro response to leukemic antigens was associated with sustained remission. In contrast, patients who did not gain, or lost in vitro reactivity suffered early relapses.

Finally, Gutterman has studied the reactivity of blood lymphocytes to autologous bone marrow of patients with acute leukemia in remission. Lymphocytes from 8 to 25 patients with acute leukemia in complete remission were stimulated to proliferate when cultured with autologous bone marrow. Five of these eight patients relapsed in an average of 4.2 months, while the 17 patients whose bone marrow cells did not significantly stimulate autologous lymphocyte proliferation (stimulation index over 3) remained in sustained remission an average of 9.7 months later. Gutterman et al.[53] believe the reactivity of lymphocytes to autologous bone marrow detected residual disease which is not apparent morphologically.

VIII. CONCLUSION

Antigens on leukemic cells have identified the lineage of leukemic cells. Some of the results of such study have been unexpected; for example, the appearance of T lymphoblasts during "blast crisis" CML. These findings have clinical as well as experimental implications. Refined diagnostic classification allows more effective chemotherapy which can be directed at the specific leukemic cell type. In addition, the knowledge of the cell which undergoes neoplastic transformation may provide insight into the etiology of the leukemic process. Finally, the leukemia-associated antigens may serve as targets for immunotherapeutic attack. The importance of the patient's immune competence to prognosis has been discussed and suggests that nonspecific, as well as specific, immunotherapy may be beneficial to the patient. It is hoped that these approaches will allow more successful therapy of leukemia in man.

ACKNOWLEDGMENT

The thorough bibliographic search and careful secretarial assistance of Ms. Carolyn Darocy made this chapter possible.

REFERENCES

1. Rapin, A. M. C. and Burger, M., Tumor cell surfaces: general alterations detected by agglutinins, in *Advances in Cancer Research*, Vol. 20, Klein, G. and Weinhouse, S., Eds., Academic Press, New York, 1974, 1.
2. International Union of Immunological Societies, Report, July 1974, Identification, enumeration and isolation of B and T lymphocytes from human peripheral blood, *Clin. Immunol. Immunopathol.*, 3, 584, 1975.
3. Fu, S. M., Winchester, R. J., Rai, K. R., and Kunkel, H. G., Hairy cell leukemia: proliferation of a cell with phagocytic and B-lymphocyte properties, *Scand. J. Immunol.*, 3, 847, 1974.
4. Preud'homme, J. L. and Seligmann, M., Surface immunoglobulins on human lymphoid cells, *Prog. Clin. Immunol.*, 2, 121, 1974.
5. Seligmann, M., Preud'homme, J. L., and Brouet, J. C. B and T cell markers in human proliferative blood diseases and primary immunodeficiencies, with special reference to membrane bound immunoglobulins, *Transplant. Rev.*, 16, 85, 1973.
6. Bentwich, Z. and Kunkel, H. H., Specific properties of human B and T lymphocytes and alterations in disease, *Transplant. Rev.*, 16, 29, 1973.
7. Ross, G. D., Polley, M. J., Rabellino, E. M., and Grey, H. M., Two different complement receptors on human lymphocytes, *J. Exp. Med.*, 138, 798, 1973.
8. Brouet, J. C., Flandrin, G., Sasportes, M., Preud'homme, J. L., and Seligmann, M., Chronic lymphocytic leukemia of T-cell origin, *Lancet*, 2, 890, 1975.
9. Insel, R. A., Melewicz, F. M., La Via, M. F., and Balch, C. M., Morphology, surface markers and *in vitro* responses of a human leukemic T cell, *Clin. Immunol. Immunopathol.*, 4, 382, 1975.
10. Abdou, N. I. and Abdou, N. L., The monoclonal nature of lymphocytes in multiple myeloma, *Ann. Int. Med.*, 83, 42, 1975.
11. Sen, L. and Borella, L., Clinical importance of lymphoblasts with T markers in childhood acute leukemia, *N. Engl. J. Med.*, 292(16), 828, 1975.
12. Flandrin, G., Brouet, J. C., Daniel, M. T., and Preud'homme, J. L., Acute leukemia with Burkitt's tumor cells: a study of six cases with special reference to lymphocyte surface markers, *Blood*, 45(2), 183, 1975.
13. Davey, F. R. and Gottlieb, A. J., Lymphocyte surface markers in acute lymphocytic leukemia, *Am. J. Clin. Pathol.*, 62, 818, 1974.
14. Winchester, R. J., Fu, S. M., Wernet, P, Kunkel, H. G., Dupont, B., and Jersild, C., Recognition by pregnancy serums of non-HL-A alloantigens selectively expressed on B lymphocytes, *J. Exp. Med.*, 141, 942, 1974.
15. Mann, D. L., Abelson, L., Harris, S., and Amos, D. B., Detection of antigens specific for B-lymphoid cultured cell lines with human alloantisera, *J. Exp. Med.*, 142, 84, 1975.
16. Fu, S. M., Winchester, R. J., and Kunkel, H. G., The occurrence of the HL-B alloantigens on the cells of unclassified acute lymphoblastic leukemias, *J. Exp. Med.*, 142, 1334, 1975.
17. Dausset, J., Degos, L., and Hors, J., The association of HL-A antigens with diseases, *Clin. Immunol. Immunopathol.*, 3, 127, 1974.
18. Lilly, F., The influence of H-2 type on gross virus leukemogenesis in mice, *Transplant. Proc.*, 3(3), 1239, 1971.
19. Sato, H., Boyse, E. A., Aoki, T., Iritani, C., and Old, L. J., Leukemia- associated transplantation antigens related to murine leukemia virus, *J. Exp. Med.*, 138, 593, 1973.
20. Zarling, J. M., Nowinski, R. C., and Bach, F. H., Lysis of leukemia cells by spleen cells of normal mice, *Proc. Natl. Acad. Sci. U.S.A.*, 72(7), 2780, 1975.
21. Gallagher, R. E. and Gallo, R. C., Type C RNA tumor virus isolated from cultured human acute myelogenous leukemia cells, *Science*, 187, 350, 1975.
22. Teich, N. M., Weiss, R. A., Zaki Salahuddin, S., Gallagher, R. E., Gillespie, D. H., and Gallo R. C., Infective transmission and characterisation of a C-type virus released by cultured human myeloid leukemia cells, *Nature*, 256, 551, 1975.
23. Mann, D. L., Halterman, R., and Leventhal, B., Acute leukemia-associated antigens, *Cancer*, 34, 1446, 1974.
24. Thorsby, E., Engeset, A., and Lie, S. O., HL-A antigens and susceptibility to diseases, *Tissue Antigens*, 1, 147, 1971.
25. Killmann, S. A., Leukocyte-auto-agglutinin in a case of acute monocytic leukemia, *Acta Haematol.*, 17, 360, 1957.
26. DeCarvalho, S., Identity of reaction of an autologous antibody in leukemic children in remission with a heterologous antibody produced with leukemic antigens, *Proc. Am. Assoc. Cancer Res.*, 5, 14, 1964.
27. Yoshida, T. O. and Imai, K., Auto-antibody to human leukemic cell membrane as directed by immune adherence, *Rev. Eur. Etud. Clin. Biol.* 15(1), 61, 1970.
28. Gutterman, J. U., Hersh, E. M., Mavligit, G. M., Freireich, E. J., Rossen, R. D., Butler, W. T., McCredie, K. B., Bodey, G. P.,Sr., and Rodriquez, V., Cell- mediated and humoral immune response to acute leukemia cells and soluble leukemia antigen – relationship to immunocompetence and prognosis, *Natl. Cancer Inst. Monogr.*, 37, 153, 1973.
29. Edynak, E. M., Old, L. J., Vrana, M., and Lardis, M. P., A fetal antigen associated with human neoplasia, *N. Engl. J. Med.*, 386(22), 1178, 1972.
30. Klein, G., Stiner, M., Wiener, F., and Klein, E., Human leukemia-associated anti-nuclear reactivity, *Proc. Natl. Acad. Sci. U.S.A.*, 71(3), 685, 1974.

31. **Mann, D. L., Halterman, R., and Leventhal B. G.,** Crossreactive antigens on human cells infected with Rauscher leukemia virus and on human acute leukemia cells, *Proc. Natl. Acad. Sci. U.S.A.,* 70(2), 495, 1973.

32. **Mann, D. L., Rogentine, G. N., Halterman, R., and Leventhal, B.,** Detection of an antigen associated with acute leukemia, *Science,* 174, 1136, 1971.

33. **Durantez, A., Zighelboim, J., Thieme, T., and Fahey, J. L.,** Antigens shared by leukemic blast cell and lymphoblastoid cell lines detected by lymphocyte-dependent antibody, *Cancer Res.,* 35, 2693, 1975.

34. **Billing, R. and Terasaki, P. I.,** Human leukemia antigen. I. Production and characterization of antisera, *J. Natl. Cancer Inst.,* 53, 1635, 1974.

35. **Greaves, M. F., Brown, G., Rapson, N. T., and Lister, T. A.,** Antisera to acute lymphoblastic leukemia cells, *Clin. Immunol. Immunopathol.,* 4, 67, 1975.

36. **Mills, B., Sen, L., and Borella, L.,** Reactivity of antihuman thymocyte serum with acute leukemic blasts, *J. Immunol.,* 115(4), 1038, 1975.

37. **Boyse, E. A., Old, L. J., and Stockert, E.,** An approach to the mapping of antigens on the cell surface, *Proc. Natl. Acad. Sci. U.S.A.,* 60, 886, 1968.

38. **Brown, G., Greaves, M. F., Lister, T. A., Rapson, N., and Papamichael, M.,** Expression of human T and B lymphocyte cell-surface markers on leukemic cells, *Lancet,* 2, 753, 1974.

39. **Yata, J., Klein, G., Kobayashi, N., Furukawa, T., and Yanagisawa, M.,** Human thymus-lymphoid tissue antigen and its presence in leukemia and lymphoma, *Clin. Exp. Immunol.,* 7, 781, 1970.

40. **Brown, G. and Greaves, M. F.,** Cell surface markers for human T and B lymphocytes, *Eur. J. Immunol.,* 4, 302, 1974.

41. **Baker, M. A., Ramachandar, K., and Taub, R. N.,** Specificity of heteroantisera to human acute leukemia-associated antigens, *J. Clin. Invest.,* 54, 1273, 1974.

42. **Mohanakumar, T., Metzgar, R. S., and Miller, D. S.,** Human leukemia cell antigens: serologic characterization with xenoantisera, *J. Natl. Cancer Inst.,* 52(5), 1435, 1974.

43. **Metzgar, R. S., Mohanakumar, T., and Miller, D. S.,** Antigens specific for human lymphocytic and myeloid leukemia cells: detection by nonhuman primate antiserums, *Science,* 178, 986, 1972.

44. **Herberman, R. B.,** Cell-mediated immunity to tumor cells, in *Advances in Cancer Research,* Vol. 19, Klein, G. and Weinhouse, S., Academic Press, New York, 1974, 207.

45. **Fridman, W. H. and Kourilsky, F. M.,** Stimulation of lymphocytes by autologous leukemic cells in acute leukemia, *Nature,* 224, 277, 1969.

46. **Viza, D. C., Bernard-Degani, O., Bernard, C., and Harris, R.,** Leukemia antigens, *Lancet,* 2, 493, 1969.

47. **Gutterman, J. U., Hersh, E. M., McCredie, K. B., Bodey, G. P., Sr., Rodriguez, V., and Freireich, E. J.,** Lymphocyte blastogenesis to human leukemia cells and their relationship to serum factors, immunocompetence, and prognosis, *Cancer Res.,* 32, 2524, 1972.

48. **Leventhal, B. G., Halterman, R. H., Rosenberg, E. B., and Herberman, R. B.,** Immune reactivity of leukemia patients to autologous blast cells, *Cancer Res.,* 32, 1820, 1972.

49. **Powles, R. L., Balchin, L. A., Hamilton Fairley, G., and Alexander, P.,** Recognition of leukemia cells as foreign before and after autoimmunization, *Br. Med. J.,* 1, 486, 1971.

50. **Leventhal, B. G., Halterman, R. H., and Herberman, R. B.,** *In Vitro* and *In Vivo* immunologic reactivity against autochthonous leukemia cells, *Proc. Am. Assoc. Cancer Res.,* 12, 51, 1971.

51. **Gutterman, J. U., Mavligit, G., McCredie, K. B., Bodey, G. P., Sr., Freireich, E. J., and Hersh, E. M.,** Antigen solubilized from human leukemia: lymphocyte stimulation, *Science,* 177, 1114, 1972.

52. **Leventhal, B. G., Mann, D. L., and Rogentine, G. N., Jr.,** Sensitization to water-soluble HL-A antigens, *Transplant. Proc.,* 3(1), 243, 1971.

53 **Gutterman, J. U., Mavligit, G., Burgess, M. A., McCredie, K. B., Hunter, C., Freireich, E. J., and Hersh, E. M.,** Immunodiagnosis of acute leukemia: detection of residual disease, *J. Natl. Cancer Inst.,* 53, 389, 1974.

54. **Han, T. and Wang, J.,** Antigenic disparity between leukemic lymphoblasts and normal lymphocytes in identical twins, *Clin. Exp. Immunol.,* 12, 171, 1972.

55. **Fefer, A., Mickelson, E., and Thomas, E. D.,** Leukemia antigens: mixed leukocyte culture tests on twelve leukemic patients with identical twins, *Clin. Exp. Immunol.,* 18, 237, 1974.

56. **Bach, M. L., Bach, F. H., and Joo, P.,** Leukemia-associated antigens in the mixed leukocyte culture test, *Science,* 166, 1520, 1969.

57. **Santos, G. W., Mullins, G. M., Bias, W. B., Anderson, P. N., Graziano, K. D., Klein, D. L., and Burke, P. J.,** Immunologic studies in acute leukemia, *Natl. Cancer Inst. Monogr.,* 37, 69, 1973.

58. **Weksler, M. E. and Birnbaum, G.,** Lymphocyte transformation induced by autologous cells: stimulation by cultured lymphoblast lines, *J. Clin. Invest.,* 51, 3124, 1972.

59. **Weksler, M. E.,** Lymphocyte transformation induced by autologous cells. III. Lymphoblast-induced lymphocyte stimulation does not correlate with EB viral antigen expression or immunity, *J. Immunol.,* 116, 310, 1976.

60. **Kuntz, M. M., Innes, J. B., and Weksler, M. E.,** Lymphocyte transformation induced by autologous cells. IV. Human T lymphocyte proliferation induced by autologous or allogeneic non-T lymphocytes, *J. Exp. Med.,* 143, 1042, 1976.

61. **Kuntz, M. M., Innes, J. B., and Weksler, M. E.,** Impaired immune surveillance in chronic lymphocytic leukemia (CLL) and systemic lupus erythematosus (SLE) (abstr.), *Clin. Res.,* 24, A448, 1976.

62.   **Fass, L., Herberman, R. B., and Ziegler, J.,** Delayed hypersensitivity reactions to autologous extracts of Burkitt-Lymphoma cells, *N. Engl. J. Med.,* 282, 776, 1970.

63.   **Fass, L., Herberman, R. B., and Kiryabwiri, J. W. M.,** Cutaneous hypersensitivity reactions to autologous extracts of malignant melanoma cells, *Lancet,* 1, 116, 1970.

64.   **Char, D. H., Lepourhiet, A., Leventhal, B. G., and Herberman, R. B.,** Cutaneous delayed hypersensitivity responses to tumor-associated and other antigens in acute leukemia, *Int. J. Cancer,* 12, 409, 1973.

65.   **Hersh, E. M., Whitecar, J. P., Jr., McCredie, K. B., Bodey, G. P., Sr., and Freireich, E. J.,** Chemotherapy, immunocompetence, immunosuppression and prognosis in acute leukemia, *N. Engl. J. Med.,* 285, 1211, 1971.

66.   **Baker, M. A., Taub, R. N., Brown, S. M., and Ramachandar, K.,** Delayed cutaneous hypersensitivity in leukemic patients to autologous blast cells, *Br. J. Haematol.,* 27, 627, 1974.

67.   **Rosenberg, E. B., Herberman, R. B., Levine, P. H., Halterman, R. H., McCoy, J. L., and Wunderlich, J. R.,** Lymphocyte cytotoxicity reactions to leukemia-associated antigens in identical twins, *Int. J. Cancer,* 9, 648, 1972.

68.   **Depuy, J. M., Kourilsky, F. M., Fradelizzi, D., Feingold, N., Bernard, J., and Dausset, J.,** Depression of immunologic reactivity of patients with acute leukemia, *Cancer,* 27, 323, 1971.

69.   **Valdimarsson, H., Agnarsdottir, G., and Lachmann, P. J.,** Measles virus receptor on human T lymphocytes, *Nature,* 255, 554, 1975.

Chapter 12
PRODUCTION OF COAGULATION FACTORS BY LEUKEMIA CELLS

Murray Nussbaum

Leucocytes and their precursors participate in both normal and abnormal hemostasis. It has been suggested that the fibroblasts within the structure of thrombi are produced by monocytes and that normal neutrophils invade thrombi, contributing to their mechanical disruption.[5] The granules of mast cells and basophils of many species are the source of heparin.[1-4] Plasminogen has been localized within the granules of normal eosinophils.[6] Both clot-promoting and anticoagulant properties are attributed to the subcellular lysosomal fractions of leucocytes.[7-9] Lysosomal cationic proteins of normal rabbit polymorphonuclear leucocytes interfered with the interaction of phospholipid with factors X and V and calcium.[10] An antiheparin activity in these fractions has also been demonstrated.[11-13]

In disorders characterized by abnormal clot formation, mature granulocytes are a source of thromboplastic and antiheparin activities[14,15] as exemplified by intravascular coagulation of the generalized Shwartzman reaction.[15,16]

In leukemia and allied disorders, hemorrhage is most often attributable to thrombocytopenia. However, other mechanisms have been less frequently implicated but may participate in ". . . a spectrum of generalized hemostatic disorders,"[17] including deficiencies of specific clotting factors, platelet dysfunction, hyperviscosity, primary fibrinolysis, disseminated intravascular coagulation (DIC), circulating anticoagulants, and liver dysfunction due to leukemic infiltration or to drug toxicity.[17-19] In many of these disorders, the exact role of the leukemic cell in the pathogenesis of bleeding is as yet unclear. Major bleeding, other than that attributable to thrombocytopenia, has been directly correlated with the "leukemic load," i.e., the elevation of the total white blood cells (WBC), hypercellularity of the marrow, hepatosplenomegaly, and/or lymphadenopathy.[17,20,21]

Hampton[22] reported his observations in a patient with subacute myelogenous leukemia and a bleeding diathesis which was attributable to a leukocyte anticoagulant. The extracted anticoagulant, neutralized by phospholipid in vitro, increased markedly during a blastic crisis and disappeared as leukopenia developed following therapy. Prolongation of the partial thromboplastin time was noted when the extract was added to known deficient plasmas. Factor VIII-deficient plasma was inhibited by 10%, factor IX-deficient plasma by 21%, and factor XI-deficient plasma by 23%. Less pronounced anticoagulant activity with prolongation of the prothrombin time was also noted in extracts of granulocytes obtained from patients with chronic granulocytic leukemia.[23] Homogenates of leucocytes obtained from patients with chronic granulocytic leukemia (CGL), chronic lymphocytic leukemia (CLL), acute leukemia (AL), and eosinophilic leukemia (EL) exhibited thromboplastic, antithrombin, and antiheparin activities of varying degree.[24] Antithrombin activity, present in normal neutrophils, is high in CGL extracts but not in other types of leukemia, suggesting that this activity is prominent only in more mature granulocytes and not in lymphocytes, blast cells, and leukemic eosinophils. Thromboplastic activity was high in leukemic eosinophils, lymphocytes, and blasts when compared to normal granulocytes and granulocytes from CGL. Antiheparin activity was high in the extracts of white cells obtained from patients with both forms of chronic leukemia and from normal donors. Cell extracts from AL and EL exhibited only traces of this activity.

Bleeding due to specific clotting-factor deficiencies or fibrinolysis is relatively rare in leukemia. Despite the known presence of proteases in leucocytes, no consistent relationship has been established between the levels of clotting factors and clinical bleeding.[19,21] Reduced levels of factors I, II, V, VII, IX, and X have been found.[19] Bleeding due to isolated factor V deficiency in a patient with acute myeloblastic leukemia (AML) and due to factor X deficiency in a patient with acute lymphocytic leukemia has been reported.[21] Each of these cases was characterized by large numbers of circulating blast cells. The authors suggested that these clotting factors were degraded by specific leukocyte proteases. In most cases, however, the clotting-factor deficiency can be attributed to liver dysfunction secondary to leukemic infiltration, sepsis, or chemotherapy.[25,26] In one reported series of 131 cases of acute and chronic leukemia, increased plasma fibrinolytic activity was found in 36% of 91 cases of acute leukemia and 25% of 40 cases of chronic leukemia.[27] The increased fibrinolysis was usually associated with bleeding. The cells of the peripheral blood and bone marrow were postulated as the source of plasminogen activator. Plasminogen activator has been demonstrated in leukocytes of myelocytic leukemia but not in lymphocytic leukemia and normal leukocytes.[28] However, others[21] could find no consistent relationship between defects in coagulation or fibrinolysis and the occurrence of bleeding among 26 patients with untreated acute leukemia.

Acute promyelocytic leukemia (APL) is characterized by the preponderance of promyelocytes densely packed with spindle-shaped azurophilic granules and Auer rods, both in the blood and marrow. The granules can also be found in the intercellular spaces of the marrow. APL is invariably associated with very severe and fatal hemorrhagic manifestations. Its reported incidence among the acute leukemias is variable from about 2 to 8%.[29,30] The severe hemorrhagic manifestations are related to the presence of the heavy granulation and Auer rods in the blast cells. Cases of acute leukemia with equally high percentages of promyelocytes which show light granulation and no Auer rods usually do not demonstrate the severe bleeding characteristic of APL. The giant granules, measuring 2 to 7 μm and the Auer rods, appear to be lysosomal in nature.[31,32] Their cytochemical characteristics are similar to the giant lysosomes of Chediak-Higashi syndrome.[33] They are positive for esterase, acid phosphatase, and peroxidase.[31] They differ from the granules of normal promyelocytes in that they are positive for PAS and are resistant to ptyaline digestion. Ultrastructural studies depict the granules as longitudinally stacked hollow tubules. The periodicity of tubular stacking is reported at 250 Å,[34] which differs from the periodicity of the Auer rods and granules of the promyelocytes in acute myelocytic leukemia.

The bleeding in APL is due to DIC.[35,36] Infused fibrinogen disappears rapidly when APL is associated with low levels of fibrinogen and factor V. While DIC is not limited to APL, its occurrence in other forms of leukemia is relatively rare.[37] The etiology of the bleeding is believed to reside in the leukemic promyelocyte. Quigley[38] first noted clot-promoting activity similar to tissue factor in the promyelocytes of patients with APL. Gralnick and Abrell[39] analyzed the procoagulant and fibrinolytic activities of disrupted white blood cells obtained from four patients with APL who had major bleeding problems attributed to DIC. The addition of lysates from three of their patients shortened the clotting times of normal plasma and plasmas deficient in factor(s) VIII, IX, and to some extent factor V, but not of factor X- or VII- and X-deficient plasmas. These findings were attributed to tissue-factor activity, which was increased by 250 to 1500% compared to the lysates of normal white cells and cells from patients with AML. The increased tissue factor activity was localized to the granular fraction of the APL cells. Fibrinolytic activity, also found in the granular fraction, was slightly increased in three of the patients, ranging from 150 to 400% when compared to normal and AML lysates. The authors suggested that this disparity between the procoagulant and fibrinolytic activities was responsible for the hemorrhagic tendency. Similar procoagulant activity has been found in mucous extracts of mucin-secreting carcinomas of patients undergoing abdominothoracic surgery.[40] In vitro it is similar to the action of Russell viper venom and trypsin in the activation of factor X.

It has been pointed out that the bleeding in APL may be intensified or initiated during chemotherapy.[41] Because of this, the treatment of APL is hazardous and remains for the most part unsatisfactory. The objective of treatment is to remove the precipitating cause of the DIC by rapid induction of hypoplasia of the marrow with chemotherapy and to correct the bleeding with the use of blood-component transfusions and heparin administration. Despite the report of disappointing results with the use of heparin in most cases of DIC,[42,43] it is advised that all patients with APL be given heparin early in the course of the disease along with the blood components and intensive antileukemia therapy.[41]

REFERENCES

1. **Amman, R. and Morton, H.**, Blutmastzellen und heparin, *Acta Haematol.*, 25, 209, 1961.
2. **Hartman, W. J.**, Histadine decarboxylase activity of basophils, *Proc. Soc. Exp. Biol. Med.*, 107, 123, 1961.
3. **Wilander, O.**, Studien über das heparin, *Scand. Arch. Physiol.*, 81, Suppl. 15, 1938.
4. **Jorpes, J. E.**, Heparin, in *Handbuch für Experimentelle Pharmakologie*, Bd XXVII, *Antikoagulantein*, Springer-Verlag, Berlin, Heidelberg, and New York, 1971.
5. **Henry, N. L.**, Leukocytes and thrombosis, *Thromb. Diath. Haemorrh.*, 13, 35, 1965.
6. **Riddle, J. M. and Barnhart, M. I.**, The eosinophil as a source for profibrinolysin in acute inflammation, *Blood,* 25, 776, 1965.
7. **Graham, R. C., Ebert, R. H., Ratnoff, O. D., and Moses, J. M.**, Pathogenesis of inflammation. II. In vivo observations of the inflammatory effects of activated Hageman factor and bradykinin, *J. Exp. Med.*, 121, 807, 1965.
8. **Rapaport, S. I. and Hjort, P. F.**, The blood clotting properties of rabbit peritoneal leukocytes in vitro, *Thromb. Diath. Haemorrh.*, 17, 222, 1967.
9. **Prokopowicz, J.**, Distribution of fibrinolytic and proteolytic enzymes in subcellular fractions of human granulocytes, *Thromb. Diath. Haemorrh.*, 19, 84, 1968.
10. **Saba, H. I., Roberts, H. R. and Herion, J. C.**, The anticoagulant activity of lysosomal cationic proteins from polymorphonuclear leukocytes, *J. Clin. Invest.*, 46, 580, 1967.
11. **Lisiewicz, J.**, Antiheparin activity of normal leucocytes, *Pol. Tyg. Lek.*, 20, 1150, 1965.
12. **Saba, H. I., Roberts, H. R., and Herion, J. C.**, Anti-heparin activity of lysosomal cationic proteins from polymorphonuclear leukocytes, *Blood,* 31, 369, 1968.
13. **Poplowski, A., Prokopowiez, J., and Niewiarowski, S.**, Antiheparin activity in subcellular fractions of human granulocytes, *Thromb. Diath. Haemorrh.*, 21, 170, 1969.
14. **Eiseman, G. and Stefanini, M.**, Thromboplastic activity of leukemic white cells, *Proc. Soc. Exp. Biol. Med.*, 86, 763, 1954.
15. **Forman, E. N., Abildgaard, C. F., Bolger, J. F., Johnson, C. A., and Shulman, I.**, Generalized Shwartzman reaction. Role of the granulocyte in intravascular coagulation and renal cortical necrosis, *Br. J. Haematol.*, 16, 507, 1969.
16. **Niemetz, J. and Fani, K.**, Thrombogenic activity of leukocytes, *Blood,* 42, 47, 1973.
17. **Gralnick, H. R., Marchesi, S., and Givelber, H.**, Intravascular coagulation in acute leukemia: clinical and subclinical abnormalities, *Blood,* 40, 709, 1972.
18. **Gralnick, H. R. and Henderson, E.**, Acquired coagulation factor deficiencies in leukemia, *Cancer,* 26, 1097, 1970.
19. **Rosner, F., Dobbs, J. V., Ritz, N. D., and Lee, S. L.**, Disturbances of hemostasis in acute myeloblastic leukemia, *Acta Haematol.*, 43, 65, 1970.
20. **Leavey, R., Kahn, S., and Brodsky, I.**, Disseminated intravascular coagulation; a complication of chemotherapy in acute myelogenous leukemia, *Cancer,* 26, 142, 1970.
21. **Brakman, P., Snyder, J., Henderson, E. S., and Astrup, T.**, Blood coagulation and fibrinolysis in acute leukemia, *Br. J. Haematol.*, 18, 135, 1970.
22. **Hampton, J. W.**, Leucocyte anticoagulant with myelogenous leukemia, *Am. J. Med.*, 48, 408, 1970.
23. **Martin, H. and Roka, L.**, Beeinflussing das blutgerinnung durch leukocyten, *Klin. Wochensch.*, 29, 510, 1951.
24. **Lisiewicz, J., Astaldi, G., Okulski, J., and Merolla, R.**, On the influence of normal and leukemic human leucocytes on blood coagulation, *Acta Haematol.*, 44, 332, 1970.
25. **Einhorn, M. and Davidsohn, I.**, Hepatotoxicity of mercaptopurine, *JAMA,* 188, 802, 1965.
26. **Corrigan, J., Ray, W., and May, N.**, Changes in the blood coagulation system associated with septicemia, *N. Engl. J. Med.*, 279, 851, 1968.
27. **Girolami, R. and Cliffton, E. E.**, Fibrinolytic and proteolytic activity in acute and chronic leukemia, *Am. J. Med. Sci.*, 251, 638, 1966.
28. **Tatarsky, I., Sinakos, Z., Larrieu, M. J., and Bernard, J.**, Leucocytes et fibrinolyse II. Etude des leucocytes pathologiques, *Nouv. Rev. Fr. Hematol.*, 7, 95, 1967.
29. **Stavem, P.**, Hypergranular acute promyelocytic leukemia with intravascular coagulation, *Scand. J. Haematol.*, 11, 249, 1973.
30. **Bernard, J., Lasneret, J., Chome, J., Levy, J. P., and Boiron, M.**, A cytological and histological study of acute promyelocytic leukemia, *J. Clin. Pathol.*, 16, 319, 1963.
31. **Mintz, U., Djaldatti, M., Rozenszajn, L., Pinkhas, J. and DeVries, A.**, Giant lysosome-like structures in promyelocytic leukemia. Ultrastructural and cytochemical observations, *Biomedicine,* 19, 426, 1973.
32. **Tan, H. K., Wages, B., and Gralnick, H. R.**, Ultrastructural studies in acute promyelocytic leukemia, *Blood,* 39, 628, 1972.
33. **White, J. G.**, The Chediak-Higashi syndrome: a possible lysosomal disease, *Blood,* 28, 143, 1966.
34. **Breton-Gorius, J. and Houssay, D.**, Auer bodies in acute promyelocytic leukemia, *Lab. Invest.*, 28, 135, 1973.
35. **Sultan, C., Heilmann-Gouault, M., and Tulliez, M.**, Relationship between blast cell morphology and occurrence of a syndrome of disseminated intravascular coagulation, *Br. J. Haematol.*, 24, 255, 1973.
36. **Didisheim, P., Trombold, J. S., Vandervoort, R. L. E., and Mibashan, R. S.**, Acute promyelocytic leukemia with fibrinogen and factor V deficiencies, *Blood,* 23, 717, 1964.

37.   Goodnight, S. H., Jr., Bleeding and intravascular clotting in malignancy, a review, *Ann. N.Y. Acad. Sci.,* 230, 271, 1974.

38.   Quigley, H. J., Peripheral leukocyte thromboplastin in promyelocytic leukemia, *Fed. Proc. Fed. Am. Soc. Exp. Biol.,* abstr., 26, 648, 1967.

39.   Gralnick, H. and Abrell, E., Studies of the procoagulant and fibrinolytic activity of promyelocytes in acute promyelocytic leukemia, *Br. J. Haematol.,* 24, 89, 1973.

40.   Pineo, G. F., Brain, M. C., Gallus, A. S., Hirsh, J., Hatton, M. W. C., and Regoeczi, E., Tumors, mucus production and hypercoagulability, *Ann. N.Y. Acad. Sci.,* 20, 262, 1974.

41.   Gralnick, H. R. and Tan, H. K., Acute promyelocytic leukemia. A model for understanding the role of the malignant cell in hemostasis, *Hum. Pathol.,* 5, 661, 1974.

42.   Al-Mondhiry, H., Disseminated intravascular coagulation. Experience in a major cancer center, *Thromb. Diath. Haemorrh.,* 34, 181, 1975.

43.   Straub, P. W., A case against heparin therapy of intravascular coagulation, *Thromb. Diath. Haemorrh.,* 33, 107, 1975.

Chapter 13

PROSPECTIVES FOR LEUKEMIA RESEARCH AND THERAPY

Samuel Waxman

TABLE OF CONTENTS

I. INTRODUCTION

The previous chapters have described some of the new approaches to the classification, definition, evaluation, manifestations, and pathogenesis of leukemia. Clearly, we are in an exciting period in the understanding of leukemia. Major therapeutic breakthroughs have developed as a result of new basic knowledge of molecular biology and cell kinetics and the introduction of new drugs used in appropriate combinations and schedules. Often, the therapeutic advances have been made through careful trial and error and seemingly at a snail's pace. However, the net result of overall leukemia therapy represents one of the major medical advances of the last 25 years. Therapeutic progress has mainly been in the treatment of the acute leukemias, but the chronic leukemias, which represent the majority of leukemias, remain more refractory to present therapeutic modalities. This experience suggests that new

therapeutic concepts or modalities are required to obtain a greater impact on the chronic leukemias, as well as the similarly refractory solid tumors. The purpose of this chapter will be to summarize the pertinent observations related to etiology and to predict the new concepts and therapeutic modalities to be tested in the next decade.

II. THE LEUKEMIC GRANULOCYTE CONCEPT

Clinically, the development of most, if not all, leukemias appears to be a two-step process. The initial step consists of a genetic defect manifesting various biologic abnormalities with various degrees of impairment of cellular differentiation and function. These are the characteristics of preleukemia and perhaps, also, more specific clinical entities such as chronic myelocytic leukemia (CML), chronic lymphocytic leukemia (CLL), paroxysmal nocturnal hemoglobinuria, and certain aplastic anemias. Progression of these disorders (other than CLL) to overt blastic leukemia is characterized by more or less progressive lack of differentiation. Thus, the preleukemic phase, whether short or prolonged, is a stage in the disease that the host is capable of dealing with until some unknown factor(s) convert the disorder to the acute, undifferentiated phase. Cytotoxic chemotherapy has not been effective in preventing this clinical transformation, whereas it has been effective in dealing with manifest blastic leukemia. Similarly, the induction cytotoxic chemotherapy of acute myelogenous leukemia is effective, whereas maintenance of the remission (a possible reversion to the preleukemic state) has been more difficult. Thus, attention to the characteristics of the preleukemic cell and the development of new concepts of treatment is to be predicted.

The preleukemic cell is a disordered cell and should be a clue to the fully undifferentiated leukemic cell. Some of the genotypic expressions can be obtained by comparing the disturbed mature cell to the normal undisturbed counterpart. For example, metabolic comparison of the morphologically normal-appearing lymphocyte in chronic lymphocytic leukemia to its normal counterpart has uncovered functional disorders. Similar comparisons are necessary in the preleukemic phases of myeloid leukemia. Here is an opportunity to compare the leukemic granulocyte to the normal granulocyte. This approach enables the investigator to overcome the logistical problem of finding a normal counterpart to the totally undifferentiated leukemic cell (blast).

How, then, would one use the leukemic granulocyte to gain insight into leukemia? A readily available source of these cells could be obtained from the peripheral blood of patients with the preleukemic state, CML, myeloproliferative disorders, and acute myelogenous leukemia in remission. Preparations (> 95% granulocytes) can be made from peripheral blood by gradient separation and dextran sedimentation with readily obtainable granulocyte levels of 1×10^{10}. Although the granulocyte is not capable of division, it is metabolically active and is functionally responsive to appropriate stimuli.

The leukemic and normal granulocyte, both abundantly available, offer fresh material for research to elucidate genotypic quantitative and qualitative expressions of the leukemic cell and the normally differentiated hematopoietic cell. Functional metabolic and antigenic differences between these two populations of cells may uncover the strategy of the neoplastic cell and may expose the key enzymes involved in the biologic advantage apparently possessed by the leukemic granulocytes.

III. DISTURBANCES IN ORGAN-SPECIFIC BIOCHEMICAL PATHWAYS

Neoplasia is manifested by transformation that is hereditable and characterizes the entire cell line. The malignant program may be expressed by different degrees of transformation that range from mild, through advanced, to the full blown pattern. The biochemical expression of malignancy should be present in the leukemic granulocyte and should contain specific enzyme patterns, as has been shown by the studies of the normal regenerating liver compared to hepatomas of varying growth rates.[1-4] Thus, the study of key enzyme systems which regulate the rate and direction of the opposing synthetic and catabolic pathways offers a method for uncovering the malignant genotype of the leukemic granulocyte.

Although the leukemic granulocyte is an end cell, it should contain some of the genotypic expression associated with the leukemic progenitor. The commitment to proliferation without differentiation and the altered control of cellular replication are the chief diagnostic signs of the biologic behavior of the undifferentiated leukemic cell. Thus, the potential for anabolic pathways of the pyrimidine, purine and DNA metabolism, and diminished catabolic enzymes should be a feature of the leukemic granulocyte as compared to the normal granulocyte.

An early discovery in cancer biochemistry was made in carbohydrate metabolism by Warburg, who demonstrated that in rapidly growing, differentiated tumors, aerobic glycolysis was increased and respiration was decreased.[5] Similarly, the rat hepatoma demonstrates the pattern of increased alcoholic glycolysis, oxidative and nonoxidative pentose phosphate production, and diminished gluconeogenesis.[4] The granulocyte is an appropriate cell for the study of carbohydrate metabolism, since this is actively stimulated during the course of phagocytosis. Waxman et al. have utilized phorbol ester to initiate phagocytosis and measure marked increases in the uptake of glucose and deoxyglucose and subsequent release of carbon dioxide.[6] Preliminary observations suggest that the leukemic granulocyte has a diminished carbon dioxide release from deoxyglucose when stimulated with phorbol ester, in contrast to the normal granulocyte. The intermediates from deoxyglucose are currently being studied to see if different patterns exist in the leukemic granulocyte.

IV. DISTURBANCES IN MEMBRANE MARKERS, ANTIGENS, AND RECEPTORS

Human leukemic cell antigens have been reviewed in the chapter by Weksler. Study of the alterations at the cell surface, resulting in the appearance of new antigenic determinants on leukemic cells, has given insight into the classification of the lymphoproliferative disorders, genetic factors which may predispose to leukemia, and a rationale for diagnostic and therapeutic approaches to leukemia. Leukemic blasts have characteristically been studied for specific antigen and marker expression. Similar studies utilizing the granulocyte are lacking and may uncover an earlier expression of initiation of malignancy in the preleukemic and chronic leukemias. Externally exposed antigens can be iodinated by lactoperoxidase-catalyzed iodination of intact granulocytes. Thereafter, solubilized granulocyte membranes from normals and various stages of hematologic malignancies can be subjected to sodium dodecyl sulfate gel electrophoresis to identify novel antigens.[7]

Studies of this type may uncover membrane markers in cells associated with the expression of initiation (preleukemia) but not total expression of malignancy (blastic transformation). This may allow earlier use of therapeutic programs and also help classify the various refractory sideroblastic anemias.

V. MAPPING OF CHROMOSOMAL REGIONS RELATED TO NEOPLASIA

The relationship of chromosomal changes to neoplasia is one of the most significant unanswered questions in cancer research. Analysis of hematologic disorders, particularly the leukemias, has provided most of the information on chromosomal patterns and, thus, on the types of nonrandom chromosomal changes that occur in malignancy. It is now becoming possible to ascribe gene loci and function to specific sites on various chromosomes. Consequently, leukemia-associated chromosomal aberrations can be functionally evaluated.

The chromosome lesions induced by virus infection might be indicators of gene loci that are important in cell regulation. If one of the effects of carcinogens (including viruses) were to activate genes that regulate host cell DNA synthesis, and if this activation could be maintained, these cells would have a proliferative advantage without the need for viral gene persistence and could appear to be chromosomally normal. This mechanism would explain the failure, with rare exceptions, to isolate C type virus from patients with human leukemia.[8] In other neoplastic cells, an imbalance in regulation may result from altered transcription of the genes in translocated, trisomic, or monosomic chromosomal regions. This imbalance could act directly on metabolic pathways, indirectly through an effect on membrane receptors, or by some unknown other mechanism.

There is evidence from hematologic disorders which suggests that only certain chromosomes carry genes that confer a proliferative advantage upon the mutant clone. Aberrations in chromosomes 1 and 17 in myeloid leukemia[9] and chromosome 14 in proliferative lymphoid diseases[10] are often found. These aberrations may provide the information required for increased rate of cell division, prolonged cell life span, or relaxation of proliferative controls which confer a selective advantage to the malignant cell. It is of interest that in normal human DNA there is evidence by in situ hybridization for a DNA sequence homologous to RNA tumor virus RNA on a D-group chromosome.[11]

In the past, a number of investigators[12-15] have considered the possibility that malignancy represents a balance phenomenon between genes related to the expression or suppression of malignancy. In some in vitro systems transformation was reversible and was related to the presence or absence of specific chromosomal segments.[14,15] A chromosomal change that promotes the expression of malignancy in such systems may be one that changes the level of some enzymes related to nucleic acid metabolism, either through a change in location or through duplication of gene loci.

Nonrandom chromosomal changes — particularly consistent, specific translocations — now seem to be an important component in the proliferative advantage of the mutant cell in neoplasia. The challenge to the cell biologist is to decipher the meaning of these changes. The elucidation of specific functional biochemical expressions of nonrandom chromosomal aberrations associated with neoplasia will open new concepts for specific cytotoxic or differentiation chemotherapy.

VI. VIRUSES AND THE PATHOGENESIS OF HUMAN LEUKEMIA

Viral leukemogenesis continues to be an exciting approach to the future understanding and management of human leukemia. This topic has been reviewed in the excellent chapters by Gabelman and Baxt. At this time, the significance of the extraordinary developments of viral genetics, infectivity, molecular biology, and immunology to human leukemia remains to be determined.

Gallo recently summarized the types of reports describing evidence for RNA tumor viruses or virus related components in human leukemia;[16] these are outlined below:

1. Intracytoplasmic virus-like particles are found frequently in the cytoplasm of fresh leukemic blood and bone marrow cells.[17,18]
2. Documented viral-like reverse transcriptase in the above mentioned particles, in some cases, show immunologic relatedness to certain primate RNA tumor viruses.
3. Viral-related nucleic acid sequences in the intracytoplasmic particles mentioned above contained nucleic acids with some homology to certain mammalian type C RNA tumor viruses.
4. Isolation of whole infectious virus from a few patients, which is related to the primate virus groups.[19-21]
5. Antibodies reactive with RNA tumor viruses (primate viruses) have been reported

in human sera. These reports vary depending on the assay used. Some investigators find antibodies in normal sera and leukemics while another reported no antibodies in normal sera or in patients with malignancy.[30-32]

The above data provide firm evidence for the presence of RNA tumor virus-related information in the human population. However, no cohesive pattern has emerged and this precludes making any etiologic inferences. The data also emphasize heterogeneity of the viral-related information, varying among normals as well as patients.

It has been proposed that subsequent to activation of endogenous viral information and the resultant transformation of the cell, cancer antigens formed on the surface of the malignant cell are recognized by the immune surveillance system and lead not only to the destruction of the affected cells and the prevention of their proliferation, but also make it possible for the cellular mediators (T cells) to recognize the tumor as nonself. Conversely, any congenital or induced defect in the thymus-dependent immune system would result in the proliferation of abnormal cells and ultimately the destruction of the organism.

It has been reported that the DNA of all humans contains viral-related endogenous sequences which appear to be related to the stable genes of various primate species. It should be noted that although immunologic data suggest widespread presence of virus information, detection of novel proviral sequences in leukemic DNA is rarely found. This constellation suggests that RNA tumor viruses and, perhaps, DNA tumor viruses are more involved in host immunologic surveillance to prevent dissemination of malignancy rather than to propagate neoplasia.[29] Clearly, tumor-associated virus production is a consequence of many carcinogens[33-35] and viral expression could provide a selective marker for the destruction of a cell initiated to malignancy by somatic mutation.

These observations are consistent with Good's speculation that evolutionarily more complex organisms require a cellular immune system primarily to defend the organism against mutational events which result in the proliferation of tissues which are nonself, thereby maintaining the evolutionary stability of the organism.[22] Therefore, whatever increases the efficiency with which immune-surveillance mechanisms recognize neoplastic and therefore nonself cells lends an adaptive advantage to the host organism and is of selective value. In short, it is postulated that viruses, rather than causing cancer, may help to prevent it.

The mechanisms of viral-mediated destruction of malignant cells could be cytopathic, such as with Herpes-like virus (Herpes simplex as an example), or immunologic. Both mechanisms would remove the source of viral expression in DNA and leave a residual of immunologic information. A clinical model which appears to demonstrate this viral role is infectious mononucleosis (IM). IM is an acute clinical disorder associated with lymphoproliferation demonstrating some morphologic features of malignancy. The disorder is self-limited and seroepidemiologically associated with E-B virus (a Herpes-like virus). IM is also associated with induction of antibodies against specific cell antigens such as the i antigen. Anti-i antibody is highly cytotoxic against cells expressing i antigen. This is rarely a problem since i antigen is a fetal antigen and I antigen is expressed in mature red blood cells. However, severe hemolytic anemia is found in patients with IM and concommitant thalessemia is found in those who express i antigen in the red cell membrane. Lymphocyte membrane contains the I/i antigen system. It is suggested that E-B virus infection of the lymphocyte also induces the expression of the fetal antigen i, causing the selective destruction of the transformed cell (mononucleosis cell). This may be a generalized phenomenon in malignancy since fetal antigens are often expressed in neoplastic conditions. These fetal antigens may be an expression of tumor virus-induced immunosurveillance. This conception may help develop insight for specific immunotherapeutic approaches to the future management of leukemia.

VII. DIFFERENTIATION CHEMOTHERAPY OF LEUKEMIA

The cellular abnormalities in human myelogenous leukemia appear to be due to an increased proliferation of stem cells generally committed to the myelogenous series. This may involve a block in differentiation. Not all undifferentiated cells in acute myelogenous leukemia are irreversibly blocked at the blast stage. Some respond partly and some completely to growth- and differentiation-promoting proteins. These differentiating-inducing proteins are derived from conditioned media from various cells and induce differentiation in solid or semisolid systems.[23,24] This solid system has the limitations of a short growth period and the difficulty of recovering cells for biochemical studies.

More recently, human hematopoietic cells have been grown in suspension culture for longer periods of time.[23,26] Myelogenous leukemia cells can be grown in suspension culture in the presence of conditioned media from certain embryonic fibroblast cell lines.[27] Some of these conditioned media contain factors which affect only the growth of myelogenous leukemia cells but not normal cells. Results from these systems suggest that myelogenous leukemic cells are not completely autonomous. There is considerable heterogeneity in the ability of these cells to differentiate in response to these factors.[23] The selectivity of the differentiating response to conditioned media suggests that there are fundamental differences, probably at the cell membrane level, in recognition of these growth and differentiation factors.

Studies in the related field of viral leukemogenesis support the concept that malignant cells retain the capacity to differentiate. Differentiation can be induced despite the persistence of the oncogenic viral genome. As discussed in Preisler's chapter, inducing differentiation of leukemic cells would have several advantages over cytotoxic chemotherapy. Partial differentiation should reduce the symptoms of leukemia regardless of etiology. Differentiation chemotherapy should have selectivity for leukemic cells.

Application of the mechanisms of in vitro differentiation of leukemic cells will provide the design for in vivo differentiation chemotherapy. Differentiation of Friend leukemia cells (FLC) in tissue culture is manifested by a decrease in nuclear:cytoplasmic ratio, a decrease in the size of the cell, the development of globin mRNA, the development of the enzymes required for heme synthesis, and then benzidine positivity. The addition of dimethylsulfoxide

(DMSO), or any of a variety of other cryoprotective compounds, or butyric acid induces the
differentiation of FLC. During this process the
number of viruses budding from the cell membrane appears to be increased. However, differentiation appears unrelated to viral production
since interferon which prevents viral production does not inhibit DMSO differentiation of
FLC.

The list of in vitro differentiating agents is
extensive and growing. A variety of physical
structures are possible for a compound to induce differentiation. No unifying mechanism
has been elucidated and perhaps these agents
operate through a variety of mechanisms. Some
agents, such as glycerol or urea, with little differentiating ability of their own, potentiate the
effects of DMSO.

Differentiation by DMSO is dose and schedule dependent. Exposure of more than 24 hr is
needed and the longer the exposure, the more
irreversible the differentiation. It appears that
FLC must be exposed to DMSO during a sensitive phase in the cell cycle if differentiation is
to occur. At least two rounds of DNA synthesis
and/or two mitoses in the presence of DMSO
are essential for differentiation of FLC to be
induced. Therefore, tumor kinetic patterns will
be important in the development of differentiation chemotherapy, as has been demonstrated
in cytotoxic chemotherapy.

Moreover, different FLC lines demonstrate
varying responses to differentiating agents.

There are individual biologic characteristics
that must also be studied in evaluating differentiation chemotherapeutic agents. During
DMSO-induced differentiation of FLC, globin
mRNA accumulates in response to the expression of DNA sequences which code for globin
mRNA. This may result from DMSO interfer-
ence with the binding of histone to DNA, thus
permitting DNA to unwind and become nicked
by accessibility to DNase.[28] Cryoprotective differentiating agents are membrane active and
this may be a mechanism whereby globin
mRNA is initiated. Differences in mechanisms
of action would explain why some combinations of inducers appear to be additive, while
others are synergistic and some lines are totally
refractory.

The complexity of in vitro differentiating
agents predicts that in vivo differentiation
chemotherapy will require an in-depth, system-
atic program such as that done with cytotoxic
chemotherapy. Preliminary in vivo studies have
revealed inhibition of FLC proliferation but no
evidence of differentiation. These have been
modest studies and clearly not conclusive. The
concept of differentiation chemotherapy is clinically appealing, biologically possible, and must
be tested in various animal tumor models. It is
possible that the development of appropriate
schedules, routes of administration, vehicles,
and inducing agents in carefully defined in vivo
tumor models will establish the clinical efficacy
of differentiating chemotherapy.

REFERENCES

1. **Weber, G.,** Behavior of liver enzymes during hepatocarcinogenisis, *Adv. Cancer Res.,* 6, 403, 1961.
2. **Weber, G.,** Behavior and regulation of enzyme systems in normal liver and in hepatomas of different growth rates, *Adv. Enzyme Regul.,* 1, 321, 1963.
3. **Weber, G.,** The molecular correlation concept: recent advances and implications, in *The Molecular Biology of Cancer,* Busch, H., Ed., Academic Press, New York, 1974, 487.
4. **Weber, G.,** Enzymology of cancer cells, *N. Engl. J. Med.,* 296, 486 and 541, 1977.
5. **Warburg, O.,** On the origin of cancer cells, *Science,* 123, 309, 1956.
6. **Waxman, S., Acs, G., Zabos, P., Mendelsohn, N., Schreiber, C., and Christman, J.,** unpublished observations.
7. **Troy, F. A., Fenyo, E., and Klein, G.,** Moloney leukemia virus-induced cell surface antigen: detection and character-ization in sodium dodecyl sulfate gels, *Proc. Natl. Acad. Sci. U.S.A.,* 74(12), 5270, 1977.
8. **Gillespie, D. and Gallo, R. C.,** RNA processing and RNA tumor virus origin and evolution, *Science,* 188, 802, 1975.
9. **Rowley, J. D.,** Mapping of human chromosomal regions related to neoplasia: evidence from chromosomes 1 and 17, *Proc. Natl. Acad. Sci. U.S.A.,* 74(12), 5729, 1977.

10. **McCaw, B. K., Hecht, F., Harnden, D. G., and Teplitz, R. L.,** Somatic rearrangement of chromosome 14 in human lymphocytes, *Proc. Natl. Acad. Sci. U.S.A.,* 72, 2071, 1975.
11. **Price, P. M., Hirschorn, K., Gabelman, N., and Waxman, S.,** *In situ* hybridization of RD114-virus RNA with human metaphase chromosomes *Proc. Natl. Acad. Sci. U.S.A.,* 70, 11, 1973.
12. **Klein, G., Bregola, V., Weiner, F., and Harris, H.,** The analysis of malignancy by cell fusion. I. Hybrids between tumor cells and L cell derivatives, *J. Cell Sci.,* 8, 659, 1971.
13. **Yamamoto, T., Hayashi, M., Rabinowitz, Z., and Sachs, L.,** Chromosomal control of malignancy in tumors from cells transformed by polyoma virus, *Int. J. Cancer,* 11, 555, 1973.
14. **Codish, S. D. and Paul, B.,** Reversible appearance of a specific chromosome which supresses malignancy, *Nature* (London), 252, 610, 1974.
15. **Azumi, J. and Sachs, L.,** Chromosome mapping of the genes that control differentiation and malignancy in myeloid leukemic cells, *Proc. Natl. Acad. Sci. U.S.A.,* 74, 253, 1977.
16. **Gallo, R. C.,** Viruses and the pathogenesis of human leukemia, *Schweiz. Med. Wochenschr.,* 107, 1436, 1977.
17. **Gallo, R. C. and Todaro, G. J.,** Oncogenic RNA viruses, in *Seminars in Oncology,* Yarbo, J. W., Bornstein, R. S., and Mastrangelo, M. J., Eds., Grune & Stratton, New York, 1976, 81.
18. **Spiegelman, S.,** Molecular evidence for the association of RNA tumor viruses with human mesenchymal malignancies, in *Modern Trends in Human Leukemia,* Vol. 2, Neth, R., Gallo, R. C., Mannweiler, K., and Moloney, W. C., Eds., J. F. Lehmanns Verlag, Munich, 1976, 391.
19. **Gallagher, R. E. and Gallo, R. C.,** Type C RNA tumor viruses isolated from cultured human acute myelogenous leukemia cells, *Science,* 187, 350, 1975.
20. **Nooter, J., Aarsen, A. M., Bentvelzen, P., Degroot, F. G., and Van Pelt, F. G.,** Isolation of infectious C-type onconoviruses from human leukemic bone marrow cells, *Nature* (London), 256, 595, 1975.
21. **Gabelman, N., Waxman, S., Smith, W., and Douglas, S. D.,** Appearance of C-type virus particles after cocultivation of human lung tumor and rat (XC) cells, *Int. J. Cancer,* 16, 355, 1975.
22. **Good, R. A.,** Disorders of the immune system, in *Immunobiology; Current Knowledge of Basic Concepts in Immunobiology and Their Clinical Applications,* Good, R. A. and Fisher, D. W., Eds., Sinauer, Stamford, Conn., 1971, 3.
23. **Sachs, L.,** Regulation of membrane changes, differentiation and malignancy in carcinogenesis, in *Harvey Lectures,* Series 68, Academic Press, New York, 1974, 1.
24. **Metcalf, D., Moore, M. A. S., Sheridan, J. W., and Spitzer, G.,** Responsiveness of human granulocytic leukemia cells to colony-stimulating factor, *Blood,* 43, 874, 1974.
25. **Morgan, D. A., Ruscetti, F. W., and Gallo, R. C.,** Selective *in vitro* growth of T-lymphocytes from normal human bone marrow, *Science,* 193, 1007, 1976.
26. **Gallagher, R. E., Salhuddin, S. Z., Hall, W. T., McCredie, K. B., and Gallo, R. C.,** Growth and differentiation in culture of leukemic leucocytes from a patient with acute myelogenous leukemia and re-identification of a type-C virus, *Proc. Natl. Acad. Sci. U.S.A.,* 72, 4137, 1975.
27. **Gallagher, R. E. and Gallo, R. C.,** Continuous production of complete type-C virus by exponentially-growing cultured leucocytes from one of sixteen patients with myelogenous leukemia, in *Proc. 2nd Int. Congr. Pathological Physiology,* Prague, 1975.
28. **Scher, W. and Friend, C.,** Breakage of DNA and alterations in folded genomes by inducers of differentiation in Friend erythroleukemic cells, *Cancer Res.,* 38, 841, 1978.
29. **Hirschhorn, K., Price, P. M., Gabelman, N., and Waxman, S.,** The evolutionary significance of the persistence of latent oncogenic information in vertebrates, *Lancet,* 1, 1158, 1973.
30. **Prowchownik, E. and Kirsten, W. H.,** Inhibition of reverse transcriptases of primate C-type viruses by 7S immunoglobulin from patients with leukemia, *Nature (London),* 260, 64, 1978.
31. **Stephenson, J. R. and Aaronson, S. A.,** Search for antigens and antibodies cross-reactive with type C viruses of the Woolly Monkey and Gibbon Ape in animal models and in humans, *Proc. Natl. Acad. Sci. U.S.A.,* 73, 1725, 1976.
32. **Gabelman, N., Robinson, A., Ong, S., and Waxman, S.,** Antibodies to an oncornavirus (v-L104) isolated from human tumor cells cocultivated with rat cells, *Proc. Am. Assoc. Cancer Res.,* 18, 135, 1977.
33. **Whitmeyer, C. E. and Heubner, R. J.,** The inhibition of chemical carcinogenesis by viral vaccines, *Science,* 177, 60, 1972.
34. **Salerno, R. A., Whitmire, C. E., Garcia, I. M., and Heubner, R. J.,** Chemical carcinogenesis in mice inhibited by interferon, *Nature (London),* 239, 31, 1972.
35. **Price, P. L. J., Bellow, T. M., King, F. V., Freeman, A. E., Gilden, R. V., and Heubner, R. J.,** Prevention of viral-chemical co-carcinogenesis in vitro by type specific antiviral antibody. *Proc. Natl. Acad. Sci. U.S.A.,* 73, 152, 1976.

INDEX

A

N-Acetyl-β-glucosamimidase, use in cytochemistry, 11, 21
Acute lymphoblastic leukemia
  antigens present in, 156
  bone marrow transplants, 111, 114
  cell characteristics, 131
  clinical significance of antigens in leukemic cells, 161
  derivation of neoplastic cells, 154
  origin of lymphoblasts, 155
  reaction in humans to animal antisera, 157
  skin test reactions as measure of cell immunity, 160
Acute lymphocytic leukemia
  cells, reaction to cytochemical stains, 13
  chromosomal abnormalities, 30
  leukocyte CFU count, 90
Acute monocytic leukemia, classification, 12
Acute myeloblastic leukemia
  antigens present in, 156
  classification, 12
  differentiation of neoplastic cells, 65, 66
  reaction in humans to animal antisera, 157
Acute myelocytic leukemia
  leucocyte CFU count, 90
Acute myelogenous leukemia, chromosomal aberrations, 28, 29
Acute myelomonocytic leukemia
  cell differentiation, 66
  classification, 12
  leucocyte CFU count, 90
Acute promyelocytic leukemia, bleeding in, 166
Agammaglobulinemia, immunoglobulin synthesis in, 146
ALL, see Acute lymphoblastic leukemia; Acute lymphocytic leukemia
AML, see Acute myeloblastic leukemia; Acute myelogenous leukemia
AMML, see Acute myelomonocytic leukemia
AMoL, classification, 12
Anemia in friend leukemia, 66
Antigens on human leukemic cells, see Human leukemia

B

Benzidine, use in cytochemistry, 8
Blood disorders in leukemia, 165
Bone marrow
  cells
    experiments to determine immunoglobulin synthesis, 138—141
    research involving, 5
    with XY karyotype, 115
  chromosomal abnormalities
    in ALL, 30
    in AML, 29
    in CML, 26
    in macroglobulinemia of Waldenström, 32
    in multiple myeloma, 32
  leukocyte CFU count in certain leukemias, 90
  oncornavirus isolated from, 55

Philadelphia chromosome finding in CML, 26
  transplants in ALL cases, 111, 114
Breast cancer virus, relationship to murine mammary tumor virus, 56
Burkitt's lymphoma, chromosomal abnormalities in, 33

C

Carbohydrate metabolism, effect of cancer on, 170
Carcinogenesis, molecular mechanisms, study of, 107—121
Cat, experiment with involving human tumor virus, 55
Cells
  effect of leukemia on, 93
  generation cycles, time of, 91
  membranes, research involving, 5
Chromosomes
  aberrations
    in acute lymphocytic leukemia, 30
    in acute myelogenous leukemia, 28
    in chronic myelogenous leukemia, 26, 27
    in Hodgkin's disease, 33
    in lymphomas, 33
    in macroglobulinemia of Waldenström, 32
    in multiple myeloma, 32
    in polycythemia vera, 31
    relationship to susceptibility to neoplasia, 34
    specific etiologic agent, possibility of, 35
  alteration as fundamental to malignancy, 26
  changes in, relationship to neoplasia, question of, 171
  inactive X, role in CML, 109, 110
  Philadelphia
    clonal origin, 27, 109
    description, 26
    duplication in acute phase of CML, 28
    finding in CML, 26
    identification, 27
    in chronic myelocytic leukemia, 95
    occurrence in sex chromosome mosaics, 109
Chronic lymphocytic leukemia
  antigens present in, 156
  β-glucuronidase values in, 14
  cell characteristics, 132
  cells, experimental use, 136
  cellular kinetics, 98
  charactistics of development, 169
  clinical significance of antigens in leukemic cells, 161
  derivation of leukemic cells, 154
  reaction in humans to animal antisera, 157
  role of lymphocyte differentiation in, 129
  studies of, 30
  unicellular origin studied, 111
Chronic myelocytic leukemia
  cellular kinetics, 98
  cellular proliferation, 96
  characteristics of development, 169
  cyclic phenomena, 77
  differentiation of malignant cells, 65
  leucocyte CFU count, 90

H

Hairy cell
  β-cell derivation of leukemic cells, 154
  characteristics, 131
  enzymatic activity, 14
HD, chromosomal abnormalities in, 33
Heary-chain diseases described, 144
hemorrhage in leukemia, 165
Histocompatibility genes, link to susceptibility to
    leukemia, 155
History of research, 1—6
Hodgkin's disease, chromosomal abnormalities in, 33
Human leukemia, see also particular leukemias
  antigens on leukemic cells
    cellular immunity as demonstration, 158
    clinical significance, 161
    delayed cutaneous hypersensitivity as demonstration,
      160
    identification, 156
  cell systems, effect of disease on, 93
  delayed cutaneous hypersensitivity as measure of cell-
    mediated immunity, 160
  development, characteristics of, 169
  immune reactivity
    correlation with prognosis, 161
    defect in, possible effect, 172
  leukemic blasts
    in peripheral blood, 92
    proliferation, 91
  leukocyte colony formation, 89, 95
  lymphocyte reactions to leukemic cells, 159
  lymphoid cell surface markers, 154
  molecular genesis
    aberrant differentiation, 119, 121
    clonal origin of malignancy, 109
    somatic mutation hypothesis, 108
    oncogenic viruses, role of, 111—114
  reaction to animal antisera, 157
  RNA tumor viruses in, evidence of, 172
  surface immunoglobulin in, 154
  therapy
    aberrant differentiation theory, 121
    differentiation chemotherapy, 173
    drugs, effect of, 94, 98
    infidelity of DNA synthesis, 121
    progress in, 169
    somatic mutation hypothesis, 120
    viral etiology, 120
  viral etiology, study, 156, 172
  virus, see Oncornaviruses; Viruses
Human lymphoreticular disease, see Lymphoreticular
    system

I

Immunoglobulin synthesis
  analysis of process, 136
  B cells, role of, 135
  inadequate primary immune response, 146
  in agammaglobulinemia, 146

  in heavy-chain disease, 144
  in macroglobulinemia, 142, 143
  in myeloma, 140—142
  labeling experiment with cells of
    hypergammaglobulinemia patient, 138
  polypeptide chains, 136, 137
  structure, 136
  suppression in myeloma, 146
  surface Ig, 144, 154
Immunology techniques, use in cell research, 5

L

LAP, see Leukocyte alkaline phosphatase
Leukemic granulocyte, use in research, 169, 170, 171
Leukemic reticuloendothelial cell, enzymatic activity, 14
Leukemic reticuloendotheliosis, cell characteristics, 131
Leukemogenic virus, see Oncornaviruses; Viruses
Leukocyte acid phosphatase, function, 10, 14, 15
Leukocyte alkaline phosphatase
  determination, method, 18
  function, 8
  score in chronic myelogenous leukemia and other
    diseases, 13
Lymphocytes, see Lymphoreticular system
Lymphoma
  cell characteristics, 132
  chromosomal abnormalities in, 33
  lymphocytic, B-cell derivation of leukemic cells, 154
Lymphoreticular system
  B cells, function, 128, 135
  cells, nature of, 127
  cell surface markers
    on malignant cells, 131, 154
    theoretical differentiation based on, 129, 130
  cellular interactions within, 127—129
  differentiation, theoretical, 129, 130
  LRE cells, characteristics, 131
  malignancies, abnormal immunologic interaction in, 129
  M-H cells, function, 127, 128
  T cells, function, 128
  viral infections, role in disorders, 129

M

Macroglobulinemia
  chromosomal changes in, 32
  immunoglobulin synthesis in, 142, 144, 146, 155
  monoclonal, B-cell derivation of leukemic cells, 154
Malignant cells
  development, 170
  differentiation
    relationship to patient survival, 65
    therapeutic potential, 66
Mast cell leukemia, cytochemical reaction, 14, 18
Monoblasts, identification procedure, 20
Monocytes, identification procedure, 20
Mouse leukemia, research, 3, 26, 35, 41, 66, 85, 156
Multiple myeloma, chromosomal abnormalities in, 32
Mutation, see also Chromosomes